ACP | MKSAP® 18

Medical Knowledge Self-Assessment Program®

Endocrinology and Metabolism

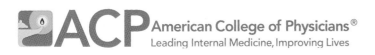

American College of Physicians®
Leading Internal Medicine, Improving Lives

Welcome to the Endocrinology and Metabolism Section of MKSAP 18!

In these pages, you will find updated information on disorders of glucose metabolism, disorders of the pituitary gland, disorders of the adrenal glands, disorders of the thyroid gland, reproduction disorders, transgender hormone therapy management, and calcium and bone disorders. All of these topics are uniquely focused on the needs of generalists and subspecialists *outside* of endocrinology.

The core content of MKSAP 18 has been developed as in previous editions–all essential information that is newly researched and written in 11 topic areas of internal medicine–created by dozens of leading generalists and subspecialists and guided by certification and recertification requirements, emerging knowledge in the field, and user feedback. MKSAP 18 also contains 1200 all-new peer-reviewed, psychometrically validated, multiple-choice questions (MCQs) for self-assessment and study, including 84 in Endocrinology and Metabolism. MKSAP 18 continues to include *High Value Care* (HVC) recommendations, based on the concept of balancing clinical benefit with costs and harms, with associated MCQs illustrating these principles and HVC Key Points called out in the text. Internists practicing in the hospital setting can easily find comprehensive *Hospitalist*-focused content and MCQs, specially designated in blue and with the 🄷 symbol.

If you purchased MKSAP 18 Complete, you also have access to MKSAP 18 Digital, with additional tools allowing you to customize your learning experience. MKSAP Digital includes regular text updates with new, practice-changing information, 200 new self-assessment questions, and enhanced custom-quiz options. MKSAP Complete also includes more than 1200 electronic, adaptive learning-enhanced flashcards for quick review of important concepts, as well as an updated and enhanced version of Virtual Dx, MKSAP's image-based self-assessment tool. As before, MKSAP 18 Digital is optimized for use on your mobile devices, with iOS- and Android-based apps allowing you to sync between your apps and online account and submit for CME credits and MOC points online.

Please visit us at the MKSAP Resource Site (mksap.acponline.org) to find out how we can help you study, earn CME credit and MOC points, and stay up to date.

On behalf of the many internists who have offered their time and expertise to create the content for MKSAP 18 and the editorial staff who work to bring this material to you in the best possible way, we are honored that you have chosen to use MKSAP 18 and appreciate any feedback about the program you may have. Please feel free to send any comments to mksap_editors@acponline.org.

Sincerely,

Patrick C. Alguire, MD, FACP
Editor-in-Chief
Senior Vice President Emeritus
Medical Education Division
American College of Physicians

Endocrinology and Metabolism

Committee

Cynthia A. Burns, MD, FACP, Section Editor[1]
Director of Undergraduate Medical Education in Internal
    Medicine
Internal Medicine Clerkship Director and Subspecialty
    Acting Internships Course Director
Associate Professor of Internal Medicine
Section of Endocrinology and Metabolism
Wake Forest School of Medicine
Winston-Salem, North Carolina

Leigh M. Eck, MD, FACP[2]
Program Director, Internal Medicine Residency Program
Associate Professor of Medicine
University of Kansas Health System
Kansas City, Kansas

Kurt A. Kennel, MD[2]
Assistant Professor of Medicine
Division of Endocrinology, Metabolism and Nutrition
Mayo Clinic College of Medicine and Science
Rochester, Minnesota

Wanda C. Lakey, MD, MHS, FACP[2]
Associate Professor of Medicine
Division of Endocrinology
Duke University Medical Center
Durham VA Medical Center
Durham, North Carolina

Sarah E. Mayson, MD[2]
Assistant Professor
Division of Endocrinology, Metabolism and Diabetes
University of Colorado School of Medicine
Aurora, Colorado

Farah Morgan, MD[1]
Assistant Professor
Cooper Medical School of Rowan University
Endocrine Fellowship Program Director
Cooper University Hospital
Camden, New Jersey

Neena Natt, MD[1]
Associate Professor, Endocrinology
Mayo Clinic College of Medicine and Science
Rochester, Minnesota

Editor-in-Chief

Patrick C. Alguire, MD, FACP[2]
Senior Vice President Emeritus, Medical Education
American College of Physicians
Philadelphia, Pennsylvania

Deputy Editor

Denise M. Dupras, MD, PhD, FACP[1]
Associate Program Director
Department of Internal Medicine
Associate Professor of Medicine
Mayo Clinic College of Medicine and Science
Rochester, Minnesota

Endocrinology and Metabolism Reviewers

Karen Barnard, MBBCh[1]
Shankar S. Bettadahalli, MD, FACP[1]
Michelle L. Cordoba Kissee, MD[1]
Benjamin A. Dennis, MD[1]
Ruban Dhaliwal, MD[1]
Antonette Brigidi Frasch, MD, FACP[2]
Peter A. Goulden, MD[2]
Dona Leslie Gray, MD, FACP[2]
Airani Sathananthan, MD, FACP[2]
Sarah H. See, MD, FACP[1]
Michael H. Shanik, MD, FACP[2]

Hospital Medicine Endocrinology and Metabolism Reviewers

Kyaw K. Soe, MD, FACP[1]
Scott M. Stevens, MD, FACP[2]

Endocrinology and Metabolism ACP Editorial Staff

Randy Hendrickson[1], Production Administrator/Editor
Julia Nawrocki[1], Digital Content Associate/Editor
Margaret Wells, Director, Self-Assessment and Educational
    Programs
Becky Krumm, Managing Editor, Self-Assessment and
    Educational Programs

ACP Principal Staff

Davoren Chick, MD, FACP[2]
Senior Vice President, Medical Education

Patrick C. Alguire, MD, FACP[2]
Senior Vice President Emeritus, Medical Education

Sean McKinney[1]
Vice President, Medical Education

Margaret Wells
Director, Self-Assessment and Educational Programs

Becky Krumm[1]
Managing Editor

Valerie Dangovetsky[1]
Administrator

Ellen McDonald, PhD[1]
Senior Staff Editor

Megan Zborowski[1]
Senior Staff Editor

Jackie Twomey[1]
Senior Staff Editor

Randy Hendrickson[1]
Production Administrator/Editor

Julia Nawrocki[1]
Digital Content Associate/Editor

Linnea Donnarumma[1]
Staff Editor

Chuck Emig[1]
Staff Editor

Joysa Winter[1]
Staff Editor

Kimberly Kerns[1]
Administrative Coordinator

---

1. Has no relationships with any entity producing, marketing, reselling, or distributing health care goods or services consumed by, or used on, patients.

2. Has disclosed relationship(s) with any entity producing, marketing, reselling, or distributing health care goods or services consumed by, or used on, patients.

Disclosure of Relationships with any entity producing, marketing, reselling, or distributing health care goods or services consumed by, or used on, patients.

Patrick C. Alguire, MD, FACP
Royalties
UpToDate

Davoren Chick, MD, FACP
Royalties
Wolters Kluwer Publishing
Consultantship
EBSCO Health's DynaMed Plus
Other
Owner and sole proprietor of Coding 101, LLC; Spouse: research consultant for Vedanta Biosciences

Leigh M. Eck, MD, FACP
Consultantship
NovoNordisk

Antonette Brigidi Frasch, MD, FACP
Consultantship
Medical Reviewers of America

Peter A. Goulden, MD
Research Grants/Contracts
NovoNordisk

Dona Leslie Gray, MD, FACP
Speakers Bureau
Janssen, Sanofi

Kurt A. Kennel, MD
Consultantship
Acupera
Honoraria
ACGME-I, American Association of Clinical Endocrinology

Wanda C. Lakey, MD, MHS, FACP
Research Grants/Contracts
Janssen, Regeneron, Amarin, Sanofi/Aventis

Sarah E. Mayson, MD
Other: Principal Investigator, Rosetta Genomics

Airani Sathananthan, MD, FACP
Research Grants/Contracts
Principal investigator for Western University for NovoNordisk/Sanofi

Michael H. Shanik, MD, FACP
Research Grants/Contracts
NovoNordisk, AstraZeneca, Boehringer Ingelheim, Eli Lilly, Amarin
Speakers Bureau
NovoNordisk, AstraZeneca, Boehringer Ingelheim, Eli Lilly, Amarin
Consultantship
NovoNordisk, Boehringer Ingelheim, Eli Lilly, Amarin

Scott M. Stevens, MD, FACP
Research Grants/Contracts
Bristol-Myers Squibb

Acknowledgments

The American College of Physicians (ACP) gratefully acknowledges the special contributions to the development and production of the 18th edition of the Medical Knowledge Self-Assessment Program® (MKSAP® 18) made by the following people:

Graphic Design: Barry Moshinski (Director, Graphic Services), Michael Ripca (Graphics Technical Administrator), and Jennifer Gropper (Graphic Designer).

Production/Systems: Dan Hoffmann (Director, Information Technology), Scott Hurd (Manager, Content Systems), Neil Kohl (Senior Architect), and Chris Patterson (Senior Architect).

MKSAP 18 Digital: Under the direction of Steven Spadt (Senior Vice President, Technology), the digital version of MKSAP 18 was developed within the ACP's Digital Products and Services Department, led by Brian Sweigard (Director, Digital Products and Services). Other members of the team included Dan Barron (Senior Web Application Developer/ Architect), Chris Forrest (Senior Software Developer/Design Lead), Kathleen Hoover (Senior Web Developer), Kara Regis (Manager, User Interface Design and Development), Brad Lord (Senior Web Application Developer), and John McKnight (Senior Web Developer).

The College also wishes to acknowledge that many other persons, too numerous to mention, have contributed to the production of this program. Without their dedicated efforts, this program would not have been possible.

MKSAP Resource Site (mksap.acponline.org)

The MKSAP Resource Site (mksap.acponline.org) is a continually updated site that provides links to MKSAP 18 online answer sheets for print subscribers; access to MKSAP 18 Digital; Board Basics® e-book access instructions; information on Continuing Medical Education (CME), Maintenance of Certification (MOC), and international Continuing Professional Development (CPD) and MOC; errata; and other new information.

International MOC/CPD

For information and instructions on submission of international MOC/CPD, please go to the MKSAP Resource Site (mksap.acponline.org).

Continuing Medical Education

The American College of Physicians is accredited by the Accreditation Council for Continuing Medical Education (ACCME) to provide continuing medical education for physicians.

The American College of Physicians designates this enduring material, MKSAP 18, for a maximum of 275 *AMA PRA Category 1 Credits*™. Physicians should claim only the credit commensurate with the extent of their participation in the activity.

Up to 19 *AMA PRA Category 1 Credits*™ are available from December 31, 2018, to December 31, 2021, for the MKSAP 18 Endocrinology and Metabolism section.

Learning Objectives

The learning objectives of MKSAP 18 are to:

- Close gaps between actual care in your practice and preferred standards of care, based on best evidence
- Diagnose disease states that are less common and sometimes overlooked and confusing
- Improve management of comorbid conditions that can complicate patient care
- Determine when to refer patients for surgery or care by subspecialists
- Pass the ABIM Certification Examination
- Pass the ABIM Maintenance of Certification Examination

Target Audience

- General internists and primary care physicians
- Subspecialists who need to remain up to date in internal medicine
- Residents preparing for the certifying examination in internal medicine
- Physicians preparing for maintenance of certification in internal medicine (recertification)

ABIM Maintenance of Certification

Check the MKSAP Resource Site (mksap.acponline.org) for the latest information on how MKSAP tests can be used to apply to the American Board of Internal Medicine (ABIM) for Maintenance of Certification (MOC) points following completion of the CME activity.

Successful completion of the CME activity, which includes participation in the evaluation component, enables the participant to earn up to 275 medical knowledge MOC points in the ABIM's MOC program. It is the CME activity provider's responsibility to submit participant completion information to ACCME for the purpose of granting MOC credit.

Earn Instantaneous CME Credits or MOC Points Online

Print subscribers can enter their answers online to earn instantaneous CME credits or MOC points. You can submit your answers using online answer sheets that are provided at mksap.acponline.org, where a record of your MKSAP 18 credits will be available. To earn CME credits or to apply for

MOC points, you need to answer all of the questions in a test and earn a score of at least 50% correct (number of correct answers divided by the total number of questions). Please note that if you are applying for MOC points, you must also enter your birth date and ABIM candidate number.

Take either of the following approaches:

1. Use the printed answer sheet at the back of this book to record your answers. Go to mksap.acponline.org, access the appropriate online answer sheet, transcribe your answers, and submit your test for instantaneous CME credits or MOC points. There is no additional fee for this service.

2. Go to mksap.acponline.org, access the appropriate online answer sheet, directly enter your answers, and submit your test for instantaneous CME credits or MOC points. There is no additional fee for this service.

Earn CME Credits or MOC Points by Mail or Fax

Pay a $20 processing fee per answer sheet and submit the printed answer sheet at the back of this book by mail or fax, as instructed on the answer sheet. Make sure you calculate your score and enter your birth date and ABIM candidate number, and fax the answer sheet to 215-351-2799 or mail the answer sheet to Member and Customer Service, American College of Physicians, 190 N. Independence Mall West, Philadelphia, PA 19106-1572, using the courtesy envelope provided in your MKSAP 18 slipcase. You will need your 10-digit order number and 8-digit ACP ID number, which are printed on your packing slip. Please allow 4 to 6 weeks for your score report to be emailed back to you. Be sure to include your email address for a response.

If you do not have a 10-digit order number and 8-digit ACP ID number, or if you need help creating a user-name and password to access the MKSAP 18 online answer sheets, go to mksap.acponline.org or email custserv@acponline.org.

Disclosure Policy

It is the policy of the American College of Physicians (ACP) to ensure balance, independence, objectivity, and scientific rigor in all of its educational activities. To this end, and consistent with the policies of the ACP and the Accreditation Council for Continuing Medical Education (ACCME), contributors to all ACP continuing medical education activities are required to disclose all relevant financial relationships with any entity producing, marketing, re-selling, or distributing health care goods or services consumed by, or used on, patients. Contributors are required to use generic names in the discussion of therapeutic options and are required to identify any unapproved, off-label, or investigative use of commercial products or devices. Where a trade name is used, all available trade names for the same product type are also included. If trade-name products manufactured by companies with whom contributors have relationships are discussed, contributors are asked to provide evidence-based citations in support of the discussion. The information is reviewed by the committee responsible for producing this text. If necessary, adjustments to topics or contributors' roles in content development are made to balance the discussion. Further, all readers of this text are asked to evaluate the content for evidence of commercial bias and send any relevant comments to mksap_editors@acponline.org so that future decisions about content and contributors can be made in light of this information.

Resolution of Conflicts

To resolve all conflicts of interest and influences of vested interests, ACP's content planners used best evidence and updated clinical care guidelines in developing content, when such evidence and guidelines were available. All content underwent review by peer reviewers not on the committee to ensure that the material was balanced and unbiased. Contributors' disclosure information can be found with the list of contributors' names and those of ACP principal staff listed in the beginning of this book.

Hospital-Based Medicine

For the convenience of subscribers who provide care in hospital settings, content that is specific to the hospital setting has been highlighted in blue. Hospital icons (H) highlight where the hospital-only content begins, continues over more than one page, and ends.

High Value Care Key Points

Key Points in the text that relate to High Value Care concepts (that is, concepts that discuss balancing clinical benefit with costs and harms) are designated by the HVC icon [HVC].

Educational Disclaimer

The editors and publisher of MKSAP 18 recognize that the development of new material offers many opportunities for error. Despite our best efforts, some errors may persist in print. Drug dosage schedules are, we believe, accurate and in accordance with current standards. Readers are advised, however, to ensure that the recommended dosages in MKSAP 18 concur with the information provided in the product information material. This is especially important in cases of new, infrequently used, or highly toxic drugs. Application of the information in MKSAP 18 remains the professional responsibility of the practitioner.

The primary purpose of MKSAP 18 is educational. Information presented, as well as publications, technologies, products, and/or services discussed, is intended to inform subscribers about the knowledge, techniques, and experiences of the contributors. A diversity of professional opinion exists, and the views of the contributors are their own and not those of the ACP. Inclusion of any material in the program does not constitute endorsement or recommendation by the ACP. The ACP does not warrant the safety, reliability, accuracy, completeness, or usefulness of and disclaims any and all liability for damages and claims that may result from the use of information, publications, technologies, products, and/or services discussed in this program.

Publisher's Information

Disclaimer Regarding Direct Purchases from Online Retailers

CME and/or MOC for MKSAP 18 is available only if you purchase the program directly from ACP. CME credits and MOC points cannot be awarded to those purchasers who have purchased the program from non-authorized sellers such as Amazon, eBay, or any other such online retailer.

Unauthorized Use of This Book Is Against the Law

MKSAP 18 ISBN: 978-1-938245-47-3
(Endocrinology and Metabolism) ISBN: 978-1-938245-54-1

Printed in the United States of America.

For order information in the U.S. or Canada call 800-ACP-1915. All other countries call 215-351-2600 (Monday to Friday, 9 AM – 5 PM ET). Fax inquiries to 215-351-2799 or email to custserv@acponline.org.

Errata

Errata for MKSAP 18 will be available through the MKSAP Resource Site at mksap.acponline.org as new information becomes known to the editors.

Table of Contents

Endocrinology and Metabolism High Value Care Recommendations

The American College of Physicians, in collaboration with multiple other organizations, is engaged in a worldwide initiative to promote the practice of High Value Care (HVC). The goals of the HVC initiative are to improve health care outcomes by providing care of proven benefit and reducing costs by avoiding unnecessary and even harmful interventions. The initiative comprises several programs that integrate the important concept of health care value (balancing clinical benefit with costs and harms) for a given intervention into a broad range of educational materials to address the needs of trainees, practicing physicians, and patients.

HVC content has been integrated into MKSAP 18 in several important ways. MKSAP 18 includes HVC-identified key points in the text, HVC-focused multiple choice questions, and, for subscribers to MKSAP Digital, an HVC custom quiz. From the text and questions, we have generated the following list of HVC recommendations that meet the definition below of high value care and bring us closer to our goal of improving patient outcomes while conserving finite resources.

High Value Care Recommendation: A recommendation to choose diagnostic and management strategies for patients in specific clinical situations that balance clinical benefit with cost and harms with the goal of improving patient outcomes.

Below are the High Value Care Recommendations for the Endocrinology and Metabolism section of MKSAP 18.

- Tight inpatient glycemic control is not consistently associated with improved outcomes and may increase mortality.
- The sole use of "sliding-scale insulin" is not recommended since it leads to large glucose fluctuations.
- Treatment with an ACE inhibitor or angiotensin receptor blocker is not recommended for patients with diabetes who have a normal blood pressure, a urine albumin-creatinine ratio level less than 30 mg/g, and an estimated glomerular filtration rate (eGFR) greater than 60 mL/min/1.73 m².

- In the evaluation of fasting or postprandial hypoglycemia, specimens for C-peptide, insulin, proinsulin, β-hydroxybutyrate are obtained but are not sent for analysis unless a simultaneous glucose is less than 60 mg/dL (3.3 mmol/L).
- A history of normal menses rules out hypogonadotropic hypogonadism and additional testing is not required.
- Elevated plasma renin activity in patients taking an ACE inhibitor or angiotensin receptor blocker rules out hyperaldosteronism.
- Fine-needle aspiration biopsy is generally not needed for isolated subcentimeter thyroid nodules.
- Measurement of triiodothyronine in the setting of hypothyroidism is not needed.
- In the evaluation of Hashimoto thyroiditis, measurement of thyroid perioxidase (TPO) antibody titer is not necessary unless the diagnosis is unclear.
- Thyroid function should not be assessed in hospitalized patients unless there is a strong clinical suspicion of thyroid dysfunction.
- Before making the diagnosis of subclinical hypothyroidism, transient elevation of serum thyroid-stimulating hormone should be ruled out by repeating the measurement of thyroid-stimulating hormone in 2 to 3 months (see Item 65).
- Screening men with nonspecific symptoms of hypogonadism is not recommended.
- Testosterone therapy in men without biochemical evidence of deficiency is not beneficial and may be associated with significant harms.
- Routine screening for vitamin D deficiency is not recommended in healthy populations.
- For low-risk osteoporotic women, treatment with antiresorptive therapy for 5 years is sufficient (see Item 20).
- Screening for osteoporosis in premenopausal women is not indicated in the absence of risk factors (see Item 70).

Endocrinology and Metabolism

Disorders of Glucose Metabolism

Hyperglycemia results from abnormal carbohydrate metabolism secondary to insulin deficiency, peripheral resistance to insulin action, or a combination of both. Hyperglycemia that exceeds the normal glucose range but does not meet the diagnostic criteria for diabetes mellitus is defined as prediabetes, which increases the risk for the development of diabetes.

Diabetes Mellitus

Screening for Diabetes Mellitus

Screening for type 2 diabetes mellitus in the general adult population is indicated because: (1) type 2 diabetes is often preceded by a prolonged asymptomatic hyperglycemic period in which microvascular and macrovascular damage may occur; (2) lifestyle interventions and medications have demonstrated the ability to delay or prevent onset of type 2 diabetes in persons with prediabetes, and (3) early intensive glucose control and management of hyperlipidemia and hypertension may prevent or reduce the progression of microvascular and macrovascular cardiovascular disease (CVD).

The American Diabetes Association (ADA) and the U.S. Preventive Services Task Force (USPSTF) include age, BMI, race/ethnicity, and other risk factors as part of their criteria for screening recommendations for type 2 diabetes (**Table 1**). These risk factors are associated with a high risk of incident diabetes.

Screening for type 1 diabetes is not recommended. Antibody screening in a high-risk person with a relative with type 1 diabetes should occur within the context of a clinical trial (www.diabetestrialnet.org).

Diagnostic Criteria for Diabetes Mellitus

Diabetes mellitus can be diagnosed by an abnormal result in one of three tests: hemoglobin A_{1c}, fasting plasma glucose (FPG), or 2-hour plasma glucose (2-hr PG) after a 75-gram carbohydrate challenge during an oral glucose tolerance test (OGTT) (**Table 2**). An abnormal result in asymptomatic persons should be confirmed with repeat testing. A single random plasma glucose value greater than or equal to 200 mg/dL (11.1 mmol/L) in the setting of symptomatic hyperglycemia is diagnostic of diabetes.

The results of testing for diabetes differ depending on which test is done, FPG, 2-hr PG, or hemoglobin A_{1c}. The 2-hr PG test has a higher sensitivity for the diagnosis of diabetes

compared with FPG or hemoglobin A_{1c}. The advantages and disadvantages of the tests must be considered when determining the best screening option for a patient (**Table 3**).

> ### KEY POINTS
>
> - Diabetes mellitus can be diagnosed by an abnormal result in one of the following screening tests: hemoglobin A_{1c}, fasting plasma glucose, or 2-hour plasma glucose after a 75-gram carbohydrate challenge during an oral glucose tolerance test.
>
> - An abnormal result in asymptomatic persons should be confirmed with repeat testing.

Classification of Diabetes Mellitus

The underlying insulin abnormality, whether absolute or relative insulin deficiency, peripheral insulin resistance, or an overlap of both abnormalities, is important for classifying the type of diabetes mellitus and has implications for treatment options (**Table 4**).

Insulin Deficiency

Type 1 Diabetes Mellitus

Type 1 diabetes mellitus is characterized by a state of insulin deficiency secondary to the destruction of the insulin-producing beta cells in the pancreas. The destruction may be secondary to autoimmunity, idiopathic, or acquired.

Immune-Mediated Diabetes Mellitus

Immune-mediated type 1 diabetes mellitus (type 1A) is the underlying cause in 5% to 10% of persons newly diagnosed with diabetes. The mechanism of the beta cell destruction is multifactorial and likely due to environmental factors in persons with genetic susceptibilities. Specific human leukocyte antigen (HLA) alleles demonstrate a strong association with immune-mediated type 1 diabetes. At diagnosis, one or more autoantibodies directed at the following targets are typically present: glutamic acid decarboxylase (GAD65), tyrosine phosphatases IA-2 and IA-2β, islet cells, insulin, and zinc transporter (Zn T-8). Owing to highly automated available assays, GAD65 and IA-2 autoantibodies are recommended for initial screening. GAD65 autoantibodies have a high prevalence (70%) at the time of diagnosis and may remain detectable for years.

Immune-mediated type 1 diabetes has a variable presentation that ranges from moderate hyperglycemia to life-threatening diabetic ketoacidosis (DKA). At the time of diagnosis, approximately 90% of the functioning beta cells have been destroyed. Initiating insulin at the time of diagnosis may decrease toxicity associated with extreme hyperglycemia allowing the beta cell

TABLE 1. Screening Guidelines for Type 2 Diabetes Mellitus in Asymptomatic Adults

	ADA (2018)[a]	USPSTF (2015)
Screening criteria	Screen overweight adults (BMI ≥25 or ≥23 in Asian Americans) with at least one additional risk factor:	Screen adults aged 40 to 70 years who are overweight or obese as part of risk assessment for cardiovascular disease.
	First-degree relative with diabetes	Other risk factors:
	High-risk race/ethnicity (black, Hispanic/Latino, American Indian, Asian, Native Hawaiian/Pacific Islander)	High percentage of abdominal fat
	History of gestational diabetes mellitus	Hyperlipidemia
	History of cardiovascular disease	Hypertension
	Physical inactivity	Physical inactivity
	Hypertension (≥140/90 or on antihypertensive therapy)	Smoking
	HDL cholesterol <35 mg/dL (0.90 mmol/L) and/or triglyceride >250 mg/dL (2.82 mmol/L)	
	Polycystic ovary syndrome	
	Hemoglobin A_{1c} ≥5.7% (39 mmol/mol), IGT, or IFG on previous testing	
	Other conditions associated with insulin resistance (severe obesity, acanthosis nigricans)	
Additional screening criteria	All adults age 45 years or older	—
Additional screening considerations	Consider screening patients on medications known to increase the risk of diabetes, such as glucocorticoids, thiazide diuretics, HIV medications, and atypical antipsychotics.	Diabetes may occur in younger patients or at a lower BMI. Consider screening earlier if one of the following risk factors is present:
		Family history of diabetes
		History of gestational diabetes
		Polycystic ovary syndrome
		High-risk race/ethnicity (black, Hispanic/Latino, Asian American, American Indian/Alaskan Native, Native Hawaiian/Pacific Islander)
Screening intervals	Rescreen every 3 years if results are normal. Yearly testing recommended if prediabetes is diagnosed (hemoglobin A_{1c} between 5.7% and 6.4%, IGT, IFG).	Data supporting optimal screening intervals are limited. Rescreening every 3 years may be reasonable.

ADA = American Diabetes Association; CVD = cardiovascular disease; IFG = impaired fasting glucose; IGT = impaired glucose tolerance; USPSTF = U.S. Preventive Services Task Force.

[a]An optional ADA screening tool for diabetes risk can be found at www.diabetes.org/are-you-at-risk/diabetes-risk-test/. Accessed May 16, 2018.

Recommendations from American Diabetes Association. 2. Classification and diagnosis of diabetes: standards of medical care in diabetes-2018. Diabetes Care. 2018;41:S13-S27. [PMID: 29222373]

Recommendations from Siu AL; U S Preventive Services Task Force. Screening for abnormal blood glucose and type 2 diabetes mellitus: U.S. Preventive Services Task Force Recommendation Statement. Ann Intern Med. 2015;163:861-8. [PMID: 26501513] doi:10. 7326/M15-2345.

to regain some ability to produce insulin. Although this "honeymoon period" can last several weeks to years, insulin use should be continued to decrease stress on the remaining functioning beta cells and prolong their lifespan. Insulin deficiency requires life-long use of insulin therapy.

Patients with immune-mediated type 1 diabetes also have an increased risk for other autoimmune disorders, including celiac disease, thyroid disorders, vitiligo, and autoimmune primary adrenal gland failure.

Late autoimmune diabetes in adults (LADA) is characterized by autoantibody development leading to beta cell destruction and ultimately insulin deficiency. Individuals with LADA are typically not insulin-dependent initially and are frequently misclassified as having type 2 diabetes. There is a slow progression toward insulin dependence over months to years after diagnosis in the setting of positive autoantibodies.

KEY POINT

- Autoantibodies glutamic acid decarboxylase (GAD65) and tyrosine phosphatase IA-2 demonstrate a strong association with immune-mediated type 1 diabetes and should be measured at initial diagnosis to determine etiology.

Idiopathic Type 1 Diabetes Mellitus

Idiopathic type 1 diabetes (type 1B) is characterized by variable insulin deficiency due to beta cell destruction without the

TABLE 2. Diagnostic Criteria for Diabetes Mellitus[a]

Test	Normal Range	Increased Risk for Diabetes (Prediabetes)	Diabetes
Random plasma glucose	—	—	Hyperglycemic symptoms plus a random glucose ≥200 mg/dL (11.1 mmol/L)
Fasting plasma glucose[b]	<100 mg/dL (5.6 mmol/L)	100-125 mg/dL (5.6-6.9 mmol/L)	≥126 mg/dL (7.0 mmol/L)
2-Hour plasma glucose during an OGTT[c]	<140 mg/dL (7.8 mmol/L)	140-199 mg/dL (7.8-11.0 mmol/L)	≥200 mg/dL (11.1 mmol/L)
Hemoglobin A$_{1c}$[d,e]	<5.7% (39 mmol/mol)	5.7%-6.4% (39-46 mmol/mol)	≥6.5% (48 mmol/mol)

OGTT = oral glucose tolerance test.

[a]In the absence of hyperglycemic symptoms, an abnormal fasting plasma glucose, OGTT, or hemoglobin A$_{1c}$ should be confirmed by repeating the same test on a separate day. If two different tests demonstrate discordant results, the American Diabetes Association recommends repeating the test with the abnormal results.

[b]Fasting for at least 8 hours.

[c]An OGTT involves the consumption of a 75-g glucose load dissolved in water.

[d]The American Diabetes Association recommends a National Glycohemoglobin Standardization Program (NGSP)-certified hemoglobin A$_{1c}$ assay that is standardized to the Diabetes Control and Complication Trial (DCCT) assay.

[e]The Veterans Affairs/Department of Defense guidelines recommend confirmation of diabetes based upon an elevated hemoglobin A$_{1c}$ value of 6.5% to 6.9% with an elevated fasting plasma glucose of ≥126 mg/dL (7.0 mmol/L) due to strong evidence supporting racial differences between glycemic control and hemoglobin A$_{1c}$ values for diagnosis and treatment.

Data from American Diabetes Association. 2. Classification and diagnosis of diabetes: Standards of Medical Care in Diabetes—2018. Diabetes Care. 2018;41 (Suppl. 1):S13-S27. [PMID: 29222373]

Data from U.S. Department of Veterans Affairs/U.S. Department of Defense. VA/DoD Clinical Practice Guidelines for the management of diabetes mellitus in primary care. 2017. www.healthquality.va.gov/guidelines/cd/diabetes. Accessed May 16, 2018.

presence of autoantibodies. Individuals with idiopathic type 1 diabetes may develop episodic DKA. There is typically a strong family history of type 2 diabetes in persons with idiopathic diabetes, and it is more common in Asian and African American patients, particularly with sub-Saharan African ancestry.

Acquired Type 1 Diabetes Mellitus

Beta cell destruction may occur from diseases affecting the pancreas or from the effect of drugs or infections (see Table 4). This may result in impaired insulin production or secretion with the subsequent development of type 1 diabetes.

Insulin Resistance

The ineffective use of insulin by the peripheral cells to utilize glucose and fatty acids characterizes insulin resistance. Blood glucose levels remain in the normal range as long as the beta cells can increase insulin production. Hyperglycemia results from a relative insulin deficiency when the pancreas can no longer produce enough insulin. Obesity increases the risk for insulin resistance, which is also a component of the metabolic syndrome and predisposes to the development of type 2 diabetes.

Metabolic Syndrome

Metabolic syndrome comprises a constellation of risk factors for development of type 2 diabetes and CVD, which includes abdominal obesity, impaired glucose metabolism, hyperlipidemia, and hypertension. Multiple organizations define

metabolic syndrome differently (**Table 5**). The Endocrine Society recommends screening patients with risk factors for metabolic syndrome every 3 years to evaluate fasting plasma glucose, fasting lipid panel, blood pressure, and waist circumference. Calculation of the 10-year cardiovascular risk, using either the Framingham Risk Score or the American College of Cardiology (ACC)/American Heart Association (AHA) risk calculator, is recommended for patients with metabolic syndrome.

Type 2 Diabetes Mellitus

Most cases of diabetes (90% to 95%) meet the criteria for type 2 diabetes. Hyperglycemia accompanied by insulin resistance and/or relative insulin deficiency defines type 2 diabetes. The extent of beta cell dysfunction determines the degree of hyperglycemia, which may worsen over time with progressive decrease in insulin production. The pathogenesis of type 2 diabetes is multifactorial with influence from both genetic and environmental factors. Type 2 diabetes is commonly present in first-degree relatives of both individuals at high risk for or diagnosed with type 2 diabetes. There is also an increased risk in several ethnicities including: Hispanic/Latino, African American, American Indian, Asian American. Additional risk factors for diabetes risk include increasing age and decreased physical activity.

Type 2 diabetes classically presents in adults, although there is an increased incidence among children and adolescents as the rate of overweight/obesity increases in these populations. Type 2 diabetes has a gradual onset with most

TABLE 3. Comparison of Screening Tests for Diabetes Mellitus

Test	Advantages	Disadvantages
Hemoglobin A$_{1c}$	Convenient: Does not require fasting and no restrictions on collection time	Lower sensitivity for diagnosis compared with FPG or 2-hr PG
	Not altered by illness, stress, etc.	Erroneous increases or decreases in hemoglobin A$_{1c}$ result secondary to factors affecting erythrocyte survival[a]:
	Measures blood glucose concentration over the prior 8-12 weeks	Iron deficiency anemia
	Minimal biological variability	Blood loss/hemolysis
	Blood sample remains stable	Kidney disease
	Standardized assay	Liver disease
	Test accuracy is monitored	Pregnancy
	Measurement correlates with microvascular and macrovascular outcomes	Hemoglobin variants in individuals with African, Southeast Asian, and Mediterranean heritage[b]
		Higher value in black compared with non-Hispanic white persons[c]
		Affected by some glucose-6-phosphate dehydrogenase variants[d]
		Unavailable in some areas of the world
		Expensive
FPG	Inexpensive	Inconvenient: ≥ 8 hour fasting required and restriction on time of collection
	Widely available	Affected by illness and stress
	Automated assay	Measures single point in time
		High biological variability within patient
		Blood sample unstable after collection
		Diurnal variation
		Diabetes complications not as closely linked to FPG compared with hemoglobin A$_{1c}$
		Sample source (capillary, venous, or arterial blood) alters the measurement
		Assay standardization incomplete
2-hr PG during an OGTT	Highly sensitive to detect risk of developing diabetes	Similar disadvantages as FPG test
	Detects early abnormalities in glucose metabolism	Prolonged patient preparation
		Risk of hypoglycemia at 4-6 hours in normal persons
		Poor reproducibility
		Expensive

2-hr PG = 2-hour prandial glucose; FPG = fasting plasma glucose; OGTT = oral glucose tolerance test.

[a]Blood glucose tests should be used instead of hemoglobin A$_{1c}$ to screen for diabetes in the setting of altered red blood cell turnover.

[b]Some methods used to measure hemoglobin A$_{1c}$ can accurately measure hemoglobin A$_{1c}$ in individuals with hemoglobin variants who are heterozygous for HbS, HbE, HbC, HbD, and increased HbF. For individuals who are homozygous for HbS, HbC, or HbSC, blood glucose should be used instead of hemoglobin A$_{1c}$ for diagnostic purposes. Blacks who are heterozygous for HbS can have a hemoglobin A$_{1c}$ 0.3% lower than individuals without the trait for any level of mean glycemia.

[c]Hemoglobin A$_{1c}$ is higher in blacks compared with non-Hispanic whites in the setting of similar FPG and postprandial glucose values. Despite this, the risk of complications associated with A$_{1c}$ remains similar in blacks and non-Hispanic white persons.

[d]There is an association between a lower hemoglobin A$_{1c}$ and hemizygous men and homozygous women with X-linked glucose-6-phosphate dehydrogenase G202A by 0.8% and 0.7%, respectively.

Data from American Diabetes Association. 2. Classification and diagnosis of diabetes: Standards of Medical Care in Diabetes—2018. Diabetes Care. 2018;41:S13-S27. [PMID: 29222373]

Data from American Diabetes Association. 6. Glycemic targets: Standards of Medical Care in Diabetes—2018. Diabetes Care. 2018;41:S55-S64. [PMID: 29222377]

Data from Sacks DB. A1C versus glucose testing: a comparison. Diabetes Care. 2011;34:518-23. [PMID: 21270207]

Data from NGSP: Harmonizing Hemoglobin A1c Testing web site. www.ngsp.org. Accessed June 2018.

Data from National Institute of Diabetes and Digestive and Kidney Diseases. Comparing tests for diabetes and prediabetes. Mar. 2014. NIH Publication No. 14-7850. www.diabetes.niddk.nih.gov. Accessed June 2018.

TABLE 4.	Classification of Diabetes Mellitus

Insulin Deficiency[a]

Immune-mediated (type 1A)

  Type 1 diabetes

  LADA

  Rare forms: "stiff man" syndrome, anti-insulin receptor antibodies

Idiopathic (type 1B) (seronegative)

Acquired

  Diseases of the exocrine pancreas: pancreatitis, trauma/pancreatectomy, neoplasia, cystic fibrosis, hemochromatosis, fibrocalculous pancreatopathy

  Drug-related: Vacor (rat poison), intravenous pentamidine

  Infections: congenital rubella, enteroviruses

Insulin Resistance

Type 2 diabetes[b]

Ketosis-prone[c]

Other or Rare Types

Genetic defects in beta-cell function (including six distinct MODY syndromes)

Genetic defects in insulin action

Endocrinopathies:

  Acromegaly, Cushing syndrome, glucagonoma, pheochromocytoma, hyperthyroidism[d]

  Somatostatinoma, aldosteronoma[d]

Drug-related:

  Glucocorticoids, thiazides, β-blockers, diazoxide, tacrolimus, cyclosporine, niacin, HIV protease inhibitors, atypical antipsychotics (clozapine, olanzapine)[e]

Genetic syndromes:

  Down syndrome[f]

  Wolfram syndrome (DIDMOAD)[g]

  Klinefelter, Turner, and Prader-Willi syndromes; myotonic dystrophy[d]

DIDMOAD = diabetes insipidus, diabetes mellitus, optic atrophy, and deafness; LADA = late autoimmune diabetes in adults; MODY= maturity-onset diabetes of the young.

[a]Beta-cell destruction usually leading to absolute insulin deficiency.

[b]Insulin resistance with progressive relative insulin deficiency.

[c]More common in nonwhite persons who present with diabetic ketoacidosis but become non-insulin-dependent over time.

[d]Impaired insulin action.

[e]Impaired insulin secretion, impaired insulin action, or altered hepatic glucose metabolism.

[f]Insulin deficiency, immune-mediated.

[g]Insulin deficiency.

Data from American Diabetes Association. 2. Classification and diagnosis of diabetes: Standards of Medical Care—2018. Diabetes Care. 2018;41:S13-S27. [PMID: 29222373]

affected persons remaining asymptomatic for several years. At the time of diagnosis, these patients may already have microvascular and/or macrovascular CVD. Although the beta cell

does not produce sufficient insulin to overcome insulin resistance and maintain euglycemia, there is adequate insulin production to suppress lipolysis and prevent DKA in type 2 diabetes. DKA in type 2 diabetes may rarely occur in the setting of extreme stress or illness.

The development of type 2 diabetes in high-risk individuals can be delayed or prevented with modifications to lifestyle (diet, exercise), pharmacologic intervention, or metabolic surgery. The goal of these interventions is weight loss and the reduction of insulin resistance. In the Diabetes Prevention Program (DPP), lifestyle modifications reduced the incidence of type 2 diabetes in persons with prediabetes by 58%. Thus, the ADA recommends the DPP goals of 7% weight loss over 6 months and at least 150 min/week of moderate-intensity exercise to reduce the risk of diabetes development. A diet rich in monounsaturated fat, whole grains, vegetables, whole fruits, and nuts is recommended.

Several pharmacologic interventions have demonstrated efficacy in diabetes risk reduction (**Table 6**). Safety data, cost, and long-term durability of each intervention must be considered for each individual patient. Metformin reduced the incidence of diabetes by 31% compared with placebo in the DPP. In addition metformin has long-term safety data. The ADA and the American Association of Clinical Endocrinologists (AACE) recommend metformin initially for diabetes risk prevention in individuals with prediabetes, particularly in those with increasing hemoglobin A_{1c} values despite lifestyle modifications who are younger than 60 years of age, are obese, or have a history of gestational diabetes.

KEY POINTS

- According to the Diabetes Prevention Program, lifestyle modifications, including weight loss, healthy diet, and exercise, reduced the incidence of type 2 diabetes in persons with prediabetes by 58%.

- The American Diabetes Association (ADA) and the American Association of Clinical Endocrinologists (AACE) recommend metformin initially for diabetes risk prevention in individuals with prediabetes, particularly in those with increasing hemoglobin A_{1c} values despite lifestyle modifications who are younger than 60 years of age, are obese, or have a history of gestational diabetes.

Ketosis-Prone Diabetes Mellitus

The term "ketosis-prone diabetes" (KPD) incorporates several glycemic syndromes also known as ketosis-prone type 2 diabetes, "Flatbush diabetes," type 1B diabetes, or atypical diabetes. These syndromes present with episodic DKA resulting from insulin deficiency but have variable periods of insulin dependence and independence.

For individuals with KPD, insulin therapy for the treatment of DKA is required until DKA has resolved and the beta cells are no longer impaired by glucose toxicity, if possible, and can produce sufficient amounts of insulin to suppress

TABLE 5. Criteria for the Definition of Metabolic Syndrome

Qualifying Criteria	NCEP ATP III 2005 (Meets at Least 3 of 5 Criteria)	International Diabetes Federation (2006) (Required Central Obesity and at Least 2 of 4 Remaining Criteria)

Waist circumference	Men ≥40 in (102 cm)
	
	Women ≥35 in (88 cm)
		Europids
		   Men ≥37 in (94 cm)
		   Women ≥31 in (80 cm)
		South Asians
		   Men ≥35 in (90 cm)[a]
		   Women ≥31 in (80 cm)
		Chinese
		   Men ≥35 in (90 cm)[a]
		   Women ≥31 in (80 cm)
		Japanese
		   Men ≥35 in (90 cm)[a]
		   Women ≥31 in (80 cm)
		South/Central Americans
		   Men ≥35 in (90 cm)[a]
		   Women ≥31 in (80 cm)
		Sub-Saharan Africans
		   Men ≥37 in (94 cm)
		   Women ≥31 in (80 cm)
		Eastern Mediterranean and Middle East
		   Men ≥37 in (94 cm)
		   Women ≥31 in (80 cm)

Fasting TG	≥150 mg/dL (1.7 mmol/L) or Drug therapy treating increased TG	≥150 mg/dL (1.7 mmol/L) or Drug therapy treating increased TG
HDL cholesterol	Men <40 mg/dL (1.0 mmol/L) Women <50 mg/dL (1.3 mmol/L) or Drug therapy targeting decreased HDL cholesterol	Men <40 mg/dL (1.0 mmol/L) Women <50 mg/dL (1.3 mmol/L) or Drug therapy targeting decreased HDL cholesterol
Blood pressure	Systolic ≥130 mmHg Diastolic ≥85 mmHg or Drug therapy for hypertension	Systolic ≥130 mmHg Diastolic ≥85 mmHg or Drug therapy for hypertension
Fasting glucose	Blood glucose ≥100 mg/dL or Drug therapy for increased glucose	Blood glucose ≥100 mg/dL or Drug therapy for increased glucose

HDL = high-density lipoprotein cholesterol; NCEP ACP III = National Cholesterol Education Program - Adult Treatment Panel III; TG = triglyceride.

[a]Waist circumference is 90 cm (35 inches) according to the International Diabetes Foundation and 88 cm (35 inches) according to the NCEP ATP III.

Data from Alberti KG, Eckel RH, Grundy SM, Zimmet PZ, Cleeman JI, Donato KA, et al; International Diabetes Federation Task Force on Epidemiology and Prevention. Harmonizing the metabolic syndrome: a joint interim statement of the International Diabetes Federation Task Force on Epidemiology and Prevention; National Heart, Lung, and Blood Institute; American Heart Association; World Heart Federation; International Atherosclerosis Society; and International Association for the Study of Obesity. Circulation. 2009;120:1640-5. [PMID: 19805654]

Data from International Diabetes Federation. The IDF consensus worldwide definition of the metabolic syndrome, 2006. www.idf.org/our-activities/advocacy-awareness/resources-and-tools/60:idfconsensus-worldwide-definitionof-the-metabolic-syndrome.html. Accessed June 2018.

lipolysis. Given the variable clinical course exhibited with KPD, uncertainty prevails regarding the need for short-term and long-term insulin treatment regimens. Four classification systems have therefore been developed to provide predictive guidance on the length of insulin therapy. A longitudinal study demonstrated greater accuracy in predicting beta-cell reserve and insulin dependence 12 months after the initial episode of DKA with the Aβ system when compared to the other classification systems, with a sensitivity of 99% and specificity of 96%. With the Aβ system, autoantibody status (A) and

TABLE 6. Strategies to Prevent or Delay Onset of Type 2 Diabetes Mellitus

Intervention	Effectiveness
Diet and exercise[a]	Shown to delay onset of diabetes by up to 10-20 years
Smoking cessation	Modestly effective as long as it does not cause weight gain, but is always recommended
Bariatric surgery	Effective if used in morbidly obese persons (BMI >40)
Metformin[a]	Shown to delay onset of diabetes by up to 10 years
Lipase inhibitors (orlistat)	Shown to delay onset of diabetes up to 4 years
α-Glucosidase inhibitors (acarbose, voglibose)	Shown to delay onset of diabetes up to 3 years
Thiazolidinediones (troglitazone, rosiglitazone, pioglitazone)	Shown to delay onset of diabetes up to 3 years
Glucagon-like peptide 1 (GLP-1) receptor agonists (exenatide, liraglutide)	Significant weight loss and improvements in glycemic control in high-risk persons in short-term studies
Insulin and insulin secretagogues (sulfonylureas, meglitinides)	Ineffective
ACE inhibitors and angiotensin receptor blockers	Ineffective
Estrogen-progestin	Modest effect only

[a]Preferred.

Data from American Diabetes Association. 5. Prevention or delay of type 2 diabetes: Standards of Medical Care in Diabetes—2018. Diabetes Care. 2018;41:S51-S54. [PMID: 29222376]

Data from Garber AJ, Abrahamson MJ, Barzilay JI, Blonde L, Bloomgarden ZT, Bush MA, et al. Consensus statement by the American Association of Clinical Endocrinologists and American College of Endocrinology on the comprehensive type 2 diabetes management algorithm—2018 Executive Summary. Endocr Pract. 2018;24:91-120. [PMID: 29368965]

CONT.

beta-cell function (β) are key determinants affecting whether an individual will require long-term insulin. Longitudinal data from KPD cohorts indicate individuals without beta-cell reserve regardless of the antibody status (A⁺β⁻ and A⁻β⁻) are more likely to have poor glycemic control and develop long-term insulin dependence after the development of DKA compared to individuals with preserved beta-cell function. ◨

Gestational Diabetes Mellitus

An increase in insulin resistance during the second and third trimester of pregnancy is a normal physiologic phenomenon driven by placental hormones. With impaired beta-cell function, insulin production will be inadequate to overcome the insulin resistance with subsequent development of hyperglycemia.

Gestational diabetes is defined as hyperglycemia during the second or third trimester in women without a prepregnancy diagnosis of type 1 or type 2 diabetes. Risk factors include age over 25 years, overweight/obesity, family history of type 2 diabetes,

and high-risk racial/ethnic groups (blacks, Hispanic/Latino Americans, South or East Asians, Pacific Islanders, and American Indians). Adverse maternal and neonatal outcomes related to gestational diabetes increase with worsening hyperglycemia. Complications include macrosomia, labor and delivery complications, preeclampsia, fetal defects, neonatal hypoglycemia, spontaneous abortion, and intrauterine fetal demise.

Given the increased prevalence of undiagnosed type 2 diabetes in the general population, the ADA recommends standard screening for any pregnant woman with diabetes risk factors at the initial prenatal visit. Women with hyperglycemia identified during the first trimester are classified as having type 2 diabetes instead of gestational diabetes. For all other pregnant women without a prior diabetes diagnosis, gestational diabetes screening should occur between gestation weeks 24 and 28. The screening method recommended varies among expert groups. The "one-step" OGTT involves blood glucose measurements at baseline (fasting) and 1 and 2 hours after a 75-g oral glucose load. One abnormal value above the cut-point is diagnostic of gestational diabetes. The "two-step" OGTT involves an initial blood glucose measurement 1 hour after a 50-g OGTT. If the blood glucose is abnormal, the second step is initiated. Glucose is measured at baseline (fasting) and 1, 2, and 3 hours after a 100-g oral glucose load. Two abnormal blood glucose values after the 100-g load are diagnostic for gestational diabetes.

Most women with gestational diabetes have glucose normalization after pregnancy, but they are at an increased risk for development of recurrent gestational diabetes and type 2 diabetes. The ADA recommends a 75-g OGTT 4 to 12 weeks postpartum to confirm resolution of hyperglycemia. If the initial postpartum screen is normal, life-long screening should continue every 1 to 3 years with a 75-g OGTT, hemoglobin A_{1c}, or fasting plasma glucose.

Uncommon Types of Diabetes Mellitus

Genetic defects impairing either insulin secretion or insulin action are rare forms of diabetes mellitus (see Table 4). Maturity-onset diabetes of the young (MODY) is characterized as an autosomal dominant monogenetic defect on different chromosomal loci resulting in six subtypes defined by the specific gene affected. Although insulin action remains normal in MODY, glucose sensing and insulin secretion are altered. Autoantibodies are absent. Individuals with MODY present with a clinical course that is frequently atypical of type 1 or type 2 diabetes. The onset of symptoms occurs before 25 years of age, and there is typically a strong family history of atypical diabetes in nonobese patients.

Excess hormone production associated with several endocrinopathies can also impair insulin secretion or insulin action-inducing hyperglycemia (see Table 4).

Management of Diabetes Mellitus

Effective diabetes management is best achieved through a patient-centered approach with patients and their caregivers developing individualized goals and treatment plans compatible with patient preferences, lifestyle requirements, comorbidities, and safety. Management should also incorporate patient education, self-monitoring of blood glucose, lifestyle modifications, and pharmacologic therapies.

- Effective diabetes management requires a patient-centered approach that individualizes goals and treatment plans, taking into consideration unique characteristics of the patient and patient preferences.

Patient Education

Diabetes self-management education and support (DSMES) provides the knowledge and skills for patients to perform diabetes-related self-care and develop effective problem-solving strategies. The ADA recommends consideration of referral for DSMES at several critical periods in care: at time of diagnosis, annually to reassess needs during care transitions, and when self-management skills are impacted by health status changes. DSMES has been shown to improve outcomes, such as hemoglobin A_{1c} and quality of life, and also reduce costs, as patients are able to reduce utilization of acute care and inpatient facilities for diabetes management.

Self-Monitoring of Blood Glucose

Self-monitoring of blood glucose (SMBG) is recommended for patients on intensive insulin regimens (multiple-dose insulin regimens or insulin pump therapy). Specific regimens for SMBG monitoring are individualized and may include prior to meals, at bedtime, before and after exercise, and before operation of machinery. SMBG may be used to detect and correct hypoglycemia. SMBG may be informative when preprandial blood glucose values are at the target goal, but the hemoglobin A_{1c} is above goal. Measuring postprandial blood glucose levels may identify undetected hyperglycemia.

In motivated patients on nonintensive insulin regimens, SMBG can be considered; however, the optimal testing frequency has not been determined in these patients.

Hemoglobin A_{1c} generally correlates with average 3-month blood glucose level in patients without hemoglobinopathies or increased erythrocyte turnover; therefore, treatment efficacy can be measured by combining SMBG and hemoglobin A_{1c} data (**Table 7** and **Table 8**).

Another option is a continuous glucose monitoring system (CGMS), which can alert the user to retrospective and current trends of hypoglycemia and hyperglycemia. In addition, the FDA has approved a CGMS for real-time insulin dosing as well as monitoring. The goals in using a CGMS are to improve diabetes care by lowering hemoglobin A_{1c} and avoiding hypoglycemia, which is critical for those with hypoglycemic unawareness. The ADA endorses CGMS use in adults (≥18 years of age) with type 1 diabetes who are not meeting glycemic targets. The Endocrine Society endorses the use of CGMS in patients with type 1 diabetes with an elevated hemoglobin A_{1c} or an A_{1c} level at goal when worn daily, since data demonstrate improved glycemic control with longer duration of CGMS use. In the future, CGMS may be indicated for patients with type 2 diabetes on intensive insulin regimens as well.

- Self-monitoring of blood glucose or a continuous glucose monitoring system is recommended for patients on intensive insulin regimens (multiple-dose insulin regimens or insulin pump therapy).

Recommended Vaccinations and Screening

Persons with diabetes should receive age-appropriate vaccinations as recommended by the Advisory Committee on Immunization Practices guidelines. Additionally, patients with diabetes should receive influenza vaccinations annually, the pneumococcal polysaccharide vaccine (PPVS23), and the series of hepatitis B vaccinations. The CDC's recommended immunization schedule can be reviewed at: https://www.cdc.gov/vaccines/schedules/hcp/imz/adult.html.

Nonpharmacologic Approaches to Diabetes Management

Lifestyle changes are essential for the long-term management of diabetes and prevention of cardiovascular complications. While they should be individualized, diet and physical activity are critical components for patients with type 1 and type 2 diabetes.

Medical nutrition therapy with a registered dietitian provides individualized diabetes-specific education to promote healthy diet choices to achieve glycemic goals and weight management and has also been associated with reductions in hemoglobin A_{1c} in patients with type 1 and type 2 diabetes. The ADA does not recommend a specific diet; however, in overweight and obese patients with type 2 diabetes, a goal of at least 5% weight loss is recommended and has been shown to improve glycemic control.

Physical activity recommendations are the same as those of the DPP program: moderate to vigorous intensity aerobic activity for 150 minutes/week, vigorous-intensity aerobic activity for 75 minutes/week, or a combination of both. This has been shown to reduce hemoglobin A_{1c}, decrease weight, improve a sense of wellbeing, and improve CAD risk factors. Resistance training is recommended two or more times per week. Older adults with diabetes should engage in flexibility and balance training two to three times per week, if possible. Prolonged sedentary behavior should be interrupted at 30-minute intervals with light activity or standing.

Weight loss medications or metabolic surgery are alternative options to consider if medical nutrition therapy and physical activity are unsuccessful (see MKSAP 18 General Internal Medicine). Metabolic surgery should be considered in obese persons with type 2 diabetes. Significant weight loss and improvements in glycemic control, including diabetes remission, can occur postoperatively.

Additional factors to consider and address in patients with diabetes mellitus include anxiety, depression, and

TABLE 7.	American Diabetes Association Recommended Outpatient Glycemic Goals for Adults with Diabetes Mellitus				
State of Health	Characteristics of Patients	Hemoglobin A$_{1c}$[a]	Preprandial Capillary Glucose	Postprandial Capillary Glucose (1-2 Hours After Meal)[c]	Bedtime Capillary Glucose
Healthy	Early in disease course Few comorbidities Preconception Patient preference Life expectancy >10 years	<7.0% <6.5% for select patients[b]	80-130 mg/dL (4.4-7.2 mmol/L)	<180 mg/dL[c] (10.0 mmol/L)	
Complex health issues	Significant comorbidities including advanced atherosclerosis or microvascular complications Longer duration of diabetes with difficulty achieving glycemic goals despite appropriate management Frequent hypoglycemia Hypoglycemia unawareness Life expectancy <10 years	<8.0%			
Older adults	Healthy Few comorbidities Extended life expectancy No impairment of cognition or function	<7.5%	90-130 mg/dL (5.0-7.2 mmol/L)		90-150 mg/dL (5.0-8.3 mmol/L)
	Complex/Intermediate Multiple comorbidities Hypoglycemia risk Fall risk Multiple instrumental ADL impairments Mild-to-moderate impairment in cognition	<8.0%	90-150 mg/dL (5.0-8.3 mmol/L)		100-180 mg/dL (5.6-10.0 mmol/L)
	Very complex/poor health Chronic comorbidities with end-stage disease Long-term care placement Moderate-to-severe impairment in cognition Multiple ADL dependencies Limited life expectancy	<8.5%	100-180 mg/dL (5.6-10.0 mmol/L)		110-200 mg/dL (6.1-11.1 mmol/L)
Pregnant women[d]	Preexisting type 1 diabetes, preexisting type 2 diabetes, or gestational diabetes	6.0-6.5% without severe hypoglycemia[e] (<6.0% may be optimal as pregnancy progresses)	Fasting ≤95 mg/dL (5.3 mmol/L)	1-hour postprandial ≤140 mg/dL (7.8 mmol/L) or 2-hour postprandial ≤120 mg/dL (6.7 mmol/L)	

ADL = activities of daily living.

[a]Recommended if goal can be met without severe recurrent hypoglycemia. If severe recurrent hypoglycemia is present, there is no recommended hemoglobin A$_{1c}$ goal, as modification of the patient's diabetes regimen to resolve severe recurrent hypoglycemia should take precedence. When severe recurrent hypoglycemia has resolved, a hemoglobin A$_{1c}$ goal can be chosen, and treatment decisions can again be made based on that individualized goal without frequent hypoglycemia. Hemoglobin A$_{1c}$ should be measured at diagnosis followed by 3-month intervals as changes to lifestyle modifications and/or pharmacologic therapies occur. Hemoglobin A$_{1c}$ measurements can be reduced to every 6 months once glycemic targets are achieved.

[b]This can be considered for patients with an early diagnosis of diabetes mellitus, no significant cardiovascular disease, long life expectancy, or managed with lifestyle modifications or metformin.

[c]When the hemoglobin A$_{1c}$ is not at goal despite meeting preprandial glucose goals, the postprandial glucose values should be targeted. Elevated postprandial glucose values have a greater impact on A$_{1c}$ values near 7%.

[d]Both preprandial and postprandial glucose monitoring are recommended in pregnant women.

[e]Preprandial and postprandial glucose measurements should be the primary evaluation of glycemic control, as hemoglobin A$_{1c}$ values decrease with increased red blood cell turnover associated with pregnancy.

Recommendations from American Diabetes Association. 6. Glycemic targets: Standards of Medical Care in Diabetes—2018. Diabetes Care. 2018;41(Suppl. 1):S55-S64. [PMID: 29222377]

Recommendations from American Diabetes Association. 11. Older adults: Standards of Medical Care in Diabetes—2018. Diabetes Care. 2018;41(Suppl. 1):S119-S125. [PMID: 29222382]

Recommendations from American Diabetes Association. 13. Management of diabetes in pregnancy: Standards of Medical Care in Diabetes—2018. Diabetes Care. 2018;41:S137-S143. [PMID: 29222384]

TABLE 8. Comparison of Hemoglobin A$_{1c}$ Value and Estimated Plasma Glucose Level

Hemoglobin A$_{1c}$	Estimated Average Plasma Glucose Level	Estimated Average Plasma Glucose Level
(%)	mg/dL (95% CI)	mmol/L (95% CI)
6	126 (100-152)	7.0 (5.5-8.5)
7	154 (123-185)	8.6 (6.8-10.3)
8	183 (147-217)	10.2 (8.1-12.1)
9	212 (170-249)	11.8 (9.4-13.9)
10	240 (193-282)	13.4 (10.7-15.7)
11	269 (217-314)	14.9 (12.0-17.5)
12	298 (240-347)	16.5 (13.3-19.3)

Data from American Diabetes Association. 6. Glycemic targets: Standards of Medical Care in Diabetes—2018. Diabetes Care. 2018;41:S55-S64. [PMID: 29222377]

diabetes-related distress. Screening for psychosocial issues and behavioral health conditions should occur at the time of diabetes diagnosis and periodically. These conditions can adversely affect glycemic control directly and through challenges with patient adherence to management plans.

Pharmacologic Therapy

Pharmacologic therapy should be individualized taking into consideration a person's age, state of health, weight, the pathophysiology of his/her hyperglycemia, specific risks/benefits of a potential therapeutic agent, medication cost, and the person's lifestyle and personal treatment goals. The hemoglobin A$_{1c}$ goals are generally not stringent in patients with significant comorbid conditions, macrovascular CVD, short life expectancy, long duration of diabetes, limited resources and social support, low health literacy/numeracy, nonadherence, and at high risk for complications from hypoglycemia. Most clinical practice guidelines, including the ADA, recommend target hemoglobin A$_{1c}$ thresholds based on a patient's state of health (see Table 7). In contrast, the VA/DoD guidelines for the management of type 2 diabetes recommend a hemoglobin A$_{1c}$ target range instead of a target threshold. The VA/DoD guidelines attempt to avoid intensification of pharmacologic therapy based solely upon marginal changes in hemoglobin A$_{1c}$ caused by known patient characteristics and laboratory limitations that could potentially cause greater harm than benefit in individuals with major comorbidities, microvascular complications, or advancing age.

The American College of Physicians (ACP) recommends a hemoglobin A$_{1c}$ level between 7% and 8% in most patients with type 2 diabetes, and clinicians should consider deintensifying pharmacologic therapy in patients who achieve hemoglobin A$_{1c}$ levels less than 6.5%. The rationale for these targets is based on evidence that collectively shows treating to targets of less than 7% compared with targets around 8% did not reduce death or macrovascular events over about 5 to 10 years of treatment but did result in substantial harms. More stringent

targets may be appropriate for patients who have a long life expectancy (>15 years) and are interested in more intensive glycemic control with pharmacologic therapy despite the risk for harms, including but not limited to hypoglycemia, patient burden, and pharmacologic costs. ACP also recommends avoiding targeting an hemoglobin A$_{1c}$ level in patients with a life expectancy less than 10 years due to advanced age (80 years or older), residence in a nursing home, or chronic medical conditions because the harms outweigh the benefits in this population.

Several landmark studies provide guidance on glycemic goals and CVD risk reduction. Intensive glycemic control compared with standard control significantly reduces the incidence and progression of microvascular complications in patients with type 1 and type 2 diabetes, as demonstrated by the Diabetes Control and Complications Trial (DCCT) and the UK Prospective Diabetes Study (UKPDS). Long-term follow-up demonstrated continued reductions in microvascular complications despite convergence in glycemic control between the study arms. Action to Control Cardiovascular Risk in Diabetes (ACCORD), Action in Diabetes and Vascular Disease: Preterax and Diamicron MR Controlled Evaluation (ADVANCE), and the Veterans Affairs Diabetes Trial (VADT) further reinforced the association of reduced microvascular complications with tight glycemic control, but also highlighted that patients and providers must balance the risks/benefits of a labor-intensive regimen with the potential morbidity and mortality in specific populations.

Long-term follow-up evaluation of participants in the intensive insulin arms of the DCCT and UKPDS trials who were early in the course of diabetes demonstrated a significant reduction in CVD and mortality. In contrast, ACCORD, ADVANCE, and VADT evaluated tight glycemic control in older persons with more advanced type 2 diabetes and preexisting CVD or CVD risk factors. CVD was not significantly reduced in the ACCORD and ADVANCE trials. VADT demonstrated a significant reduction in cardiovascular events, but no change in cardiovascular or overall mortality.

Recently, the EMPA-REG Outcome trial, a randomized controlled trial (RCT), found that in patients with established CVD, empagliflozin, a sodium-glucose cotransporter 2 (SGLT2) inhibitor, reduced the composite outcome (cardiovascular death, nonfatal myocardial infarction, or nonfatal stroke); it was primarily driven by a significant relative risk reduction in rates of cardiovascular death by 38%. There was also a significant reduction in all-cause mortality by 32% and hospitalization for heart failure by 35%. As a result of this trial, empagliflozin received FDA approval for reduction of cardiovascular death in adults with type 2 diabetes and CVD. Another SGLT2 inhibitor, canagliflozin, also demonstrated a reduction in cardiovascular events, but not cardiovascular death, in patients with type 2 diabetes at high risk for cardiovascular disease when compared to placebo in the CANVAS (Canagliflozin Cardiovascular Assessment Study) Program.

CONT.

The Liraglutide Effect and Action in Diabetes: Evaluation of Cardiovascular Outcome Results (LEADER) RCT included subjects at risk for CVD and found that liraglutide, a glucagon-like peptide 1 (GLP-1) analogue, significantly reduced the primary composite outcome (cardiovascular death, nonfatal MI, or nonfatal stroke) by 13% compared with placebo (relative risk reduction). Liraglutide also significantly reduced cardiovascular death (22%) and all-cause mortality (15%) relative to placebo. Based on the LEADER data, the FDA approved liraglutide for the reduction of major cardiovascular events and cardiovascular deaths in adults with type 2 diabetes and CVD. **H**

KEY POINT

HVC
- Pharmacologic therapy should be individualized taking into consideration a person's age, state of health, weight, the pathophysiology of his/her hyperglycemia, specific risks/benefits of a potential therapeutic agent, medication cost, and the person's lifestyle and personal treatment goals.

H

Therapy for Type 1 Diabetes Mellitus

Due to destruction of the beta cells and subsequent insulin deficiency, life-long insulin therapy is required for persons with type 1 diabetes mellitus. Ideally, an intensive insulin regimen should be prescribed, which includes multiple daily doses of insulin (MDI) to mimic the physiologic action of the pancreas. The insulin regimen should include basal coverage to maintain glycemic control while fasting and between meals, prandial coverage, and supplemental insulin for correction of hyperglycemia. This can be accomplished with subcutaneous insulin injections, inhaled insulin preparations, or continuous subcutaneous insulin infusions (CSII) with an insulin pump.

Initial total daily insulin dosing ranges from 0.4 to 1.0 U/kg/day in patients with type 1 diabetes. Basal insulin typically encompasses approximately 50% of the total daily dose of insulin, with prandial insulin covering the remaining 50%. The available insulin formulations and their activity profiles are summarized in **Table 9**.

The timing and mode of prandial insulin delivery varies based on patient needs/preferences and dietary habits. MDI prandial dosing can be accomplished with fixed-dosing, carbohydrate counting, or modified carbohydrate counting. In general, 1 unit of insulin covers 10 to 20 grams of carbohydrates consumed. A modified carbohydrate counting method can be used when the grams of carbohydrates consumed cannot be accurately counted. With this method, regular or analogue insulin doses can be adjusted by 50% based on the portion of food consumed. For example, the dose for the size of the meal would be as follows: small (50%), regular (100%), large (150%). MDI should also incorporate supplemental insulin to correct hyperglycemia. A common method to calculate the correction dose of insulin is to give an additional 1 unit of regular or analogue insulin at the time of the premeal measurement for every glucose value 50 mg/dL (2.8 mmol/L) above the target glucose value in insulin-sensitive individuals and

1 unit for every 25 mg/dL (1.4 mmol/L) in insulin-resistant individuals. The supplemental insulin can be given with the prandial insulin in one injection. For example, an additional 3 units of insulin would be given with the prandial insulin if the target glucose was 120 mg/dL (6.7 mmol/L) and the current glucose was 270 mg/dL (15.0 mmol/L) in someone with type 1 diabetes.

TABLE 9.	Pharmacokinetic Properties of Insulin Products[a]		
Insulin Type	**Onset**	**Peak**	**Duration**
Rapid-acting analogues			
Lispro, aspart, glulisine	5-15 min	45-90 min	2-4 h
Inhaled insulin	5-15 min	50 min	2-3 h
Concentrated rapid-acting analogue			
Lispro (200 U/mL)	5-15 min	45-90 min	2-4 h
Short-acting			
Human regular	0.5 h	2-5 h	4-8 h
Intermediate-acting			
NPH insulin	1-3 h	4-10 h	10-18 h
Concentrated human regular			
Human regular U-500 (500 U/mL)	0.5 h	2-5 h	13-24 h
Long-acting basal analogues			
Detemir	1-2 h	None[b]	12-24 h[c]
Glargine	2-3 h	None[b]	20-24+ h
Degludec	1-3 h	None	24-42 h
Concentrated basal analogue (ultra long-acting)			
Glargine (300 U/mL)	6 h	None	24-36 h
Degludec (200 U/mL)	1-3 h	None	24-42 h
Premixed insulins[d]			
70% NPH/30% regular	0.5-1 h	2-10 h	10-18 h
75% NPL/25% lispro	10-20 min	1-6 h	10-18 h
50% NPL/50% lispro	10-20 min	1-6 h	10-18 h
70% NPA/30% aspart	10-20 min	1-6 h	10-18 h
70% degludec/30% aspart	10-30 min	0.5-2 h	24+ h

NPA = neutral protamine aspart; NPH = neutral protamine Hagedorn; NPL = neutral protamine lispro.

[a]The time course of each insulin varies significantly between persons and within the same person on different days. Therefore, the time periods listed should be considered general guidelines only.

[b]Both detemir insulin and glargine insulin can produce a peak effect in some persons, especially at higher doses.

[c]The duration of action for detemir insulin varies depending on the dose given.

[d]Premixed insulins containing a larger proportion of rapid- or short-acting insulin tend to have larger peaks occurring at an earlier time than mixtures containing smaller proportions of rapid- and short-acting insulin.

Premixed insulin formulations combine intermediate-acting or long-acting basal insulin and rapid-acting or short-acting insulin in fixed concentrations. These formulations are typically administered twice daily and should be considered for those who are unable or unwilling to perform more frequent daily insulin injections. Premixed formulations can increase glycemic excursions, including hypoglycemia, since this is a nonphysiologic regimen.

Inhaled insulin is a rapid-acting formulation for prandial dosing. The availability of inhaled insulin in cartridges with preset doses of insulin (4, 8, and 12 units) limits the flexibility of insulin dosing. Pulmonary function should be assessed at baseline and monitored because lung function may decline with use of inhaled insulin.

CSII provides continuous delivery of basal insulin and uses a bolus calculator programmed to achieve individual glycemic goals to calculate prandial and bolus correction doses. The Endocrine Society recommends CSII over MDI for all adults with type 1 diabetes who have not attained their hemoglobin A_{1c} goal and for those who have attained their A_{1c} goal but have large glycemic variability, severe hypoglycemia, or hypoglycemia unawareness. Additional considerations include a need for flexibility in insulin delivery, early morning hyperglycemia ("dawn phenomenon"), active lifestyle, or patient preference. There are CSII systems that will decrease or stop delivery of insulin if glucose levels fall below a threshold value that is set within the CSII system and will increase delivery if glucose levels are above a threshold value. Insulin delivery will be reinitiated or increased/decreased back to baseline when the threshold is no longer met.

Hypoglycemia and weight gain are risks associated with insulin use. The risk of hypoglycemia is lower with analogue insulin compared with regular insulin due to a shorter duration of action. Hypoglycemia caused by insulin stacking occurs when insulin dosing is too frequent and overlaps with the duration of action of a prior insulin injection. This can be avoided by allowing at least 3 to 4 hours between sequential injections of analogue insulin.

An adjunctive therapy approved for use with insulin in type 1 diabetes is pramlintide, an amylin analogue. Pramlintide can lead to improved glycemic control, decreased insulin doses, and weight loss through delayed gastric emptying, increased satiety, and decreased glucagon secretion. **H**

KEY POINTS

- Life-long insulin therapy is required for persons with type 1 diabetes mellitus.
- The Endocrine Society recommends continuous subcutaneous insulin infusions over multiple daily doses of insulin for all adults with type 1 diabetes who have not attained their hemoglobin A_{1c} goal and for those who have attained their A_{1c} goal but have large glycemic variability, severe hypoglycemia, or hypoglycemia unawareness.

Therapy for Type 2 Diabetes Mellitus

As beta cell function declines, pharmacologic therapies must often be combined with lifestyle modifications to obtain glycemic control. Therapeutic options may include monotherapy or a combination of oral agents with injectable agents (**Table 10**).

The ADA recommends initiation of monotherapy if the A_{1c} is less than 8% at the time of diagnosis. Metformin is the recommended first-line oral agent for newly diagnosed type 2 diabetes due to known effectiveness and low hypoglycemia risk. Gastrointestinal side effects of metformin are common and may be reduced by slow titration of doses, administration with food, and/or use of an extended release formulation. Lactic acidosis is a rare, potential risk associated with metformin use. Heart failure requiring pharmacologic treatment and hepatic dysfunction may increase the risk. An estimated glomerular filtration rate (eGFR) greater than 45 mL/min/1.73 m^2 is recommended for metformin initiation to avoid potential lactic acidosis with kidney dysfunction. Clinicians should assess benefits and risks of continuing therapy in patients whose eGFR falls below 45 mL/min/1.73 m^2 during therapy. Metformin is contraindicated at eGFR less than 30 mL/min/1.73 m^2.

If an iodinated contrast agent is administered with an eGFR between 30 and 60 mL/min/1.73 m^2, metformin should be held until kidney function is stable for 48 hours. Metformin should also be held in situations that may induce dehydration, such as vomiting or diarrhea. A reduction in vitamin B_{12} intestinal absorption occurs in up to 30% of patients on metformin whereas 5% to 10% develop vitamin B_{12} deficiency. Periodic monitoring may be warranted, particularly in the setting of anemia or peripheral neuropathy.

Glycemic control should be assessed every 3 months with adjustments to therapy until the glycemic target is achieved, and every 6 months if at goal. There are limited data on comparative effectiveness to guide the addition of additional agents when glycemic goals are not met with metformin and lifestyle modifications; thus, many guidelines are based on expert opinion. If the hemoglobin A_{1c} level is 9% or higher at the time of diagnosis or after 3 months of metformin therapy, the ADA recommends advancing to dual therapy defined as metformin combined with another therapeutic agent (see Table 9 and Table 10). For individuals with CVD, therapeutic agents that have been shown to reduce major adverse cardiovascular events (canagliflozin, empagliflozin, and liraglutide) and cardiovascular mortality (empagliflozin and liraglutide) should be considered for dual therapy. AACE/ACE recommends initiation of metformin if the hemoglobin A_{1c} level is less than 7.5% at diagnosis.

Dual therapy should be initiated if the hemoglobin A_{1c} level is 7.5% or higher at diagnosis or after 3 months of monotherapy. The ADA and AACE/ACE both recommend advancement to triple therapy if dual therapy fails to meet glycemic goals after 3 months. Triple therapy should be advanced to combination injectable therapy if glycemic goals are still

TABLE 10.	Pharmacologic Agents Used to Lower Blood Glucose Levels in Type 2 Diabetes Mellitus[a,b]			
Class	Mechanism of Action	Effect on Weight	Disadvantages	Long-Term Studies on Definitive Outcomes
Insulin	Decreases hepatic glucose production Increases peripheral glucose uptake Suppresses ketogenesis	Increase	Hypoglycemia, weight gain, training required, injectable forms, pulmonary toxicity with inhaled insulin	Decrease in microvascular events (UKPDS)[c,d]
Sulfonylureas (tolbutamide, chlorpropamide, glipizide, glyburide, gliclazide, glimepiride	Stimulates insulin secretion	Increase	Hypoglycemia (especially in drugs with long half-lives or in older populations); weight gain; lacks glucose-lowering durability	Decrease in microvascular events (UKPDS)[c]; possible increase in CVD events
Biguanides (metformin)	Decreases hepatic glucose production Increases insulin-mediated uptake of glucose in muscles	Neutral	Diarrhea and abdominal discomfort, vitamin B_{12} deficiency, lactic acidosis (rare). Contraindicated with progressive liver, kidney, or cardiac failure.	Decrease in CVD events (UKPDS)[d]
α-Glucosidase inhibitors (acarbose, miglitol)	Inhibits polysaccharide absorption	Neutral	Flatulence, abdominal discomfort	Possible decrease in CVD events in prediabetes (STOP-NIDDM)[e]
Thiazolidinediones (rosiglitazone, pioglitazone)	Increases peripheral uptake of glucose	Increase	Fluid retention, heart failure, edema, fractures, possible increased risk of bladder cancer with pioglitazone	Possible decrease in CVD events with pioglitazone (PROactive)[f]
Meglitinides (repaglinide, nateglinide)	Stimulates insulin release	Increase	Hypoglycemia, weight gain, frequent dosing	None
Amylin mimetic (pramlintide)	Slows gastric emptying Suppresses glucagon secretion Increases satiety	Decrease	Nausea, vomiting, exacerbates gastroparesis, increased hypoglycemia risk with concomitant use of insulin, training required, injectable, frequent dosing	None
GLP-1 receptor agonists (exenatide, exenatide extended release, liraglutide, albiglutide, lixisenatide, dulaglutide, semaglutide)	Glucose-dependent increase in insulin secretion Slows gastric emptying Glucose-dependent suppression of glucagon secretion Increases satiety	Decrease	Hypoglycemia when used in combination with sulfonylureas, nausea, vomiting, diarrhea, exacerbates gastroparesis, increased heart rate, possible pancreatitis, animal studies demonstrate C-cell hyperplasia and medullary thyroid tumors, training required, injectable	Decrease in CVD events and mortality in high-risk individuals with type 2 diabetes with liraglutide (LEADER)[g]
DPP-4 inhibitors (sitagliptin, saxagliptin, linagliptin, alogliptin)	Glucose-dependent increase in insulin secretion Glucose-dependent suppression of glucagon secretion	Neutral	Hypoglycemia when used in combination with sulfonylureas, increased risk of infections, possible increased risk of pancreatitis, dermatologic reactions, requires dose adjustments for decreasing kidney function except for linagliptin	Increased heart failure hospitalizations [saxagliptin (SAVOR-TIMI 53)][h]

(Continued on the next page)

TABLE 10. Pharmacologic Agents Used to Lower Blood Glucose Levels in Type 2 Diabetes Mellitus[a,b] *(Continued)*

Class	Mechanism of Action	Effect on Weight	Disadvantages	Long-Term Studies on Definitive Outcomes
SGLT2 inhibitors (canagliflozin, dapagliflozin, empagliflozin, ertugliflozin)	Increases kidney excretion of glucose	Decrease	Hypoglycemia with insulin secretagogues, dehydration/hypotension, acute kidney injury (canagliflozin, dapagliflozin), hypersensitivity reactions, increased candida infections and urinary tract infections, "euglycemic" DKA, possible increase in amputations (canagliflozin), hyperkalemia (canagliflozin), fractures (canagliflozin), bladder cancer (dapagliflozin)	Decrease in CVD events and mortality in high-risk individuals with type 2 diabetes with empagliflozin (EMPA-REG OUTCOME)[i] Decreases incident or worsening nephropathy in high CVD risk individuals with type 2 diabetes (EMPA-REG OUTCOME)[i] Decrease in CVD events in high-risk individuals with type 2 diabetes with canagliflozin (CANVAS Program)[j]
Bile acid sequestrants (colesevelam)	Incompletely understood: Possible decrease in hepatic glucose production Possible increase in incretin levels	Neutral	Constipation, dyspepsia, increased triglycerides, possible interference with absorption of other medications	None
Dopamine-2 agonists (bromocriptine quick release)	Increases insulin sensitivity Alters metabolism via hypothalamus	Neutral	Nausea, orthostasis, fatigue	Possible decrease in CVD events (Cycloset Safety Trial)[k]

CVD = cardiovascular disease; DKA = diabetic ketoacidosis; DPP-4 = dipeptidyl peptidase-4; GLP-1 = glucagon-like peptide-1; SGLT2 = sodium-glucose cotransporter-2.

[a]Data from American Diabetes Association. 8. Pharmacologic approaches to glycemic treatment: Standards of Medical Care in Diabetes—2018. Diabetes Care. 2018;419Suppl. 1):S73-S85. [PMID: 29222379]

[b]Recommendations from Garber AJ, Abrahamson MJ, Barzilay JI, Blonde L, Bloomgarden ZT, Bush MA, et al; American Association of Clinical Endocrinologists (AACE). Consensus Statement by the American Association of Clinical Endocrinologists and American College of Endocrinology on the Comprehensive Type 2 Diabetes Management Algorithm—2018 Executive Summary. Endocr Pract. 2018;24:91-120. [PMID: 29368965]

[c]Data from Intensive blood-glucose control with sulfonylureas or insulin compared with conventional treatment and risk of complications in patients with type 2 diabetes (UKPDS 33). UK Prospective Diabetes Study (UKPDS) Group. Lancet. 1998;352:837-53. [PMID: 9742976]

[d]Data from Effect of intensive blood-glucose control with metformin on complications in overweight patients with type 2 diabetes (UKPDS 34). UK Prospective Diabetes Study (UKPDS) Group. Lancet. 1998;352:854-65. [PMID: 9742977]

[e]Data from Chiasson JL, Josse RG, Gomis R, Hanefeld M, Karasik A, Laakso M; STOP-NIDDM Trial Research Group. Acarbose treatment and the risk of cardiovascular disease and hypertension in patients with impaired glucose tolerance: the STOP-NIDDM trial. JAMA. 2003;290:486-94. [PMID: 12876091]

[f]Data from Dormandy JA, Charbonnel B, Eckland DJ, Erdmann E, Massi-Benedetti M, Moules IK, et al; PROactive Investigators. Secondary prevention of macrovascular events in patients with type 2 diabetes in the PROactive Study (PROspective pioglitAzone Clinical Trial In macroVascular Events): a randomised controlled trial. Lancet. 2005;366:1279-89. [PMID: 16214598]

[g]Data from Marso SP, Daniels GH, Brown-Frandsen K, Kristensen P, Mann JF, Nauck MA, et al; LEADER Steering Committee. Liraglutide and cardiovascular outcomes in type 2 diabetes. N Engl J Med. 2016;375:311-22. [PMID: 27295427]

[h]Data from Scirica BM, Bhatt DL, Braunwald E, Steg PG, Davidson J, Hirshberg B, et al; SAVOR-TIMI 53 Steering Committee and Investigators. Saxagliptin and cardiovascular outcomes in patients with type 2 diabetes mellitus. N Engl J Med. 2013;369:1317-26. [PMID: 23992601]

[i]Data from Zinman B, Wanner C, Lachin JM, Fitchett D, Bluhmki E, Hantel S, et al; EMPA-REG OUTCOME investigators. Empagliflozin, cardiovascular outcomes, and mortality in type 2 diabetes. N Engl J Med. 2015;373:2117-28. [PMID: 26378978]

[j]Data from Neal B, Perkovic V, Mahaffey KW, de Zeeuw D, Fulcher G, Erondu N, et al; CANVAS Program Collaborative Group. Canagliflozin and cardiovascular and renal events in type 2 diabetes. N Engl J Med. 2017;377:644-657. [PMID: 28605608]i

[k]Data from Gaziano JM, Cincotta AH, O'Connor CM, Ezrokhi M, Rutty D, Ma ZJ, et al. Randomized clinical trial of quick-release bromocriptine among patients with type 2 diabetes on overall safety and cardiovascular outcomes. Diabetes Care. 2010;33:1503-8. [PMID: 20332352]

unmet. This includes continued metformin and initiation of a GLP-1 receptor agonist or basal insulin if not already prescribed, initiation of basal insulin on background GLP-1 receptor agonist therapy, or initiation of a GLP-1 receptor agonist or prandial insulin on optimized background basal insulin.

Algorithms from the ADA and AACE/ACE provide guidance on initiation and dosing of basal and prandial insulin regimens (**Table 11**). The ADA recommends combination injectable therapy initially in the setting of symptomatic hyperglycemia (polydipsia, polyuria), hemoglobin A_{1c} 10% or higher, or a glucose level of 300 mg/dL (16.6 mmol/L) or higher.

AACE/ACE recommends initiating insulin therapy with other agents if the initial hemoglobin A_{1c} is more than 9% in a

TABLE 11.	Comparison of Insulin Dosing Algorithms from the ADA and AACE/ACE	
Insulin Initiation or Modification	**ADA**	**AACE/ACE**
Basal insulin	Starting dose: 10 U/d or 0.1-0.2 U/kg/d	Starting dose: If A$_{1c}$ <8%: 0.1-0.2 U/kg/d If A$_{1c}$ >8%: 0.2-0.3 U/kg/d
Basal insulin dose titration	For hyperglycemia: Increase dose 1-2 times/week until glycemic goal met Increase dose by: 10%-15% or 2-4 U For hypoglycemia: Decrease dose by: 10%-20% or 4 U	For hyperglycemia: Increase dose every 2-3 days until glycemic goal met Increase dose by: 2 U or 20% if FBG >180 mg/dL (10 mmol/L) 10% if FBG 140-180 mg/dL (7.8-9.9 mmol/L) 1 U if FBG is 110-139 mg/dL (6.1-7.7 mmol/L) For hypoglycemia: Decrease dose by: 10%-20% if FBG <70 mg/dL (3/9 mmol/L) 20%-40% if FBG <40 mg/dL (2.2 mmol/L)
Prandial insulin plus basal insulin (1 meal)	Initiate prandial insulin at largest meal Starting dose: 4 U, 10% of basal dose, or 0.1 U/kg To avoid hypoglycemia, consider decreasing basal dose by same amount if A$_{1c}$ <8%.	Initiate prandial insulin at largest meal Starting dose: 5 U or 10% of basal dose
Basal-bolus insulin regimen (≥ 2 or more meals)	Prandial insulin starting dose: 4 U, 10% of basal dose, or 0.1 U/kg/meal To avoid hypoglycemia, consider decreasing basal dose by same amount if A$_{1c}$ <8%.	Prandial insulin starting dose: 0.3-0.5 U/kg = TDD 50% of TDD = basal insulin 50% of TDD = prandial insulin Each meal-time dose = 1/3 prandial insulin dose
Prandial insulin dose titration	For hyperglycemia: Increase dose 1-2 days/week until glycemic goal met Increase dose by: 10%-15% or 1-2 U If hyperglycemia persists at other meals, add additional meal-time insulin doses (basal-bolus) For hypoglycemia: Decrease dose by: 10%-20% or 2-4 U	For hyperglycemia: Increase dose every 2-3 days until glycemic goal met Increase dose by: 10% or 1-2 U if BG >140 mg/dL (7.8 mmol/L) 2 hours after meal or at next meal. If hyperglycemia persists at other meals, add additional meal-time insulin doses (basal-bolus). For hypoglycemia: Decrease TDD dose (basal and/or prandial) by: 10%-20% if BG <70 mg/dL (3.9 mmol/L) 20%-40% if BG <40 mg/dL (2.2 mmol/L)
Premixed insulin 2× daily	Starting dose: Current basal dose given at breakfast and dinner distributed as 2/3 AM and 1/3 PM or 1/2 AM and 1/2 PM	
Premixed analog insulin 3× daily	Add additional insulin dose at lunch	
Premixed insulin dose titration	For hyperglycemia: Increase dose 1-2 days/week until glycemic goal met Increase dose by: 10%-15% or 1-2 U For hypoglycemia: Decrease dose by: 10%-20% or 2-4 U	

ADA = American Diabetes Association; AACE = American Association of Clinical Endocrinologists; ACE = American College of Endocrinology; BG = blood glucose; FBG = fasting blood glucose; TDD = total daily dose.

Data from American Diabetes Association. 8. Pharmacologic approaches to glycemic treatment: Standards of Medical Care in Diabetes—2018. Diabetes Care. 2018;40(Suppl. 1): S73-S85. [PMID: 2922379]

Data from Garber AJ, Abrahamson MJ, Barzilay JI, Blonde L, Bloomgarden ZT, Bush MA, et al; American Association of Clinical Endocrinologists (AACE). Consensus statement by the American Association of Clinical Endocrinologists and American College of Endocrinology on the comprehensive type 2 diabetes management algorithm—2018 Executive Summary. Endocr Pract. 2018;24:91-120. [PMID: 29368965]

CONT. symptomatic individual. After optimizing the basal insulin dose, prandial insulin should be added prior to the largest meal if hyperglycemia persists. A basal-bolus insulin regimen, with prandial insulin prior to two or more meals, should be employed for continued hyperglycemia.

Ultralong-acting basal analogue insulins may be advantageous compared with long-acting basal analogue insulins due to a prolonged action profile (>24 hours), peakless insulin delivery, and decreased variability in action between and within individuals. The pharmacodynamic profile may decrease hypoglycemia in high-risk patients, improve glycemic fluctuations, and allow for flexibility in dosing beyond 24-hour time periods.

In patients with type 2 diabetes not at glycemic goal despite adherence to glucose monitoring and multiple treatment modalities, CSII may be considered. **H**

KEY POINTS

- Metformin is the recommended first-line oral agent for newly diagnosed type 2 diabetes due to known effectiveness and low hypoglycemia risk.

- Glycemic control should be assessed every 3 months with subsequent adjustments to therapeutic agents until the glycemic target is achieved, and every 6 months if at goal.

Therapy for Gestational Diabetes Mellitus

Pharmacologic therapy should be prescribed for patients with gestational diabetes to improve perinatal outcomes if lifestyle interventions do not achieve glycemic targets. Insulin is the recommended therapy. While metformin or sulfonylurea therapy may be considered, both therapies cross the placenta, and there is no long-term safety data for their use during pregnancy. Additionally, sulfonylurea therapy has been associated with higher rates of neonatal macrosomia and hypoglycemia.

Drug-Induced Hyperglycemia

Several drugs can induce hyperglycemia through multiple mechanisms: increased hepatic glucose production, impaired insulin action, or decreased insulin secretion (**Table 12**). Whereas hyperglycemia with temporary drug therapies may resolve after discontinuation, many of these drugs are used indefinitely for chronic medical conditions. Persons at risk for hyperglycemia and the development of diabetes due to medications should be monitored periodically.

H Inpatient Management of Hyperglycemia

Tight inpatient glycemic control (80-110 mg/dL [4.4-6.1 mmol/L]) is not consistently associated with improved outcomes and may increase mortality. As a result, current inpatient glycemic

goals strive to avoid complications from severe hypoglycemia and hyperglycemia, such as electrolyte abnormalities and dehydration.

Modifications to diet are necessary with consistent values above 140 mg/dL (7.8 mmol/L). If hyperglycemia persists, therapy should be initiated. Clinical status changes may increase the risk of adverse events associated with noninsulin therapies. Insulin is therefore preferred for inpatient management of hyperglycemia 180 mg/dL (10.0 mmol/L) and higher and adjusted to maintain a glucose level between 140 and 180 mg/dL (7.8-10.0 mmol/L) for most patients. Glucose values less than 140 mg/dL (7.8 mmol/L) may be reasonable in select noncritically ill patients if hypoglycemia is avoided, according to the ADA and AACE. In contrast, the American College of Physicians (ACP) does not recommend glucose values less than 140 mg/dL (7.8 mmol/L) due to increased hypoglycemia risk. Several factors may lead to inpatient hypoglycemia: altered mental status, fasting (expected or unexpected), illness, insulin-meal timing mismatch, poor oral intake, and alterations in hyperglycemia-inducing therapies. **H**

KEY POINT

- Tight inpatient glycemic control (80-110 mg/dL [4.4-6.1 mmol/L]) is not consistently associated with improved outcomes and may increase mortality. **HVC**

Hospitalized Patients with Diabetes Mellitus **H**

In critically ill patients with type 1 and type 2 diabetes mellitus, intravenous insulin therapy is recommended. Intravenous insulin dose adjustments should be based on a validated algorithm that incorporates point-of-care (POC) monitoring every 1 to 2 hours.

For noncritically ill patients, subcutaneous insulin is appropriate. Persons with type 1 diabetes require continuous insulin therapy. Basal insulin must be provided to avoid development of DKA. Persons with type 2 diabetes with glucose values 180 mg/dL (10.0 mmol/L) or higher should also receive insulin therapy.

If the patient is eating, the ideal insulin regimen is a basal-bolus regimen with prandial coverage and correction boluses for premeal hyperglycemia. POC measurements and prandial insulin injections should occur prior to meal consumption. Postprandial insulin administration may be appropriate to allow for dose reduction with decreased oral intake for some persons or those with delayed gastric emptying. Overnight POC measurements are warranted if there are concerns for undetected hypoglycemia; otherwise glucose checks overnight should be avoided due to sleep disruption and increased risk of insulin stacking. The sole use of correction insulin ("sliding-scale insulin") is not recommended since it is a reactive, nonphysiologic approach that leads to large glucose fluctuations.

Continuation of outpatient CSII therapy may be appropriate for those patients with normal mental status who can

TABLE 12. Drug-Induced Hyperglycemia		
Drug Category	**Drug**	**Mechanism of Hyperglycemia**
Glucocorticoid	All systemic glucocorticoids	Decreased insulin production
		Increased peripheral insulin resistance
		Increased hepatic glucose production
Immunosuppressants	Calcineurin inhibitors	Decreased insulin production and release
	Sirolimus	
	Tacrolimus	
	Cyclosporine	
Antiretrovirals	Protease inhibitors	Increased peripheral insulin resistance
	NRTIs	Pancreatic damage through drug-induced pancreatitis (didanosine)
Cardiovascular medications	Niacin	Increased hepatic glucose production
	Statins	Impaired pancreatic beta-cell function
		Increased peripheral resistance
	β-blockers	Decreased insulin release
	Atenolol	Increased peripheral insulin resistance
	Metoprolol	Carvedilol (α-blocking) has a neutral effect on glucose
	Propranolol	
	Thiazides	Decreased insulin secretion secondary to hypokalemia
	Hydrochlorothiazide	Increased insulin resistance
	Chlorthalidone	
	Chlorothiazide	
	Indapamide	
	Vasopressors	Decreased insulin secretion
	Epinephrine	Increased glycogenolysis
	Norepinephrine	Increased hepatic glucose production
		Stimulation of glucagon and cortisol
Hormonal medications	Oral contraceptives	Abnormal hepatic glucose metabolism
	Combined estrogen-progestin	Increased peripheral insulin resistance
	Progestin only	Decreased risk of hyperglycemia with low-dose pills containing ≤35 μg ethinyl estradiol
	Progestin	Increased peripheral insulin resistance
	Megestrol acetate	
	Growth hormone	Increased peripheral insulin resistance
Atypical antipsychotics (second generation)	Clozapine	Unclear
	Olanzapine	Possible increased peripheral insulin resistance
	Ziprasidone	
	Quetiapine	
	Risperidone	
	Iloperidone	
	Paliperidone	
Antibiotics	Moxifloxacin	Altered insulin secretion
	Gatifloxacin	

NRTI = nucleoside reverse transcriptase inhibitors.

Data from Fathallah N, Slim R, Larif S, Hmouda H, Ben Salem C. Drug-induced hyperglycaemia and diabetes. Drug Saf. 2015;38:1153-68. [PMID: 26370106]

Data from Thomas Z, Bandali F, McCowen K, Malhotra A. Drug-induced endocrine disorders in the intensive care unit. Crit Care Med. 2010;38:S219-30. [PMID: 20502175]

CONT.

manage the device under the supervision of health care providers proficient in this technology. If a hospitalized patient becomes unable to safely manage CSII therapy, it should be discontinued and replaced with either a subcutaneous insulin regimen or intravenous insulin.

Continuation of outpatient oral or noninsulin injectable agents is not recommended when patients are admitted due to potential hemodynamic and/or nutritional changes that may occur. Insulin therapy should be initiated for glycemic management. As a patient nears hospital discharge with stability in nutritional status and hemodynamics, reinitiation of these agents may be considered if organ function has returned to baseline. **H**

KEY POINTS

- Critically ill patients with type 1 and type 2 diabetes mellitus require intravenous insulin therapy with dosing based on a validated algorithm incorporating point-of-care monitoring every 1 to 2 hours.

- Noncritically ill persons with type 1 diabetes require basal insulin in addition to prandial insulin therapy; persons with type 2 diabetes with glucose values 180 mg/dL (10.0 mmol/L) or higher should also receive insulin therapy.

HVC
- The sole use of correction insulin ("sliding-scale insulin") is not recommended since it is a reactive, nonphysiologic approach that leads to large glucose fluctuations.

H ### Hospitalized Patients Without Diabetes Mellitus

Stress associated with acute illness, enteral/parenteral nutrition, and hyperglycemia-inducing medications in the inpatient setting may induce glucose abnormalities in persons without diabetes.

Hyperglycemia management should follow the same guidelines as hospitalized patients with diabetes.

It is important to recognize that inpatient hyperglycemia may occur in the setting of previously unrecognized diabetes. An inpatient hemoglobin A_{1c} measurement of 6.5% or higher is indicative of glucose abnormalities prior to the hospitalization, and these patients require discharge planning for management of newly diagnosed diabetes.

Acute Complications of Diabetes Mellitus

Diabetic Ketoacidosis/Hyperglycemic Hyperosmolar Syndrome

Diabetic ketoacidosis (DKA) and hyperglycemic hyperosmolar syndrome (HHS) occur with extreme hyperglycemia and must be treated early and aggressively to avoid life-threatening consequences from dehydration and electrolyte abnormalities. Severe hyperglycemia is a consequence of insufficient insulin levels coupled with an increase in counterregulatory hormones. This impairs efficient glucose utilization and subsequently drives glycogenolysis and gluconeogenesis for fuel production.

DKA typically occurs in individuals with type 1 diabetes younger than 65 years of age. It is a relative or absolute insulin deficiency state resulting in unsuppressed lipolysis. Fatty acid oxidation occurs with subsequent ketone body production and development of metabolic acidosis. HHS typically occurs in individuals with type 2 diabetes who are older than 65 years of age. It is associated with a higher mortality rate compared with DKA. It is characterized as a partial insulin deficiency that is able to suppress lipolysis and prevent ketone body production, but unable to correct hyperglycemia or prevent the subsequent dehydration and electrolyte abnormalities. Younger patients with type 1 diabetes have a higher glomerular filtration rate, which allows a higher level of glucosuria compared with those with type 2 diabetes. As a result, HHS is associated with more extreme hyperglycemia compared to DKA (**Figure 1**).

Inciting factors for the development of DKA or HHS include infection, myocardial infarction, accidental or deliberate nonadherence to diabetes therapy, stress, trauma, and confounding medications (atypical antipsychotics, glucocorticoids, and SGLT2 inhibitors). DKA or HHS may be the initial presentation of a person with undiagnosed diabetes.

DKA and HHS may present with a multitude of symptoms and plasma glucose levels that can be normal to very high. Symptoms from DKA typically occur within 24 hours of onset, whereas symptoms from HHS may not appear for several days. DKA and HHS symptoms may include abdominal pain, nausea, polyuria, polydipsia, vomiting, weight loss, or shortness of breath. Extreme glucosuria causes an osmotic diuresis and severe volume depletion, which may be exacerbated by gastrointestinal losses of volume and electrolytes. The condition may progress to lethargy, obtundation, and death if the hyperglycemia, dehydration, and electrolyte abnormalities are not treated aggressively and early.

Initial evaluation includes the measurement of serum glucose levels, serum electrolytes, serum ketones, blood urea nitrogen and serum creatinine, plasma osmolality, complete blood count, arterial blood gases, urinalysis, and urine ketones. An electrocardiogram should also be reviewed. Cultures (blood, sputum, urine) and a chest radiograph may be obtained if an infection is suspected after a history is gathered and examination performed.

Multiple laboratory abnormalities are present with DKA and HHS. An increased anion gap metabolic acidosis is present in DKA secondary to production of acetoacetic acid and β-hydroxybutyrate. Although some patients with HHS may have an increased anion gap, typically with glucose levels above 400 to 600 mg/dL (22.2-33.3 mmol/L), they do not develop significant ketoacidosis as seen in DKA.

A moderate to severe reduction in serum bicarbonate levels is present in DKA, but levels may remain normal or mildly reduced (>20 mEq/L [20 mmol/L]) in HHS. Serum pH is typically

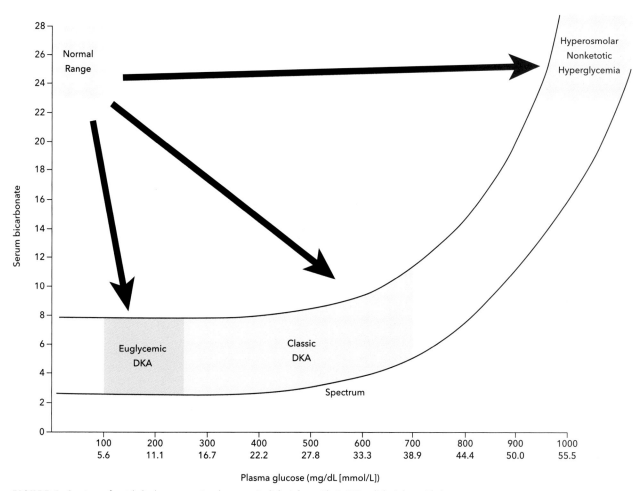

FIGURE 1. Spectrum of metabolic decompensation that occurs in diabetic ketoacidosis. DKA = diabetic ketoacidosis.

greater than 7.3 in HHS. Pseudohyponatremia may occur in DKA and HHS with extreme hyperglycemia and osmotic shifts of water from intracellular to extracellular compartments. A normal or elevated sodium level indicates severe dehydration. Increased osmolality, frequently greater than 320 mOsm/kg H_2O, is often present in HHS secondary to more severe hyperglycemia and water loss from osmotic diuresis compared with type 1 diabetes. Serum potassium levels may be elevated due to shifts from the intracellular to extracellular spaces due to ketoacidosis and the absence of sufficient insulin. Normal or low serum potassium levels indicate a depletion of body stores and require supplementation prior to insulin therapy to avoid cardiac arrhythmias. Stress may induce mild leukocytosis, but higher levels may indicate an infectious cause for DKA or HHS.

A multi-pronged approach is required to treat DKA and HHS (**Table 13**). Intravenous hydration is necessary for volume repletion. Electrolyte deficits, such as potassium, should be repleted. Hyperglycemia should be corrected preferably with intravenous insulin with hourly glucose measurements to guide dose adjustments. Frequent electrolyte measurements are necessary to guide repletion as hydration and insulin therapy continues. Most patients with DKA or HHS are managed in the ICU due to the high complexity of care required. Other conditions that contributed to the development of DKA or HHS, such as infection, should be treated.

KEY POINTS

- Diabetic ketoacidosis and hyperglycemic hyperosmolar syndrome occur with extreme hyperglycemia and must be treated early and aggressively to avoid life-threatening consequences from dehydration and electrolyte abnormalities.

- Inciting factors for the development of diabetic ketoacidosis and hyperglycemic hyperosmolar syndrome include infection, myocardial infarction, accidental or deliberate nonadherence to diabetes therapy, stress, trauma, and confounding medications (SGLT2 inhibitors, atypical antipsychotics, and glucocorticoids).

- Treatment of diabetic ketoacidosis and hyperglycemic hyperosmolar syndrome requires correction of hyperglycemia, intravenous hydration, electrolyte repletion, and treatment of suspected infections.

TABLE 13. Management of Hyperglycemic Crisis: Diabetic Ketoacidosis and Hyperglycemic Hyperosmolar Syndrome

Fluids	Insulin (Regular)	Potassium	Correction of Acidosis
Assess for volume status, then give 0.9% saline IV at 1 L/h initially in all patients, and continue if patient is severely hypovolemic. Switch to 0.45% normal saline at 250-500 mL/h if corrected serum sodium level becomes normal or high. When the plasma glucose level reaches 200 mg/dL (11.1 mmol/L) in patients with DKA or 300 mg/dL (16.7 mmol/L) in HHS in the setting of continued IV insulin, switch to 5% dextrose with 0.45% normal saline at 150-250 mL/h to maintain the blood glucose and avoid hypoglycemia.	Give regular insulin, 0.1 U/kg, as an IV bolus followed by 0.1 U/kg/h as an IV infusion. If the plasma glucose level does not decrease by 10% in the first hour, give an additional bolus of 0.14 U/kg and resume previous infusion rate. When the plasma glucose level reaches 200 mg/dL (11.1 mmol/L) in DKA and 300 mg/dL (16.7 mmol/L) in HHS, reduce to 0.02-0.05 U/kg/h, and maintain the plasma glucose level between 150-200 mg/dL (8.3-11.1 mmol/L) until anion gap acidosis is resolved in DKA. The plasma glucose should be maintained between 250-300 mg/dL in HHS until the patient is alert and the hyperosmolar state resolves.	Assess for adequate kidney function, with adequate urine output (approximately 50 mL/h). If serum potassium is <3.3 mEq/L (3.3 mmol/L), do not start insulin but instead give IV potassium chloride, 20-30 mEq/h, through a central line catheter until the serum potassium level is >3.3 mEq/L (3.3 mmol/L). Then add 20-30 mEq of potassium chloride to each liter of IV fluids to keep the serum potassium level in the 4.0-5.0 mEq/L (4.0-5.0 mmol/L) range. If the serum potassium level is >5.2 mEq/L (5.2 mmol/L), do not give potassium chloride, but instead start insulin and IV fluids, and check the serum potassium level every 2 hours.	If pH is <6.9, consider sodium bicarbonate, 100 mmol in 400 mL of water, and potassium chloride, 20 mEq, infused over 2 hours. If pH is 6.9 or greater, do not give sodium bicarbonate.

DKA = diabetic ketoacidosis; HHS = hyperglycemic hyperosmolar syndrome; IV = intravenous.

Recommendations from Kitabchi AE, Umpierrez GE, Miles JM, Fisher JN. Hyperglycemic crises in adult patients with diabetes. Diabetes Care. 2009;32:1335-43. [PMID: 19564476]

Chronic Complications of Diabetes Mellitus

Cardiovascular Morbidity

A major cause of morbidity and mortality in persons with diabetes mellitus is cardiovascular disease (CVD). Diabetes is an independent risk factor for CVD. Other significant risk factors for CVD include hypertension, dyslipidemia, tobacco use, family history, and albuminuria. Simultaneous management of CVD risk factors is recommended to decrease morbidity and mortality. Screening interval guidelines for risk factors are listed in **Table 14**.

Hypertension contributes to the development of macrovascular and microvascular complications. The American Diabetes Association (ADA) defines hypertension as sustained blood pressures 140/90 mm Hg or higher. Citing concerns for increased treatment complications with a lower blood pressure target below 130/80 mm Hg, the ADA treatment goal for most persons is below 140/90 mm Hg. Those persons at high risk for CVD may aim for lower blood pressure targets if this can be achieved safely. In contrast, guidelines from the American Association of Clinical Endocrinologists/American College of Endocrinology (AACE/ACE) and the American College of Cardiology/American Heart Association (ACC/AHA) and nine other organizations advocate for a treatment target below 130/80 mm Hg for most patients with diabetes. ADA recommended treatment strategies include lifestyle modifications (for blood pressure >120/80 mm Hg) and pharmacologic therapies (for blood pressure >140/90 mm Hg). Initial recommended antihypertensive regimens include ACE inhibitors, angiotensin receptor blockers (ARBs), dihydropyridine calcium channel blockers, and thiazide diuretics. Multiple agents are frequently required to reach the blood pressure target. Underlying comorbidities should guide selection of therapeutic agents, such as the use of an ACE inhibitor or ARB in the presence of microalbuminuria.

Lipid management in diabetes frequently requires a combination of lifestyle modifications and pharmacologic agents. The ACC/AHA risk calculator can determine the 10-year atherosclerotic cardiovascular disease (ASCVD) risk to guide therapeutic management. Statin therapy is the recommended initial pharmacologic treatment for all qualifying persons with diabetes (see MKSAP 18 General Internal Medicine).

Antiplatelet therapy with aspirin (75-162 mg/day) is recommended by the ADA for secondary prevention in those persons with diabetes and ASCVD. Aspirin therapy for primary prevention of ASCVD in persons with type 1 and type 2 diabetes may not provide universal benefit, so aspirin therapy (75-162 mg/day) may be considered in persons 50 years of age and older with at least one additional ASCVD risk factor. The ADA does not recommend aspirin therapy for persons younger than 50 years of age at low risk for ASCVD.

TABLE 14. Screening Recommendations for Chronic Complications of Diabetes Mellitus

Chronic Complication	Clinical Situation	When to Start Screening	Screening Frequency	Preferred Screening Test
Retinopathy	Type 1 diabetes	At 5 years after diagnosis	Annually[a]	Dilated and comprehensive eye examination[b]
	Type 2 diabetes	At diagnosis	Annually[a]	Dilated and comprehensive eye examination[b]
	In pregnant women with either type of diabetes	First trimester	Every trimester and then closely for 1 year postpartum	Dilated and comprehensive eye examination[b]
	In women with either type of diabetes planning to conceive	During preconception planning	Same as recommendations for pregnant women once conception occurs	Dilated and comprehensive eye examination[b]
Nephropathy	Type 1 diabetes	At 5 years after diagnosis	Annually[c]	Albumin-creatinine ratio on random spot urine, eGFR
	Type 2 diabetes	At diagnosis	Annually[c]	Albumin-creatinine ratio on random spot urine, eGFR
Neuropathy (distal symmetric polyneuropathy)[d]	Type 1 diabetes	At 5 years after diagnosis	Annually	Skin assessment, evaluate for foot deformities, lower extremity pulse assessment, neurologic assessment (10-g monofilament plus 128-Hz tuning fork, ankle reflexes, pinprick, or temperature)
	Type 2 diabetes	At diagnosis	Annually	Skin assessment, evaluate for foot deformities, lower extremity pulse assessment, neurologic assessment (10-g monofilament plus 128-Hz tuning fork, ankle reflexes, pinprick, or temperature)
Cardiovascular disease	Hypertension	At diagnosis	Every visit	Blood pressure measurement
	Dyslipidemia	At diagnosis and prior to initiating statin therapy	Annually[e]	Lipid profile

eGFR = estimated glomerular filtration rate.

[a]It is reasonable to screen every 1 to 2 years if no diabetic retinopathy is present and to screen more often than annually if diabetic retinopathy is advanced or progressing rapidly.

[b]Retinal photography is a possible alternative means of screening for diabetic retinopathy that may improve access to care and reduce costs. Retinal photography, when interpreted by eye care specialists, can detect most clinically significant diabetic retinopathy.

[c]The American Diabetes Association guidelines state that it is reasonable to assess progression of disease and response to therapeutic interventions with continued monitoring of urinary albumin-creatinine excretion.

[d]Although diabetes commonly causes peripheral neuropathy, other differential diagnoses to consider during the screening process include vitamin B_{12} deficiency, alcoholism, hypothyroidism, renal disease, malignancy and chemotherapies, vasculitis, and inherited neuropathies.

[e]Annual or periodic screening to monitor therapeutic response after initiation of statin therapy. May screen every 5 years if not on statin therapy.

Recommendations from American Diabetes Association. 9. Cardiovascular disease and risk management: Standards of Medical Care in Diabetes—2018. Diabetes Care. 2018;41(Suppl. 1):S86-S104. [PMID: 29222380]

Recommendations from American Diabetes Association. 10. Microvascular complications and foot care: Standards of Medical Care in Diabetes—2018. Diabetes Care. 2018; 41 (Suppl. 1):S105-S118. [PMID: 29222381]

Recommendations from Garber AJ, Abrahamson MJ, Barzilay JI, Blonde L, Bloomgarden ZT, Bush MA, et al; American Association of Clinical Endocrinologists (AACE). Consensus Statement by the American Association of Clinical Endocrinologists and American College of Endocrinology on the comprehensive type 2 diabetes management algorithm—2018 executive summary. Endocr Pract. 2018;24:91-120. [PMID: 29368965]

KEY POINTS

- The American Diabetes Association (ADA) recommends a blood pressure treatment goal below 140/90 mm Hg or lower for persons at high risk for CVD if this can be achieved safely; the American Association of Clinical Endocrinologists/American College of Endocrinology (AACE/ACE) and the American College of Cardiology/American Heart Association (ACC/AHA) and nine other organizations recommend a target below 130/80 mm Hg for most patients with diabetes.

(Continued)

KEY POINTS *(continued)*

- Lipid management in diabetes frequently requires a combination of lifestyle modifications and pharmacologic agents; statin therapy is the recommended initial pharmacologic treatment for all qualifying persons with diabetes.

- The American Diabetes Association (ADA) does not recommend aspirin therapy for persons younger than 50 years of age at low risk for atherosclerotic cardiovascular disease.

HVC

Diabetic Retinopathy

Retinopathy is the leading cause of preventable blindness among persons with diabetes between 20 and 74 years of age in developed countries. Risk factors for retinopathy include duration of diabetes, degree of hyperglycemia, hypertension, albuminuria, and dyslipidemia.

Diabetic retinopathy changes are classified as nonproliferative (occurs within the retina) or proliferative (occurs in the vitreous or retinal inner surface). Nonproliferative retinopathy findings may include microaneurysms, dot and blot hemorrhages, hard exudates (lipid deposition), soft exudates or cotton-wool spots (ischemic superficial nerve fibers), venous bleeding, and intraretinal microvascular abnormalities. Neovascularization due to chronic ischemia characterizes proliferative retinopathy, which may cause intraocular hemorrhage, retinal detachment, and vision loss.

Macular edema may occur with nonproliferative and proliferative retinopathy.

Screening guidelines were developed for early detection of asymptomatic abnormalities to allow for treatment interventions to prevent vision loss (see Table 14).

Optimal control of blood pressure, glucose, and lipid parameters can prevent and delay the progression of retinopathy. Panretinal laser photocoagulation can treat high-risk proliferative diabetic retinopathy and severe nonproliferative retinopathy. In addition, intravitreal injections with anti-vascular endothelial growth factor (anti-VEGF) to reduce vision loss associated with proliferative retinopathy is not inferior to panretinal laser photocoagulation. Retinopathy may develop or accelerate during pregnancy or with rapid glycemic improvements, and may require laser photocoagulation to decrease the risk of vision loss. Macular edema is preferentially treated with anti-VEGF intravitreal injections to improve vision loss. Anti-VEGF injections require monthly injections for at least 12 months followed by intermittent injections to prevent recurrent macular edema.

KEY POINTS

- Patients with type 2 diabetes should have an eye examination at the time of diagnosis.
- Optimal control of glucose, blood pressure, and lipid parameters can prevent and delay the progression of retinopathy.
- Panretinal laser photocoagulation or intravitreal injections of anti-vascular endothelial growth factor can treat high-risk proliferative diabetic retinopathy and severe nonproliferative retinopathy.

Diabetic Nephropathy

Diabetic nephropathy is the leading cause of end-stage kidney disease (ESKD). Diabetes is typically present for 5 to 10 years prior to the development of nephropathy. Individuals with a first-degree relative with ESKD due to diabetic nephropathy have increased risk of progressing to ESKD themselves.

Measurement of estimated glomerular filtration rate (eGFR) and screening for the presence of microalbuminuria is recommended for early detection of kidney disease (see Table 14). Urinary albumin excretion can be determined from a random urine collection as an albumin-creatinine ratio (UACR). An elevated UACR level (≥ 30 mg/g creatinine) should be confirmed by multiple measurements over 3 to 6 months due to possible temporary elevations from biological variability, illness, hyperglycemia, heart failure, hypertension, exercise, and menstruation. Annual measurements of eGFR and UACR may identify progression of nephropathy and guide therapeutic decisions. More frequent assessments may be necessary with worsening kidney function. An eGFR less than 30 mL/min/1.73 m^2 warrants a referral to a nephrologist.

Uncontrolled hyperglycemia and hypertension are risk factors for diabetic nephropathy; thus treatment to attain glucose and blood pressure goals is recommended. The ADA recommends an ACE inhibitor or an angiotensin receptor blocker (ARB) as first-line therapy to slow progression of nephropathy and prevent CVD in nonpregnant persons with diabetes, hypertension, a reduced eGFR (<60 mL/min/1.73 m^2), and an elevated UACR (≥ 300 mg/g creatinine). An ACE inhibitor or an ARB is also recommended for treatment of an elevated UACR between 30 and 299 mg/g creatinine in nonpregnant persons with hypertension. Treatment with an ACE inhibitor or ARB is not recommended for patients with diabetes who have a normal blood pressure, a UACR level less than 30 mg/g creatinine, and an eGFR level greater than 60 mL/min/1.73 m^2.

KEY POINTS

- Measurement of estimated glomerular filtration rate and screening for the presence of microalbuminuria are recommended for early detection of kidney disease.
- The American Diabetes Association recommends an ACE inhibitor or an angiotensin receptor blocker as first-line therapy to slow progression of nephropathy and prevent cardiovascular disease in nonpregnant persons with diabetes, hypertension, a reduced estimated glomerular filtration rate (<60 mL/min/1.73 m^2), and an elevated urine albumin-creatinine ratio (≥ 300 mg/g creatinine).
- Treatment with an ACE inhibitor or angiotensin receptor blocker is not recommended for patients with diabetes who have a normal blood pressure, a urine albumin-to-creatinine ratio level less than 30 mg/g creatinine, and an estimated glomerular filtration rate level greater than 60 mL/min/1.73 m^2. **HVC**

Diabetic Neuropathy

Diabetic neuropathy involves damage to nerves or nerve roots due to hyperglycemia. Symptoms are dependent on the affected nerve(s) and may be focal or diffuse in nature. Neuropathy may occur peripherally and/or affect the autonomic nervous system. Glycemic control may prevent peripheral neuropathy and cardiac autonomic neuropathy in individuals with type 1 diabetes and can delay progression of neuropathy in type 2 diabetes.

Diabetic peripheral neuropathy (distal symmetric polyneuropathy) typically has an ascending presentation with a "stocking and glove" distribution. It may involve damage to both small and large nerve fibers. Symptoms from small nerve fiber damage include pain, burning, and tingling. Small nerve fiber abnormalities can be detected on examination by assessment of pinprick and temperature sensations. Abnormalities in position sense, vibration, and light touch are indicative of large nerve fiber damage and convey an increased risk for foot ulcerations. Assessment of large nerve fiber damage can be achieved by assessing ankle reflexes and with a 128-Hz tuning fork and a 10-g monofilament. Since diabetic peripheral neuropathy may be asymptomatic, screening should occur for early detection to prevent limb loss (see Table 14).

Autonomic neuropathy may affect one or multiple organs with symptoms varying based on the affected organ. Symptoms may include hypoglycemia unawareness, gastroparesis, constipation, diarrhea, erectile dysfunction, and bladder dysfunction. Symptoms from cardiac autonomic dysfunction may include orthostatic hypotension, resting sinus tachycardia, and exercise intolerance. Cardiac autonomic neuropathy is an independent risk factor for sudden death.

The goal of treatment of diabetic neuropathy is symptom control. Two FDA-approved medications, pregabalin or duloxetine, are recommended as initial therapy. Other agents may provide symptom relief but are not FDA approved and include tricyclic antidepressants, venlafaxine, carbamazepine, capsaicin, and gabapentin. The primary treatment of orthostatic hypotension is nonpharmacologic and includes diet, use of compression stockings, and changing positions slowly. Medications that cause or worsen the orthostatic changes should be discontinued and other agents (fludrocortisone, midodrine, or droxidopa) added for refractory symptoms. Small and frequent low-fat, low-fiber meals may improve symptoms of gastroparesis. Metoclopramide is the only prokinetic agent approved by the FDA for the treatment of gastroparesis. Given the risk of side effects, including dystonia, careful assessment of risks and benefits should be undertaken before prescribing (see MKSAP 18 Gastroenterology and Hepatology).

Diabetic amyotrophy is a rare condition affecting the lumbosacral plexus that may occur secondary to infarction or immune vasculopathy. Presentation is acute and associated with severe asymmetric pain or proximal weakness in a leg with associated muscle wasting. Partial remission may occur over many months. Treatment is supportive.

Mononeuropathies and nerve compression syndromes (carpal tunnel syndrome, peroneal palsy) can occur in patients with diabetes. Mononeuropathies frequently resolve without intervention within a few months. Compression syndromes may respond to conservative management, or surgery may be necessary for symptom relief.

KEY POINTS

- Diabetic peripheral neuropathy (distal symmetric polyneuropathy) presents with a "stocking and glove" distribution, involving damage to both small and large nerve fibers; symptoms include pain, burning, and tingling.
- Glycemic control can delay progression of neuropathy in type 2 diabetes.

Diabetic Foot Ulcers

Significant morbidity and mortality are associated with lower extremity ulcers and amputations (see MKSAP 18 Infectious Disease). Lower extremities should be inspected at every visit and a comprehensive foot examination, including 10-g monofilament testing, should be performed at least annually. Risk factors for ulcer include: hyperglycemia, peripheral artery disease, history of foot ulcer or amputation, foot deformity, peripheral neuropathy, impaired vision, tobacco use, and diabetic nephropathy. Vascular assessment should occur in persons with absent pedal pulses or symptoms concerning for claudication. Foot care specialists should be involved in the care of high-risk individuals. Patients should be educated on the importance of daily foot inspections and properly fitting footwear.

Hypoglycemia

Hypoglycemia is defined as a glucose value less than 70 mg/dL (3.9 mmol/L). Glucose values less than 54 mg/dL (3.0 mmol/L) are serious and clinically significant. Severe hypoglycemia is any glucose value at which a person requires external assistance to correct the glucose.

Hyperadrenergic symptoms (sweating, tremors, anxiety, tachycardia) are the normal physiologic response to the development of hypoglycemia. Counterregulatory hormones (glucagon, epinephrine, norepinephrine, cortisol, and growth hormone) are subsequently released by the body to correct hypoglycemia. Neuroglycopenic signs (altered mental status, dysarthria, confusion) are associated with severe hypoglycemia. Obtundation, seizures, and death may occur if severe hypoglycemia is not corrected rapidly.

Hypoglycemia in Patients with Diabetes Mellitus

Hypoglycemia can become a rate-limiting step in achieving glycemic goals for many persons. Severe recurrent hypoglycemia is

H
CONT.

associated with acquired cognitive deficits and can lead to dementia. Therapies must be adjusted to eliminate hypoglycemia, and glycemic goals should be individualized to accommodate targets that can be safely achieved.

Several factors contribute to hypoglycemia including a mismatch of food consumption and insulin delivery, increased physical exertion, weight loss, worsening kidney impairment, abnormalities in gastrointestinal motility and absorption, and accidental/intentional overdose of insulin. Older adults are also at an increased risk for hypoglycemia.

Hypoglycemia can also occur with the use of oral antidiabetic agents due to incorrect dosages, drug-drug interactions, and intercurrent illnesses that alter the metabolism or excretion of drugs.

Hypoglycemia treatment in an alert person includes consumption of 15 to 20 grams of a fast-acting carbohydrate followed by a self-monitored blood glucose (SMBG) measurement 15 to 20 minutes later. If the glucose has not improved, repeat treatment with 15 grams of carbohydrates should occur. After glucose normalization (>70 mg/dL [3.9 mmol/L]), a meal or snack should be consumed to avoid recurrent hypoglycemia. Glucagon should be provided to those persons at risk for developing clinically significant hypoglycemia (<54 mg/dL [3.0 mmol/L]) and used intramuscularly by close contacts if the person is not able to safely consume carbohydrates to correct hypoglycemia.

Relative hypoglycemia characterizes symptoms of hypoglycemia in the setting of plasma glucose values greater than 70 mg/dL (3.9 mmol/L). This may occur with a large, rapid decrease in glucose or rapid normalization of glucose with treatment intensification in an individual with prolonged plasma glucose values above 200 mg/dL (11.1 mmol/L). Relative hypoglycemia can be prevented by avoiding large glycemic excursions and by slow correction of long-standing hyperglycemia to goal to allow a longer adjustment period. H

KEY POINTS

- Hypoglycemia is defined as a glucose value less than 70 mg/dL (3.9 mmol/L) and serious hypoglycemia as less than 54 mg/dL (3.0 mmol/L).

- Initial treatment of hypoglycemia requires oral consumption of carbohydrates or administration of glucagon with a goal of increasing the glucose to greater than 70 mg/dL (3.9 mmol/L).

- Relative hypoglycemia can be prevented by avoiding large glycemic excursions and by slow correction of long-standing hyperglycemia to goal to allow a longer adjustment period.

H Hypoglycemia in Patients Without Diabetes Mellitus

Hypoglycemia without concomitant diabetes is uncommon and warrants further assessment. A hypoglycemia evaluation should commence if the criteria for Whipple triad are met: neuroglycopenic symptoms, hypoglycemia at or below 55 mg/dL (3.1 mmol/L), and resolution of symptoms with glucose ingestion. Laboratory measurement of glucose must confirm true hypoglycemia, as point-of-contact (POC) glucose values are not reliable in this scenario. Hypoglycemia in persons without diabetes may be attributable to the following causes: drugs, alcohol, illness, organ dysfunction (kidney or liver), hormonal deficiencies (adrenal insufficiency), malnutrition, and pancreatogenous insulinoma or noninsulinoma (endogenous hyperinsulinemic hypoglycemia that is not caused by an insulinoma).

Although there may be overlap in presentation, hypoglycemia typically occurs in the fasting or in the postprandial state. Diagnostic blood and urine studies should be obtained during a hypoglycemic episode in which Whipple triad has been demonstrated. If a spontaneous episode is not witnessed, measures should be implemented to recreate circumstances that normally induce hypoglycemia (fasting or ingestion of a typical meal that causes an episode in that particular patient). Imaging studies for tumor localization should only occur after confirmation of endogenous hyperinsulinism from the diagnostic blood and urine studies. H

KEY POINT

- Imaging studies for tumor localization should only occur after confirmation of endogenous hyperinsulinism from the diagnostic blood and urine studies.   **HVC**

Fasting Hypoglycemia   H
A prolonged fast, up to 72 hours, should be initiated if the hypoglycemia typically occurs while fasting.

Five blood specimens are drawn simultaneously every 6 hours: glucose, C-peptide, insulin, proinsulin, β-hydroxybutyrate. Insulin antibodies and an oral hypoglycemic agent screen should also be measured at the beginning of the fast. Blood specimen collection should increase to every 1 to 2 hours when the glucose measurement is less than 60 mg/dL (3.3 mmol/L).

Testing is complete when one of the following parameters is met: plasma glucose 45 mg/dL (2.5 mmol/L) or below with neuroglycopenia, or plasma glucose less than 55 mg/dL (3.1 mmol/L) if Whipple triad was documented previously. POC glucose values and hyperadrenergic symptoms should not be used to determine the end of the fast. Blood specimens should be collected again at the end of the 72-hour time period if neither of the above criteria has been met.

The interpretation of the diagnostic testing results is found in **Table 15**. To decrease the cost of this procedure, the plasma glucose should be sent to the laboratory as soon as possible, and if it is less than 60 mg/dL (3.3 mmol/L), the other four blood samples should be sent. H

TABLE 15. Differential Diagnosis of Spontaneous Fasting Hypoglycemia[a] in a Person Without Diabetes Mellitus

Diagnosis	Serum Insulin	Plasma C-Peptide[b]	Plasma Proinsulin[b]	Serum β-hydroxybutyrate[c]	Serum Insulin Antibodies	Urine or Blood Metabolites of Sulfonylureas or Meglitinides
Insulinoma[d, e]	↑	↑	↑	↓	Negative	Negative
Surreptitious use of sulfonylureas or meglitinides	↑	↑	↑	↓	Negative	Positive
Surreptitious use of insulin	↑	↓	↓	↓	Negative	Negative
Insulin autoimmune hypoglycemia	↑	↑	↑	↓	Positive	Negative
IGF-II[f]	↓	↓	↓	↓	Negative	Negative

[a]Symptomatic hypoglycemia, fasting plasma glucose 55 mg/dL (3.1 mmol/L) or lower, and prompt symptomatic relief with correction of hypoglycemia (Whipple triad).

[b]C-peptide and proinsulin are indicative of endogenous insulin production.

[c]β-hydroxybutyrate will be suppressed in the presence of insulin, but elevated with hypoglycemia that is not mediated by insulin.

[d]Blood specimens should be collected at the end of testing and glucagon should be administered followed by serial glucose measurements over 30 minutes. Insulin suppresses glycogenolysis and preserves glycogen stores. In the setting of an insulinoma, glucose will increase in response to glucagon as the glycogen stores are utilized.

[e]Similar results can also be seen with non-insulinoma pancreatogenous hypoglycemia syndrome or post-gastric bypass hypoglycemia.

[f]Insulin-like growth factor (IGF)-II or its precursors may be produced by tumors and induce hypoglycemia by stimulating the insulin receptors with subsequent increases in glucose use.

Data from Cryer PE, Axelrod L, Grossman AB, Heller SR, Montori VM, Seaquist ER, et al; Endocrine Society. Evaluation and management of adult hypoglycemic disorders: an Endocrine Society Clinical Practice Guideline. Clin Endocrinol Metab. 2009;94:709-28. [PMID: 19088155]

KEY POINT

HVC • For fasting hypoglycemia, five blood specimens are drawn simultaneously every 6 hours: glucose, C-peptide, insulin, proinsulin, β–hydroxybutyrate; to decrease the cost of this procedure, the plasma glucose should be sent to the laboratory as soon as possible, and if it is less than 60 mg/dL (3.3 mmol/L), the other four blood samples should be sent.

Postprandial Hypoglycemia

Postprandial hypoglycemia typically occurs within 5 hours of the last meal. Altered gastrointestinal anatomy, as occurs after Roux-en-Y gastric bypass surgery, is frequently the cause of the postprandial hypoglycemia. Meals consisting of simple carbohydrates (pancakes, syrup, juice) are frequently the culprit. A mixed-meal test consisting of the types of food that normally induce the hypoglycemia should be performed to determine the cause. Baseline laboratory studies including glucose, C-peptide, insulin, and proinsulin should be obtained prior to meal consumption. These tests should be repeated every 30 minutes for 5 hours. If neuroglycopenia occurs, the tests should be repeated prior to administration of carbohydrates. To decrease the cost of this procedure, the plasma glucose should be sent to the laboratory as soon as possible, and if it is less than 60 mg/dL (3.3 mmol/L), the other three blood samples should be sent.

Screening should also occur for insulin antibodies and oral hypoglycemic agents if symptomatic hypoglycemia occurs. Interpretation of the results is similar to those obtained during fasting hypoglycemia (see Table 15).

Treatment generally consists of small frequent mixed meals with a balance of protein, fat, and carbohydrates.

KEY POINT

• For postprandial hypoglycemia, baseline laboratory studies including glucose, C-peptide, insulin, and pro-insulin should be obtained prior to meal consumption; to decrease the cost of this procedure, the plasma glucose should be sent to the laboratory as soon as possible, and if it is less than 60 mg/dL (3.3 mmol/L), the other three blood samples should be sent.   HVC

Hypoglycemia Unawareness

Hypoglycemia unawareness is characterized by insufficient release of counterregulatory hormones and an inadequate autonomic response to hypoglycemia. Prior episodes of hypoglycemia increase the risk of developing hypoglycemia unawareness. Treatment involves relaxation of glycemic targets and modifications of hypoglycemia-inducing diabetes therapies to avoid continued hypoglycemia. Avoidance of hypoglycemia for several weeks may reverse hypoglycemia unawareness in some persons and result in the return of adrenergic symptoms with glucose levels less than 70 mg/dL (3.9 mmol/L). A continuous glucose monitoring system may be beneficial in appropriate individuals to provide early detection of impending severe hypoglycemia for early intervention.

Disorders of the Pituitary Gland

Hypothalamic and Pituitary Anatomy and Physiology

The pituitary gland is located in the sella turcica posterior to the sphenoid sinus. The optic chiasm is located superior to the pituitary gland, and the carotid arteries are lateral (**Figure 2**). The gland is composed of the anterior pituitary (adenohypophysis), which is glandular tissue, and the posterior pituitary gland (neurohypophysis), which arises from neural tissue. A rich portal vascular network connects the hypothalamus to the anterior pituitary, whereas the posterior pituitary gland consists of nerve endings projected from neurons in the supraoptic and paraventricular nuclei in the hypothalamus. Both the portal network and hypothalamic neurons travel from the hypothalamus to the pituitary through the pituitary stalk. The carotid arteries provide blood to the pituitary through the hypophysial arteries, and venous drainage occurs by means of the petrosal sinuses to the jugular vein.

Stimulatory and inhibitory hormones, secreted into the portal blood by the hypothalamus, regulate the anterior pituitary, and the posterior pituitary hormones are synthesized in the hypothalamic nuclei and travel through neurons to be released by the posterior pituitary gland.

The anterior pituitary secretes six pituitary hormones: luteinizing hormone (LH), follicle-stimulating hormone (FSH), adrenocorticotrophic hormone (ACTH), prolactin, thyroid-stimulating hormone (TSH), and growth hormone (GH). Gonadotropin-releasing hormone (GnRH) is released from the hypothalamus in pulses, which in turn control the release of LH and FSH. LH and FSH regulate male and female reproduction including stimulation of the gonads to produce testosterone and estrogen, as well as stimulation of ovarian

follicles and spermatogenesis (see Reproductive Disorders). Corticotropin-releasing hormone (CRH), produced in the hypothalamus, stimulates the production of ACTH in the pituitary, which then stimulates cortisol production from the adrenal glands. Prolactin is synthesized in the lactotroph cells. Its synthesis and secretion is suppressed by hypothalamic dopamine, which traverses the pituitary stalk through the portal circulation. TSH is released in response to stimulation from thyrotropin-releasing hormone (TRH) produced in the hypothalamus. TSH binds to receptors on the thyroid, resulting in synthesis and secretion of thyroid hormone. GH release is regulated by two hypothalamic hormones, growth hormone-releasing hormone (GHRH), which stimulates GH release, and somatostatin, which inhibits GH release.

The posterior pituitary gland secretes oxytocin, necessary for parturition and lactation, and antidiuretic hormone (ADH), which maintains water balance.

Table 16 lists the pituitary hormones and the initial evaluation for suspected pituitary excess or deficiency of each hormone.

Pituitary Abnormalities

Incidentally Noted Pituitary Masses

When a pituitary lesion is discovered incidentally on imaging obtained for an unrelated reason, the lesion is termed a "pituitary incidentaloma." Small incidentally noted pituitary lesions are quite common. In patients undergoing MRI for nonpituitary reasons, microadenomas are found in 10% to 38%, whereas incidental macroadenomas are seen in 0.2%. Most pituitary incidentalomas are benign nonfunctional pituitary adenomas; however, a small percentage may be Rathke cleft cysts, craniopharyngiomas, or meningiomas. In patients with a history of malignancy, metastatic disease should be considered. Pituitary adenomas measuring 1 cm or larger are

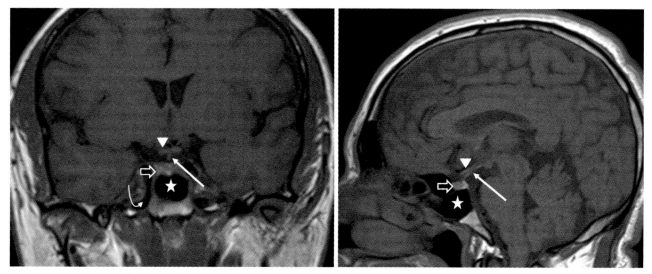

FIGURE 2. A coronal MRI (*left*) and sagittal MRI (*right*) showing the pituitary gland (*open arrow*), pituitary stalk (*thin arrow*), optic chiasm (*arrowhead*), sphenoid sinus (*star*), and carotid artery (*curved arrow*).

TABLE 16. Initial Testing for Pituitary Hormone Deficiency and Excess

Pituitary Hormone Excess			
Pituitary Hormone	**Peripheral Hormone**	**Initial Test(s)**	
ACTH	Cortisol	24-Hour urine free cortisol (×2) OR nocturnal salivary cortisol (×2) OR overnight low-dose dexamethasone test	
ADH	ADH	Simultaneous serum sodium, serum osmolality, urine sodium, and urine osmolality	
GH	IGF-1	IGF-1	
TSH	Thyroxine, triiodothyronine	TSH, free (or total) thyroxine	
PRL	Prolactin	Serum prolactin	
Pituitary Hormone Deficiency			
Pituitary Hormone	**Peripheral Hormone**	**Initial Test(s)**	**Confirmatory Test[a]**
ACTH	Cortisol	Simultaneous ACTH, cortisol	ACTH stimulation test
ADH	ADH	Simultaneous serum sodium, urine and serum osmolality	Water deprivation test
LH and FSH[b]	Testosterone or estradiol	Simultaneous LH, FSH, total testosterone (male), estradiol (female)	
TSH	Thyroxine, triiodothyronine	Simultaneous TSH, free (or total) thyroxine	
GH	IGF-1	IGF-1	GHRH-arginine test Insulin-tolerance test

ACTH = adrenocorticotropic hormone; ADH = antidiuretic hormone; FSH = follicle-stimulating hormone; GH = growth hormone; GHRH = growth hormone-releasing hormone; IGF-1 = insulin-like growth factor 1; LH = luteinizing hormone; PRL = prolactin; TSH = thyroid-stimulating hormone.

[a]See Table 18 for additional information on confirmatory testing for pituitary dysfunction.

[b]Routine testing for deficiency is not recommended without specific signs of deficiency, such as amenorrhea, gynecomastia, or impotence.

macroadenomas; those measuring less than 1 cm are microadenomas (see Evaluation of Pituitary Tumors).

KEY POINT

- Most incidentally noted pituitary masses are benign nonfunctional pituitary adenomas; however, a small percentage may be Rathke cleft cysts, craniopharyngiomas, or meningiomas.

Empty Sella

Empty sella is also typically an incidental finding on imaging done for a nonpituitary-related reason. It is a radiologic finding, rather than a medical condition. This term is used when the sella turcica is enlarged and not entirely filled with pituitary tissue. No gland may be visualized, or it is inordinately small. Primary empty sella is the result of herniation of subarachnoid space into the sella, compressing the normal pituitary gland. Primary empty sella is caused by incompetence of the sellar diaphragm, increased intracranial pressure, or volumetric changes in the pituitary gland (as can occur in pregnancy, particularly in multiparous women). Secondary empty sella can be related to infarction of a pituitary tumor or other causes including infection, autoimmune disease, trauma, or radiotherapy.

Patients with an empty sella usually have normal pituitary function because there is gland present, but it is lining the enlarged sella, like the rind of an orange. All patients with empty sella should have clinical assessment for signs and symptoms of pituitary deficiencies. Hyperprolactinemia, the most common pituitary abnormality in empty sella, can be treated with dopamine agonist therapy when needed. Asymptomatic patients should be screened with 8 AM cortisol level measurement, as well as TSH and free T_4 measurement. Additional testing should be targeted to the pituitary axes if there are signs or symptoms of deficiency.

Patients with no initial abnormalities are unlikely to develop hormonal or radiologic changes. Because of the theoretical risk of progression, however, it is recommended that asymptomatic patients with empty sella have repeat endocrine, radiologic, and ophthalmologic evaluation in 24 to 36 months. If no progression, further evaluation can be limited to those who require it clinically.

KEY POINT

- Empty sella is diagnosed when the sella turcica is enlarged and not entirely filled with pituitary tissue; all patients with empty sella should have clinical assessment for signs and symptoms of pituitary deficiencies.

Other Abnormalities

The pituitary gland can also be affected by other pathologic processes, such as autoimmune disease, infection, infiltrative diseases, metastatic disease, or infarction (**Table 17**).

Drug-Induced Abnormalities

There are a number of drugs that can affect pituitary gland function. Any hormone administered exogenously provides negative feedback to the normal cells in the pituitary gland. Exogenous estrogen or testosterone will suppress the gonadotropins, LH and FSH, whereas excess exogenous thyroid hormone will suppress TSH. Likewise, physiologic and supraphysiologic doses of glucocorticoids will suppress ACTH. Opiates have a number of effects. Most notably, chronic opioid use suppresses gonadotroph function, resulting in hypogonadotropic hypogonadism, and is increasingly recognized as a cause of ACTH deficiency.

A relatively new class of drugs, checkpoint-blocking antibodies, has been associated with pituitary abnormalities related to hypophysitis. These drugs, including nivolumab, ipilimumab, tremelimumab, and pembrolizumab, are used to treat metastatic melanoma, renal cell carcinoma, non–small cell lung cancer, and head and neck cancers. Hypophysitis occurs in 0.5% to 5% of patients and often presents with headache and fatigue. Endocrine evaluation usually reveals secondary adrenal insufficiency (ACTH deficiency) and secondary hypothyroidism (TSH deficiency), as well as low levels of LH, GH, and prolactin. Imaging demonstrates enhancement and/or enlargement of the pituitary gland with thickening of the pituitary stalk. Diabetes insipidus is uncommon. Treatment includes replacement of the hormone deficiencies along with high-dose glucocorticoids to treat the inflammatory process. Despite resolution of the inflammation, hormone deficiencies often persist.

Mass Effects of Pituitary Tumors

Mass effects of pituitary tumors most commonly include compression of the pituitary gland resulting in hormone deficiencies or compression of the optic chiasm most commonly resulting in bitemporal hemianopsia; other patterns of visual loss can also occur. Stalk compression can lead to hyperprolactinemia. Headaches can be a symptom of pituitary tumors but do not correlate well with tumor size. Headache alone is not an indication for surgery.

Pituitary deficiencies related to compression of the gland can vary from an isolated hormone deficiency, most often gonadotropin deficiency, to panhypopituitarism (deficiency of all anterior pituitary hormones).

Similarly, pituitary tumors can have variable effects on compression of surrounding structures. A rapidly growing

TABLE 17. Other Pituitary Abnormalities				
Pathology	**Cause**	**Mass Effect**	**Hormone Abnormalities**	**Clinical Context**
Inflammation				
Lymphocytic hypophysitis	Autoimmune	Possible	Most common is ACTH deficiency	Pregnancy, postpartum
Malignancy				
Pituitary metastasis	Metastasis of malignant tumor to pituitary gland	Optic nerve dysfunction occurs in 24% Can also have cranial nerve palsies and headache	Diabetes insipidus most common Also can have anterior pituitary deficits	Patients with the following primary malignancies: breast (most common), lung, lymphoma, renal cell
Pituitary carcinoma (rare) 0.1% of all pituitary tumors	Malignant pituitary tumor	Often present initially as macroadenoma	Most often there is some pituitary hypersecretion rather than deficiency	Patients found to have pituitary adenoma with significant cavernous sinus invasion or suprasellar extension
Infiltrative				
Sarcoidosis	Pituitary infiltration	Possible	Combination of anterior and posterior pituitary abnormalities	Occurs in up to 10% of patients with sarcoidosis
Hemochromatosis	Iron deposition	No	Gonadotropin deficiency	*HFE* gene mutation
Langerhans cell histiocytosis	Deposition of Langerhans cells within the pituitary gland	No	Diabetes insipidus Less likely anterior pituitary deficiencies	Rarely occur in adults
ACTH = adrenocorticotropic hormone.				

pituitary tumor or rapid expansion due to pituitary apoplexy (sudden hemorrhage or infarction of a pituitary adenoma) causing compression of the optic chiasm may result in complete bitemporal hemianopsia or even blindness. Pituitary apoplexy may even result in cranial nerve (CN) palsies of CNs III, IV, and VI, whereas a slowly growing pituitary tumor that abuts the optic chiasm may cause minimal or no loss in peripheral vision. All patients with pituitary tumors that abut or compress the optic chiasm should have an evaluation by an ophthalmologist (preferentially a neuro-ophthalmologist). Any abnormality on visual examination is an indication for surgery, unless the tumor is a prolactinoma.

Pituitary tumors can invade the cavernous sinus but rarely cause mass effect on brain tissue or narrowing of the carotid within the cavernous sinus.

KEY POINT

- Mass effects of pituitary tumors most commonly include compression of the pituitary gland resulting in hormone deficiencies or compression of the optic chiasm most commonly resulting in bitemporal hemianopsia; stalk compression can lead to hyperprolactinemia.

Evaluation of Pituitary Tumors

In patients with a pituitary tumor on CT imaging, a dedicated pituitary MRI with and without contrast with dynamic cuts through the sella should be obtained. A formal visual field examination is required for any tumor that abuts or compresses the optic chiasm.

Pituitary hypersecretion should be ruled out by measurement of prolactin and insulin-like growth factor 1 (IGF-1). Evaluation for Cushing disease is not necessary in patients without signs or symptoms of cortisol excess.

Pituitary tumors can also cause hypopituitarism. Screening for hypopituitarism is recommended in all pituitary tumors regardless of symptoms with measurement of FSH, LH, cortisol, TSH, free thyroxine (T_4), and additionally total testosterone in men. Hypogonadotropic hypogonadism can be assessed in premenopausal women through menstrual history. A history of oligomenorrhea or amenorrhea would raise concern for hypogonadotropic hypogonadism and require further hormone testing, whereas a history of normal menses would essentially rule out hypogonadotropic hypogonadism. Abnormal baseline testing may prompt further stimulatory testing to confirm hypopituitarism (**Table 18**), and referral to an endocrinologist is recommended.

If a patient does not require surgical intervention for mass effect or pituitary hypersecretion, repeat pituitary hormone assessment and imaging is performed in 6 months for macroadenomas and then yearly if no change.

Microadenomas should be reassessed with imaging in 1 year and then every 1 to 2 years thereafter. Repeat evaluation of pituitary function is not necessary in microadenomas if initial testing is normal and there has been no change clinically or in the pituitary MRI.

After 3 years of imaging follow up for a pituitary tumor (both microadenomas and macroadenomas), imaging can be performed less frequently, as long as clinical status of the patient remains stable.

KEY POINTS

- Pituitary hypersecretion should be ruled out by measurement of prolactin and insulin-like growth factor 1; evaluation for Cushing disease is not necessary in patients without signs or symptoms of cortisol excess. **HVC**

- A history of oligomenorrhea or amenorrhea would raise concern for hypogonadotropic hypogonadism and require further hormone testing, whereas a history of normal menses would essentially rule out hypogonadotropic hypogonadism. **HVC**

Treatment of Clinically Nonfunctioning Pituitary Tumors

Patients with a nonfunctioning pituitary tumor should be referred for neurosurgical evaluation if any of the following are present: visual deficits related to the tumor, a lesion abuts or compresses the chiasm or optic nerves on pituitary MRI, or pituitary apoplexy with visual disturbance. Surgery should also be considered for a tumor with clinically significant growth, such as growth toward the optic chiasm, and for patients with new loss of endocrine function. Women with a macroadenoma close to the optic chiasm who are planning pregnancy may benefit from surgical decompression of the pituitary tumor due to the risk of enlargement during pregnancy. Microadenomas rarely increase in size during pregnancy. The most common surgical approach for these tumors is transsphenoidal through the nares or mouth. Occasionally, craniotomy is needed for very large tumors. Most nonfunctioning macroadenomas will have immunocytochemistry consistent with a gonadotroph adenoma and are clinically "silent" (without hypersecretion of functional gonadotropins).

KEY POINTS

- Patients with a nonfunctioning pituitary tumor should be referred for neurosurgical evaluation if there are visual deficits related to the tumor, a lesion abuts or compresses the chiasm or optic nerves on pituitary MRI, or pituitary apoplexy with visual disturbance is present.

- Surgery should be considered for a tumor with clinically significant growth, such as growth potentially affecting vision, and for patients with new loss of endocrine function.

Pituitary Hormone Deficiency

Hypopituitarism is defined as one or more pituitary hormone deficiencies. It can occur as a result of compression of the normal pituitary cells by a tumor or as a complication of cranial surgery or radiation therapy. Somatotrophs and gonadotrophs

TABLE 18. Dynamic Testing for Pituitary Dysfunction

Indication	Test	Technique	Interpretation
ACTH (cortisol) deficiency	ACTH stimulation test	Measure baseline serum cortisol level. Administer 250 µg of synthetic ACTH IM or IV. Measure cortisol levels at 30 and 60 minutes.	Serum cortisol level >18 µg/dL (496.8 nmol/L) at any measurement indicates a normal response.
ADH deficiency (DI)	Water deprivation test, followed by desmopressin challenge, if indicated	Patient empties bladder, and baseline weight is measured. Measure urine volume and osmolality hourly. Measure serum sodium, osmolality, and weight every 2 h. *The test is stopped when one of the following occurs:* Urine osmolality/plasma osmolality is >2 Patient has lost >3% of body weight Urine osmolality is stable for 2-3 h while serum osmolality rises Plasma osmolality >295 mOsm/kg H_2O Serum sodium >145 mEq/L (145 mmol/L) *Desmopressin challenge:* If final urine osmolality <600 mOsm/kg, serum osmolality >295 mOsm/kg H_2O, or serum sodium >145 mEq/L (145 mmol/L): give desmopressin 2 µg subcutaneously. Measure urine osmolality and urine volume hourly for 4 hours after desmopressin.	*Water deprivation test interpretation:* Urine osmolality >750-800 mOsm/kg H_2O is a normal response to water deprivation, indicating ADH production and peripheral effect are intact. Serum osmolality >295 mOsm/kg H_2O and/or serum sodium >145 mEq/L (145 mmol/L) with inappropriately dilute urine (urine osmolality/plasma osmolality <2) is diagnostic of DI. *Desmopressin challenge interpretation:* Urine osmolality >800 mOsm/kg after desmopressin is consistent with complete central DI. No increase in urine osmolality (remains <300 mOsm/kg) is diagnostic of complete nephrogenic DI. Urine osmolality between 300 and 800 mOsm is consistent with partial DI
Growth hormone excess (acromegaly)	Glucose tolerance test	75-g oral glucose tolerance test. Measure glucose and GH at 0, 30, 60, 90, 120, and 150 minutes.	GH <0.2 ng/mL (0.2 µg/L) is a normal response. GH nadir ≥1.0 ng/mL (1.0 µg/L) (or ≥0.3 ng/mL [0.3 µg/L] on an ultrasensitive assay) is diagnostic of acromegaly.

ACTH = adrenocorticotropic hormone; ADH = antidiuretic hormone; DI = diabetes insipidus; GH = growth hormone.

appear to be the most sensitive to injury, so GH as well as LH and FSH are the most common pituitary deficiencies. ACTH and TSH deficiency are less common, but more serious.

Pituitary apoplexy and Sheehan syndrome (pituitary infarction associated with postpartum hemorrhage) can cause acute life-threatening hypopituitarism due to ACTH deficiency.

A full list of causes of hypopituitarism can be found in **Table 19**.

Panhypopituitarism

Panhypopituitarism occurs when a patient lacks adequate production of all anterior pituitary hormones, usually due to a large tumor or complications of pituitary surgery. These patients require daily replacement of thyroxine and cortisol. Replacement of sex steroids and GH is individualized, based on the clinical situation and evaluation of risks and benefits of treatment. Patients with panhypopituitarism should wear

medical alert identification as a deficiency of glucocorticoids can be life threatening.

Adrenocorticotropic Hormone Deficiency (Secondary Cortisol Deficiency)

The most common cause of adrenocorticotropic hormone (ACTH) deficiency is iatrogenic following administration of exogenous glucocorticoids and suppression of ACTH production. Oral, injectable (intraarticular, intramuscular), and even occasionally topical glucocorticoids can suppress ACTH. Inhaled glucocorticoids attenuate the recovery of endogenous ACTH production but rarely cause suppression of ACTH production directly. Patients with iatrogenic adrenal insufficiency have intact renin-aldosterone systems; they are at lower risk for hypotension and adrenal crisis.

Glucocorticoids prescribed in supraphysiologic doses for 3 weeks or longer should be tapered off to allow recovery of the pituitary-adrenal axis. Once the glucocorticoid dose is

TABLE 19. Causes of Hypopituitarism

Neoplastic
Pituitary adenoma
Meningioma
Craniopharyngioma
Metastatic cancer
Lymphoma
Infiltrative Disease
Sarcoidosis
Hemochromatosis
Langerhan cell histiocytosis
Inflammation
Lymphocytic hypophysitis
Iatrogenic
Surgery
Radiation
Congenital Deficiencies
Vascular
Pituitary infarction
Pituitary apoplexy
Empty Sella
Hypothalamic Disease
Traumatic Brain Injury
Medications
Opiates
Checkpoint inhibitors (nivolumab, ipilimumab, tremelimumab, pembrolizumab)

close to physiologic (equivalent of 15-20 mg hydrocortisone), hydrocortisone should be substituted. The dose can then be reduced by 5 mg every 1 to 2 weeks as tolerated. AM-only dosing may facilitate recovery of the adrenal axis.

Once on physiologic AM-only hydrocortisone, the adrenal axis can then be tested for recovery. An 8 AM cortisol level higher than 10 µg/dL (276 nmol/L) after withholding glucocorticoids for 24 hours suggests recovery of the pituitary-adrenal axis. This should be confirmed with an ACTH stimulation test. Despite recovery of the pituitary-adrenal axis, patients may take longer to recover their ability to respond to stress and may require stress-dose or sick-day dosing of glucocorticoids in the setting of an illness for up to a year.

ACTH deficiency can also occur in the setting of damage to the pituitary gland. Symptoms of secondary cortisol deficiency can include fatigue, malaise, weight loss, nausea, vomiting, asymptomatic hypoglycemia, dizziness, and hyponatremia. Because only cortisol production is affected (mineralocorticoid

production is intact), patients do not develop hyperkalemia and are less likely to have hypotension. Furthermore, patients with secondary adrenal insufficiency do not develop hyperpigmentation. Nonetheless, patients with secondary adrenal insufficiency do require physiologic glucocorticoid replacement and stress dosing during illness.

Morning cortisol levels less than 3 µg/dL (82.8 nmol/L) are diagnostic of cortisol deficiency; however, a morning cortisol level greater than 15 µg/dL (414 nmol/L) likely rules it out. Patients with cortisol levels between 3 and 15 µg/dL (82.8-414 nmol/L) should undergo an ACTH stimulation test (see Table 18). A peak cortisol level greater than or equal to 18 µg/dL (496.8 nmol/L) at 0, 30, or 60 minutes rules out cortisol deficiency. Once diagnosed, secondary adrenal insufficiency should be treated with hydrocortisone 15 to 20 mg in two divided doses, such as 10 to 15 mg in the morning and 5 mg in the afternoon. In the setting of an emergency such as pituitary apoplexy, an immediate intravenous dose of 100 mg hydrocortisone should be administered.

Glucocorticoid dosing must be adjusted in the setting of physiologic stress or acute illness. Administering two to three times the baseline dose of cortisol replacement for 2 to 3 days is usually sufficient for minor to moderate illness including minor or moderate surgery. In patients with major physiologic stress including major surgery or active labor, 100 mg hydrocortisone should be administered by intravenous injection followed by a continuous infusion of 200 mg every 24 hours or 50 mg intravenous injection every 6 hours (see Disorders of the Adrenal Glands).

KEY POINTS

- The most common cause of adrenocorticotropic hor- **HVC** mone deficiency is iatrogenic following administration of exogenous glucocorticoids and suppression of adrenocorticotropic hormone production.

- Glucocorticoids prescribed in greater than physiologic doses for 3 weeks or longer should be tapered off to allow recovery of the pituitary-adrenal axis.

- Glucocorticoid dosing must be adjusted in the setting of physiologic stress or acute illness.

Thyroid-Stimulating Hormone Deficiency

Deficiency of thyroid-stimulating hormone (TSH) results in the inability of the thyroid gland to produce thyroxine (T_4). The result is insufficient T_4 production with low or inappropriately normal TSH. The clinical symptoms of secondary hypothyroidism are the same as seen with primary hypothyroidism.

The treatment is daily administration of levothyroxine. TSH cannot be used to monitor therapy and should not be measured. Dosing based on TSH level can lead to underdosing. Free T_4 should be used to monitor dose adequacy and should be maintained in the mid to upper half of the normal range. While it takes 6 to 8 weeks for TSH to accurately reflect thyroid hormone status in primary hypothyroidism, free T_4 levels can be checked 2 to 3 weeks after a dose change to assess for adequacy in secondary hypothyroidism.

- Treatment of thyroid-stimulating hormone deficiency is daily administration of levothyroxine; only free thyroxine can be used to monitor dose adequacy, and free thyroxine should be maintained in the mid to upper half of the normal range.

Gonadotropin Deficiency

Gonadotropin deficiency can be a result of pituitary disease or a result of gonadotropin-releasing hormone (GnRH) deficiency as is seen in Kallmann syndrome and hypothalamic amenorrhea. Certain drugs, including opiates, can also suppress GnRH. Deficiency of gonadotropins, LH and FSH, results in deficiency of male and female sex hormones. The combination of low or inappropriately normal LH and FSH with low sex steroids is termed "central" or "hypogonadotropic" hypogonadism.

Treatment of hypogonadotropic hypogonadism can usually be achieved by replacing sex steroids in those with no contraindication and who do not desire fertility; testosterone treatment in men and combined estrogen-progesterone treatment in premenopausal women are used. While oral contraceptive pills may be more acceptable in young women for this purpose, other forms of estrogen and progesterone (such as estradiol patch with cycled oral progesterone) may be preferred in certain cases. In men and women who desire fertility, replacement of gonadotropins is necessary because exogenous testosterone and estrogen suppresses spermatogenesis in men and ovulation in women, respectively.

Growth Hormone Deficiency

Growth hormone (GH) is necessary for linear growth. Deficiency of GH in children causes short stature. Symptoms of growth hormone deficiency in adults are more subtle and include fatigue, loss of muscle mass, and increased ratio of fatty tissue to lean mass.

While isolated GH deficiency can occur in children, idiopathic isolated GH deficiency in adults is quite rare. Only patients with a history of hypothalamic or pituitary disease, surgery or radiation to these areas, head trauma, or other pituitary hormone deficiencies should be considered for evaluation of adult-onset isolated GH deficiency.

Owing to the pulsatile nature of GH, direct measurement is uninterpretable and GH deficiency should be assessed through measurement of insulin-like growth factor 1 (IGF-1). An IGF-1 level below the normal range for gender and age is highly suggestive of GH deficiency, whereas a normal IGF-1 level does not completely rule out growth hormone deficiency if pretest suspicion is high. Provocative tests such as an insulin tolerance test or GnRH-arginine test can be performed in consultation with an endocrinologist to establish the diagnosis of adult GH deficiency.

Benefits of treatment in those with GH deficiency include improvement in exercise capacity, body composition, and bone density. The decision to start growth hormone replacement should be individualized. It is contraindicated in the setting of malignancy or with an untreated pituitary tumor because of the potential for stimulation of tumor growth. Additionally, caution should be used in those with diabetes mellitus as it may worsen hyperglycemia. When therapy is indicated in adults, GH can be replaced with a low-dose daily injection titrated to a normal IGF-1 level and clinical assessment.

- Idiopathic isolated growth hormone deficiency in adults **HVC** is rare; only adults with a history of hypothalamic or pituitary disease, surgery or radiation to these areas, head trauma, or other pituitary hormone deficiencies should be evaluated.

Central Diabetes Insipidus

Inability of the posterior pituitary gland to produce adequate antidiuretic hormone (ADH) results in central diabetes insipidus (DI). Absent antidiuretic hormone (ADH) (complete DI) and reduced ADH (partial DI) prevent the reabsorption of water in the kidneys resulting in polyuria and polydipsia. Although significant hypernatremia is rare in patients with an intact thirst mechanism and free access to water, it can be severe if patients cannot drink to thirst.

An inappropriately low urine osmolality in the setting of an elevated serum osmolality and hypernatremia in a patient with polyuria (>50 mL/kg/24 hours in the absence of glucosuria) is diagnostic of DI. A water deprivation test can be performed when the diagnosis is uncertain (see Table 18).

DI is treated with desmopressin (DDAVP) administered intranasally, orally, or subcutaneously. Bioavailability of oral DDAVP is much lower and doses are considerably higher than with intranasal and subcutaneous routes. Despite this, oral preparations may be preferred in certain circumstances as intranasal absorption of DDAVP may be altered by changes in nasal mucosa. Doses are usually administered once nightly to prevent nocturia and ensure uninterrupted sleep, or twice daily if symptoms interfere with daily function. Caution should be taken to avoid overreplacement as this can result in hyponatremia, water intoxication, and volume overload.

- An inappropriately low urine osmolality in the setting of an elevated serum osmolality and hypernatremia in a patient with polyuria (>50 mL/kg/24 hours in the absence of glucosuria) is diagnostic of diabetes insipidus.

- Diabetes insipidus is treated with desmopressin administered intranasally, orally, or subcutaneously; caution should be taken to avoid overreplacement as this can result in hyponatremia, water intoxication, and volume overload.

Pituitary Hormone Excess

Pituitary tumors are considered functional when they secrete pituitary hormones in excess. The most common functional pituitary tumors are prolactinomas. Although pituitary tumors that produce ACTH or GH are less common, they are important to recognize because of the clinical consequences. TSH-secreting adenomas are a very rare cause of hyperthyroidism. Pituitary tumors rarely cosecrete more than one excess hormone. Cosecretion most commonly occurs with GH and prolactin.

Hyperprolactinemia and Prolactinoma

The most common cause of hyperprolactinemia is physiologic, related to pregnancy and lactation. Physiologic stress, coitus, sleep, and nipple stimulation are other nonpathologic causes of mild hyperprolactinemia. A comprehensive list of causes of hyperprolactinemia is provided in **Table 20**. Symptoms of hyperprolactinemia include amenorrhea, and sometimes galactorrhea, in premenopausal women. Men often present later with symptoms of mass effect or hypogonadism, such as decreased libido or difficulty with erections; less commonly, they experience gynecomastia and breast tenderness.

The most common cause of pathologic non–tumor-related hyperprolactinemia is medications. Of patients taking typical antipsychotics (see Table 20), 40% to 90% will have hyperprolactinemia caused by the dopamine antagonist effect of these medications. While medication-induced hyperprolactinemia most often results in prolactin levels of 25 to 100 ng/mL (25-100 µg/L), drugs such as metoclopramide, risperidone, and phenothiazines can lead to prolactin levels above 200 ng/mL (200 µg/L). Confirming that the hyperprolactinemia is related to medication can be challenging. If possible, the offending medication should be withheld for 3 days to determine whether prolactin levels return to normal.

Discontinuation of any psychotropic drug should be done only in consultation with the patient's psychiatrist. If the medication cannot be withheld and the prolactin elevation cannot be correlated to the timing of the drug initiation, a pituitary MRI should be performed to rule out prolactinoma. Antipsychotic medication–induced hyperprolactinemia is best treated in consultation with the patient's psychiatrist by switching to a drug that is less likely to cause hyperprolactinemia. While asymptomatic hyperprolactinemia related to medication does not require treatment, patients with hypogonadism should be treated with estrogen or testosterone to preserve bone mass. Treating medication-induced hyperprolactinemia with a dopamine agonist (cabergoline or bromocriptine) is controversial as it can exacerbate psychosis.

An MRI of the pituitary is indicated in all patients with unexplained hyperprolactinemia. Assessment and treatment decisions are then based on the prolactin level and MRI findings.

A prolactin level above 500 ng/mL (500 µg/L) is diagnostic of a macroprolactinoma. While levels greater than 250 ng/mL (250 µg/L) are suggestive of a macroprolactinoma, there are some medications that can raise prolactin to this level. Prolactin levels generally correlate with tumor size. Therefore when a macroadenoma is present with a prolactin level below 100 ng/mL (100 µg/L), pituitary stalk compression from a nonfunctioning tumor should be suspected for the cause of the hyperprolactinemia, rather than prolactinoma.

Patients with asymptomatic microadenomas do not require treatment. Women with hypogonadism related to a microadenoma can be treated with a combined oral contraceptive if they do not desire fertility or with a dopamine agonist if they do. Postmenopausal women with microadenomas do not require treatment.

In patients with macroadenomas, dopamine agonist therapy is recommended to lower prolactin, reduce tumor size, and restore gonadal function. Cabergoline is the preferred agent because of its superior efficacy in lowering prolactin and

TABLE 20.	Causes of Hyperprolactinemia	
Physiologic	**Medication**	**Other**
Coitus	Antipsychotics	Chest wall trauma
Exercise	Typical antipsychotics	Chronic kidney disease
Lactation	Chlorpromazine	Cirrhosis
Nipple stimulation	Fluphenazine	Cocaine
	Haloperidol	
Pregnancy	Prochlorperazine	Empty sella syndrome
Sleep	Atypical antipsychotics	Herpes zoster
Stress	Amisulpride	Polycystic ovary syndrome
	Olanzapine (rarely)	
	Paliperidone	Prolactinoma
	Risperidone	Seizures
	Ziprasidone (rarely)	Severe hypothyroidism
	SSRIs	
	Citalopram	Stalk compression
	Escitalopram	
	Fluoxetine	
	Paroxetine	
	Sertraline	
	Antihypertensives	
	Methyldopa	
	Verapamil	
	Other	
	Cimetidine	
	Domperidone	
	Estrogen	
	Metoclopramide	
	Opiates	

SSRI = selective serotonin reuptake inhibitor.

tumor shrinkage compared with bromocriptine. In addition, cabergoline dosing is twice per week compared with 1 to 3 times daily for bromocriptine. Prolactin can be monitored 2 to 4 weeks after initiation of therapy and then every 3 to 4 months once stable. MRI should be repeated for a microadenoma in 1 year. If both the tumor and prolactin are stable at 1 year follow up, no further imaging is needed. A macroadenoma should be reimaged 3 months after medical therapy and then every 6 to 12 months until stability is confirmed. Reimaging should be performed if the prolactin level rises despite therapy.

Surgery is not first-line therapy because up to 50% of prolactinomas recur after resection. Surgery should only be considered for prolactinomas in symptomatic patients who cannot tolerate dopamine agonist therapy or whose tumors do not shrink or even grow while on dopamine agonist therapy.

KEY POINTS

HVC • The most common cause of hyperprolactinemia is physiologic, related to pregnancy and lactation.

HVC • The most common cause of pathologic non–tumor-related hyperprolactinemia is medications.

HVC • Patients with asymptomatic microadenomas do not require treatment; for patients with macroadenomas, dopamine agonist therapy is recommended to lower prolactin, reduce tumor size, and restore gonadal function.

HVC • Surgery is not first-line therapy because up to 50% of prolactinomas recur after resection.

Prolactinomas and Pregnancy

Due to lactotroph hyperplasia in pregnancy, there is concern for enlargement of prolactinomas in pregnancy. Because microadenomas are not likely to enlarge during pregnancy, dopamine agonist therapy should be discontinued when pregnancy is discovered. However, patients who have macroadenomas without prior surgical or radiation therapy have a significant risk of tumor growth. Surgical tumor debulking prior to pregnancy or dopamine agonist therapy throughout pregnancy may be required in these patients. Bromocriptine is the preferred agent in pregnancy.

Patients with macroadenomas should be monitored with visual field testing each trimester while those with microadenomas can be monitored clinically. Headaches or visual field changes should prompt a noncontrast pituitary MRI.

Acromegaly

Acromegaly is caused by excess secretion of GH from a pituitary tumor in 95% of patients. In fewer than 5% of patients with GH excess, a growth hormone–releasing hormone (GHRH)-secreting tumor or neuroendocrine tumor is the cause of acromegaly. When GH-secreting pituitary tumors are present in children prior to puberty, the result is increased longitudinal growth resulting in gigantism. While gigantism is easily recognized in children, features of excess growth hormone are more subtle in adults, often not recognized for many years. A list of clinical features of acromegaly can be found in **Table 21**.

An IGF-1 level should be obtained to screen for suspected acromegaly. In those with an elevated level, an oral glucose tolerance test should be performed to confirm the diagnosis (see Table 18). A level above 1 ng/mL (1 µg/L) confirms the diagnosis of acromegaly. Once GH excess is demonstrated, a pituitary MRI should be obtained.

Transsphenoidal resection (TSR) of the GH-secreting tumor is the mainstay of therapy. Those who do not achieve remission with surgery can be treated with medical therapy and/or stereotactic radiation. Somatostatin analogues are the medications of choice as they result in reduction of tumor size as well as reduction in GH levels. Pegvisomant, a GH receptor antagonist, can be used in combination with a somatostatin analogue when needed; cabergoline can sometimes be used as well. Stereotactic radiotherapy (gamma knife) is used in certain cases. Once remission is achieved, MRI and IGF-1 levels are followed annually.

Patients with acromegaly can have increased mortality due to heart disease, sleep apnea, and cancer, but risk returns to baseline when IGF-1 is kept in the normal range. Appropriate screening and treatment for comorbidities are as important as managing the IGF-1 level.

TABLE 21. Features of Acromegaly
Clinical Signs and Symptoms
Prognathism
Macroglossia
Wide-spaced teeth (typically the first sign of growth hormone excess)
Wide nose
Enlarged and swollen hands and feet
Increased sweating
Skin tags
Joint pain
Headache
Disease Associations
Sleep apnea
Hypertension
Insulin resistance
Hypertrophic cardiomyopathy
Colon polyps and colon cancer
Thyroid nodules and thyroid cancer
Valvular heart disease
Arthropathy
Carpal tunnel syndrome

- An insulin-like growth factor 1 level should be obtained to screen for suspected acromegaly; in those with an elevated level, an oral glucose tolerance test should be performed to confirm the diagnosis followed by a pituitary MRI.

- Transsphenoidal resection of the growth hormone-secreting tumor is the mainstay of therapy; however, somatostatin analogues reduce the tumor size as well as growth hormone levels in those who do not achieve remission with surgery.

Thyroid-Stimulating Hormone-Secreting Tumors

Thyroid-stimulating hormone (TSH)-secreting pituitary tumors are extremely rare. Signs and symptoms of a TSH-secreting adenoma are those seen in hyperthyroidism, although laboratory evaluation reveals elevated T_4 and T_3 levels with an inappropriately normal or elevated TSH level. Once other causes of the laboratory abnormalities have been excluded (thyroid assay interference, thyroid hormone resistance, or familial dysalbuminemic hyperthyroxinemia), a pituitary MRI should be performed. TSR of the TSH-producing tumor is the treatment of choice. Medical therapy with somatostatin analogues can be used to control hyperthyroidism prior to surgery and following surgery in those who do not achieve remission.

Excess Antidiuretic Hormone Secretion

The syndrome of inappropriate antidiuretic hormone secretion (SIADH) results in water retention with resultant hyponatremia, often severe. CNS disorders (trauma, stroke, brain metastases, infection) drugs, pulmonary disease, and pituitary surgery (3-7 days postoperatively) can result in excess release of ADH. SIADH is a diagnosis of exclusion. Treatment involves correcting the underlying pathology, fluid restriction, vasopressin receptor antagonists, and hypertonic saline in severe hyponatremia. If hypertonic saline is being considered, consultation with an endocrinologist or nephrologist is recommended (see MKSAP 18 Nephrology).

Excess Adrenocorticotropic Hormone from Pituitary Source (Cushing Disease)

Cushing syndrome is a term used to describe hypercortisolism regardless of the cause; Cushing disease (the most common cause of endogenous Cushing syndrome) is the term used to describe hypercortisolism as a result of excess ACTH secretion from a pituitary tumor. Symptoms and signs of Cushing syndrome are listed in **Table 22**.

The diagnosis of Cushing syndrome is made by first establishing evidence of hypercortisolism (see Disorders of Adrenal Glands). Measuring ACTH establishes whether it is ACTH-dependent or ACTH-independent.

Once diagnosis of ACTH-dependent Cushing syndrome is established, a pituitary MRI should be performed for

TABLE 22.	Symptoms and Signs of Cushing Syndrome
Symptoms	
Depression	
Fatigue	
Rapid weight gain	
Decreased libido	
Menstrual abnormalities	
Signs	
Striae (especially if reddish purple and >1 cm in width)[a]	
Easy bruising[a]	
Facial plethora[a]	
Muscle weakness (proximal myopathy)	
Abdominal obesity	
Skin tears (secondary to thinning of the epidermis)	
Acne	
Hirsutism	
Dorsocervical fat pad (buffalo hump)[a]	
Supraclavicular fad pad[a]	
Hypokalemia	
Hypertension	
Diabetes	

[a]Features that best discriminate Cushing syndrome from the general population.

confirmation. If no pituitary tumor is seen or if the tumor is less than 6 mm, a high-dose 8-mg dexamethasone suppression test (DST) is done to evaluate for the presence of an ectopic ACTH-producing tumor (lung, pancreas, thymus carcinoma most commonly), which is highly resistant to dexamethasone suppression. Inferior petrosal sinus sampling (IPSS) is often recommended prior to TSR to confirm a pituitary source of ACTH excess due to low sensitivity and specificity of the high-dose DST.

The treatment of choice is TSR of the pituitary adenoma. Remission is generally defined by a morning serum cortisol level less than 5 μg/dL (138 nmol/L) within 7 days of surgery. Patients require glucocorticoid replacement postoperatively until the normal corticotroph cells recover from prolonged cortisol suppression. Recovery can take up to a year, and occasionally there is no recovery and the patient will require life-long cortisol replacement therapy.

If remission is not achieved following surgery, radiation or medical therapy (**Table 23**) may be required. Rarely, bilateral adrenalectomy is needed in patients unresponsive to all other therapies; these patients will require life-long glucocorticoid and mineralocorticoid replacement for acquired primary adrenal insufficiency. In addition, there is the risk of pituitary tumor enlargement following adrenalectomy (Nelson syndrome) due to unfettered stimulation of ACTH production.

Patients with Cushing disease require imaging and biochemical follow-up (urine free cortisol or late-night salivary

TABLE 23. Medication Management for Treatment of Cushing Syndrome

Steroidogenesis Inhibitors (Inhibits Cortisol Synthesis)	Pituitary Directed (Inhibits ACTH Secretion)	Glucocorticoid Receptor Antagonist (Inhibits Cortisol Action)
Ketoconazole	Pasireotide	Mifepristone
Metyrapone	Cabergoline	
Mitotane		
Etomidate		

ACTH = adrenocorticotropic hormone.

cortisol measurement) every year for several years, and then on a less frequent basis. The first biochemical sign of recurrence is often elevated late-night salivary cortisol levels. Recurrences are managed by repeat TSR, radiation, and/or medical therapy.

KEY POINTS

- The diagnosis of Cushing syndrome is made by first establishing evidence of hypercortisolism; once adrenocorticotropic hormone-dependent Cushing disease is confirmed, a pituitary MRI should be performed.

- The treatment of choice for adrenocorticotropic hormone-dependent Cushing disease is transsphenoidal resection of the pituitary adenoma, followed by glucocorticoid replacement until the normal corticotroph cells recover from cortisol suppression.

Disorders of the Adrenal Glands

Adrenal Anatomy and Physiology

Although considered one organ, the adrenal glands have two functionally distinct regions: an outer cortex and an inner medulla. The cortex secretes hormones that are classified as mineralocorticoid (aldosterone), glucocorticoid (cortisol), and androgen (dehydroepiandrosterone [DHEA]). The medulla secretes catecholamines.

The adrenal cortex is composed of three zones: the zona glomerulosa (outer), zona fasciculate (middle), and zona reticularis (inner). Aldosterone production in the zona glomerulosa is regulated by the renin-angiotensin system and promotes sodium reabsorption and potassium excretion across the distal tubule of the kidney. The resultant expansion of extracellular volume increases blood pressure. Aldosterone also has direct inflammatory and fibrotic effects on other organs that are independent of its effects on blood pressure. Major stimuli to aldosterone secretion include hypotension, hypovolemia, and hyperkalemia.

Cortisol production in the zona fasciculata is regulated by release of adrenocorticotropic hormone (ACTH) from the pituitary gland. Cortisol exhibits a distinct diurnal rhythm characterized by peak levels on awakening that decrease to very low levels by bedtime. Superimposed on this diurnal rhythm are small oscillations of cortisol secretion while awake. Most cortisol circulates in the blood attached to cortisol-binding protein, with only a small fraction circulating as biologically active, free hormone. Cortisol is crucial to the body's adaptive response to physiologic stress, and levels increase in response to psychological stress, as well as physical illness. Cortisol actions are diverse and include immune, vascular, anti-inflammatory, and metabolic effects.

DHEA, produced in the zona reticularis, and its sulfate DHEAS, are weak adrenal androgens that mediate their effects through peripheral conversion to testosterone. In women the adrenal gland is a significant contributor to circulating androgen levels. In men the adrenal contribution to androgen effect is negligible.

The adrenal medulla secretes the catecholamines norepinephrine and epinephrine in response to hypotension, hypoglycemia, fear, anxiety, acute illness, and other causes of psychological and physical stress. Catecholamines interact with α- and β-adrenergic receptors to increase pulse and blood pressure, relax smooth muscle, dilate bronchioles, and increase metabolic rate. A small fraction of norepinephrine and epinephrine is excreted in the urine as free hormone; the rest is degraded in the liver to metanephrine and normetanephrine prior to urinary excretion.

Adrenal Hormone Excess

Cortisol Excess (Cushing Syndrome Due to Adrenal Mass)

Cortisol-secreting adrenal adenomas and, rarely, carcinomas account for 20% of endogenous causes of Cushing syndrome. Excess cortisol secretion from these tumors suppresses ACTH production from the pituitary gland, resulting in a form of Cushing syndrome classified as ACTH-independent. ACTH-dependent Cushing syndrome is more common and is most commonly caused by pituitary adenomas (see Disorders of the Pituitary Gland). While many of the symptoms and signs of Cushing syndrome are common in the general population, some, including supraclavicular fat pads, proximal muscle weakness, facial plethora, and wide violaceous striae (**Figure 3**), are considered more discriminatory (see Disorders of the Pituitary Gland). Diagnosis of Cushing syndrome is challenging because patients present along a spectrum ranging from mild disease with subtle findings to severe, life-threatening disease. In addition, hypercortisolemia from psychological stress and physical illness can also occur in the absence of Cushing syndrome. In severe stress states such as major depression, anxiety, psychosis, poorly controlled diabetes mellitus, and severe visceral obesity, a pseudo-Cushing state may occur in which

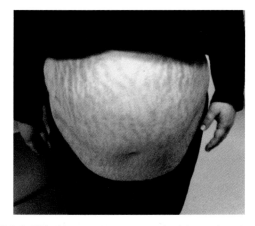

FIGURE 3. Wide violaceous striae are seen on the abdomen of a patient with Cushing syndrome. Striae larger than 1 cm in width are highly specific for hypercortisolism.

hypercortisolemia and nonspecific clinical features of Cushing syndrome coexist.

Evaluation for Cushing syndrome in patients without specific signs of Cushing syndrome is not recommended.

The evaluation of Cushing syndrome involves (1) initial testing followed by confirmatory testing for Cushing syndrome; (2) determining Cushing syndrome as ACTH-independent or -dependent; and (3) localizing the source of ACTH in ACTH-dependent disease or confirming the presence of adrenal mass (or masses) in ACTH-independent disease. It is imperative that biochemical Cushing syndrome be confirmed with certainty prior to looking for the source, as misdiagnosis may lead to unnecessary testing and treatment.

The diagnosis of Cushing syndrome necessitates a combination and repetition of tests (**Figure 4**). Measurement of morning or random serum cortisol is unreliable, due to overlap of serum cortisol levels among normal patients, those with Cushing syndrome, and those with mild hypercortisolism/pseudo-Cushing state in the absence of Cushing syndrome. In addition, total cortisol levels are unreliable when binding proteins are affected by oral estrogen, acute illness, and low protein states.

Initial tests for Cushing syndrome have similar diagnostic accuracy and include measurement of 24-hour urine free cortisol, serial late night salivary cortisols, and the 1-mg overnight dexamethasone suppression test. When suspicion for Cushing syndrome is low, a single test, if negative, makes Cushing syndrome unlikely. When there is a higher index of suspicion for Cushing syndrome, two different initial tests are recommended.

Urine free cortisol and late night salivary cortisol represent the serum free cortisol fraction and avoid pitfalls in interpretation related to changes in cortisol-binding proteins. Spurious elevation of urine free cortisol can result from hypercortisolemia not related to Cushing syndrome/pseudo-Cushing state or when significant polyuria (>5 L/d) is present. False-negative results can occur in advanced kidney disease or in patients with variable secretory rates of cortisol.

Late-night salivary cortisol is collected at home by the patient between 11 PM and midnight on at least two different nights. This test assesses for the normal diurnal rhythm of cortisol, which is lost in Cushing syndrome, and the cortisol level will not be low as expected. This test is not recommended in patients who do shift work or have an inconsistent sleep pattern. Recent cigarette smoking or contamination of the sample by topical glucocorticoids can falsely increase results.

The 1-mg (low-dose) dexamethasone suppression test depends on the principle that autonomous cortisol secretion is not subject to feedback suppression with exogenous glucocorticoids. Dexamethasone is taken at 11 PM and serum total cortisol is measured at 8 AM the following morning.

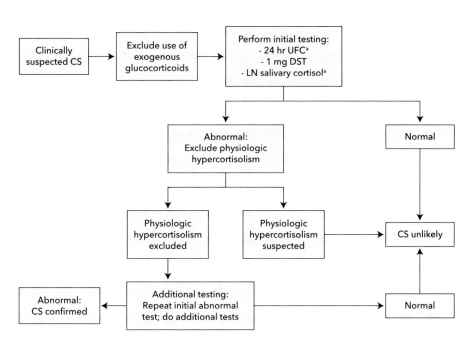

FIGURE 4. Algorithm to confirm or rule out the diagnosis of Cushing syndrome. CS = Cushing syndrome; DST = dexamethasone suppression test; LN salivary cortisol = late-night salivary cortisol; UFC = urine free cortisol.

[a]Must be performed at least twice.

A post-dexamethasone cortisol level of greater than 5 µg/dL (138 nmol/L) is considered a positive test. A lower cut-off cortisol value of greater than 1.8 µg/dL (49.7 nmol/L) has been advocated to improve test sensitivity, but this occurs at the expense of reduced specificity. False-positive results may occur with concomitant use of medications (carbamazepine, phenytoin, and pioglitazone) that induce hepatic CYP3A4 enzymes and accelerate dexamethasone metabolism. Simultaneous measurement of serum dexamethasone can confirm patient adherence or altered dexamethasone metabolism.

Many factors can raise cortisol levels in the absence of Cushing syndrome, so test interpretation should incorporate the pretest probability of Cushing syndrome. A urine free cortisol level greater than 3 times the upper normal range in the setting of clinical manifestations of Cushing syndrome is considered diagnostic of the disorder, whereas a positive test in the setting of low suspicion for Cushing syndrome does not support the diagnosis. If initial testing is positive, confirmation and further evaluation should involve consultation with an endocrinologist. Once the diagnosis of Cushing syndrome is established, the next step is measurement of ACTH; if suppressed (<5 pg/mL [1.1 pmol/L]) indicating an ACTH-independent cause of Cushing syndrome, a dedicated adrenal CT or MRI is indicated. If adrenal glands appear normal on imaging, the diagnosis of Cushing syndrome should be questioned.

Surgical resection is the definitive treatment for benign and malignant cortisol-secreting adrenal tumors.

Following adrenalectomy, patients require daily hydrocortisone therapy to allow recovery from prolonged ACTH suppression due to hypercortisolism. Recovery of adrenal fasciculate function may take up to 1 year or longer depending on the severity of Cushing syndrome (see Disorders of the Pituitary Gland).

KEY POINTS

- The evaluation of Cushing syndrome involves (1) initial testing followed by confirmatory testing for Cushing syndrome; (2) determining Cushing syndrome as adrenocorticotropic hormone (ACTH)-independent or -dependent; and (3) localizing the source of ACTH in ACTH-dependent disease or confirming the presence of adrenal mass (or masses) in ACTH-independent disease.

- Initial tests for Cushing syndrome have similar diagnostic accuracy and include measurement of 24-hour urine free cortisol, serial late-night salivary cortisols, and the 1-mg overnight dexamethasone suppression test.

- **HVC** Evaluation for Cushing syndrome in patients without specific signs of Cushing syndrome is not recommended.

Primary Aldosteronism

Primary aldosteronism (PA) is a common cause of secondary hypertension. Traditionally, hypokalemia was considered to be a biochemical prerequisite for the diagnosis of PA, but it is now recognized that more than 60% of patients have normal potassium levels. As hypertension is often the only sign of primary aldosteronism, the condition frequently goes undiagnosed. Identification of patients with primary aldosteronism is important because aldosterone has deleterious effects on the cardiovascular system and treatment prevents progression and can sometimes reverse changes. Higher cardiovascular morbidity and mortality have been noted in patients with primary aldosteronism compared to those with primary hypertension with similar blood pressure control. The potential health impact of untreated primary aldosteronism and the importance of recognizing primary aldosteronism is reflected in updated guidelines on case-detection testing for primary aldosteronism (**Table 24**).

Primary aldosteronism is caused by hyperplasia of both adrenal glands (idiopathic hyperaldosteronism) in two-thirds of cases, and a unilateral aldosterone-producing adenoma (APA) in one-third of cases. The diagnosis of primary aldosteronism involves performing stepwise case detection, as well as confirmatory and localization studies. The most reliable case-detection test is calculation of an plasma aldosterone-plasma renin ratio (ARR) by measuring plasma aldosterone concentration and plasma renin activity (or

TABLE 24. Case Detection Indications for Primary Aldosteronism and Pheochromocytoma
Primary Aldosteronism
Untreated hypertension with sustained BP >150/100 mm Hg
Hypertension (>140/90 mm Hg) on three-drug therapy
Hypertension and an incidentally discovered adrenal mass
Hypertension associated with spontaneous or diuretic-induced hypokalemia
Hypertension in the setting of a first-degree relative with PA
Hypertension in the setting of family history of hypertension onset age <40 years
Pheochromocytoma
Adrenergic-type spells (headache, sweating, and tachycardia) with or without hypertension
Incidentally discovered adrenal mass with or without hypertension
Hypertension (>140/90 mm Hg) on three-drug therapy
Hypertension with onset age <20 years
Idiopathic cardiomyopathy
Hypertensive episode induced by anesthesia, surgery, or angiography
Paraganglioma
Familial syndromes that predispose to pheochromocytoma: VHL, NF-1, and MEN 2
Family history of pheochromocytoma or paraganglioma

BP = blood pressure; MEN 2 = multiple endocrine neoplasia type 2; NF-1 = neurofibromatosis type 1; PA = primary aldosteronism; VHL = von Hippel-Lindau.

direct renin concentration) in a mid-morning seated sample. In patients taking an ACE inhibitor or an angiotensin receptor blocker, renin should be elevated, so in these patients, a simple initial test is plasma renin activity measurement. If the plasma renin activity is suppressed, the likelihood of primary aldosteronism is high and an ARR should be performed; if not, hyperaldosterone state is ruled out. Mineralocorticoid receptor antagonists (spironolactone and eplerenone) and high-dose amiloride can significantly interfere with interpretation of ARR and should be discontinued 6 weeks prior to evaluation.

Other antihypertensive agents can be continued, but because some may have minor effects on aldosterone and/or renin levels (**Table 25**), the results of the ARR should be interpreted with these effects in mind. Hydralazine, a selective α-adrenergic receptor blocker, and slow-release verapamil have minimal effects on aldosterone and renin secretion, and they can be substituted when feasible for other agents if the ARR is equivocal. An ARR greater than 20 with a plasma aldosterone concentration of at least 15 ng/dL (414 pmol/L) is considered a positive result, and patients should be referred to an endocrinologist, who may perform additional testing to confirm inappropriate aldosterone secretion in a salt-replete state.

The localization study of choice for primary aldosteronism is a dedicated adrenal CT. Findings may include normal adrenal glands or unilateral or bilateral adenoma(s)/hyperplasia. In one third of patients, the CT may not identify the cause of primary aldosteronism because some APAs are too small to see or there is an incidental adrenal mass unrelated to primary aldosteronism. Consequently, most patients with confirmed primary aldosteronism should undergo adrenal vein sampling to confirm the source of the hyperaldosteronism.

Medical therapy with an aldosterone receptor antagonist (spironolactone or eplerenone) is the treatment of choice for primary aldosteronism due to idiopathic hyperaldosteronism, or when patients with APA are not candidates for, or do not wish to undergo, surgery. Spironolactone is often preferred over eplerenone because it is less expensive and more potent. However, patients on spironolactone are more likely to develop dose-dependent side effects of gynecomastia and erectile dysfunction in men and menstrual irregularities in women. Hypokalemia almost always resolves with treatment, but blood pressure control may require additional agents. No studies clearly show superiority of adrenalectomy compared to medical therapy for APA, but surgery may be more cost-effective in the long term.

Laparoscopic adrenalectomy is effective for unilateral disease and reduces plasma aldosterone and its attendant increased risk of cardiovascular disease. Hypertension is improved in most patients and cured in about 40% of patients. Persistent hypertension following adrenalectomy may be due to vascular changes caused by chronic hypertension or coexistent primary hypertension. Patients are more likely to achieve resolution of hypertension if they were taking fewer than three antihypertensive agents preoperatively, and if they have one or fewer first-degree relatives with hypertension. Serum potassium should be monitored weekly for the first month postoperatively, and patients should be instructed to eat a high-salt diet due to risk of hyperkalemia from transient reduction in aldosterone production in the remaining adrenal gland due to chronic suppression of the renin-angiotensin system during the period of hyperaldosteronism. Short-term mineralocorticoid replacement is required in those patients who develop hyperkalemia.

KEY POINTS

- The most reliable case-detection test for primary aldosteronism is calculation of a plasma aldosterone-plasma renin ratio by measuring plasma aldosterone concentration and plasma renin activity (or direct renin concentration) in a mid-morning seated sample; if the plasma renin activity is suppressed, the likelihood of primary aldosteronism is high.

- In patients taking an ACE inhibitor or an angiotensin receptor blocker, renin should be elevated, so in these patients, a simple initial test is a plasma renin activity measurement; if the plasma renin activity is suppressed, the likelihood of primary aldosteronism is high and a plasma aldosterone-plasma renin ratio should be performed; if not, hyperaldosterone state is ruled out. **HVC**

(Continued)

TABLE 25. The Effect of Commonly Prescribed Medications on Measurements of Plasma Renin Activity and Plasma Aldosterone Concentration				
Effect on Test Results	Medication Class	PRA	PAC	PAC/PRA
False-Positive	α₂-Adrenoceptor agonist	↓↓	↓	↑
	β-Adrenoceptor blocker	↓↓	↓	↑
	Direct renin inhibitor	↓	↓	↑
	NSAID	↓↓	↓	↑
False-Negative	ACE inhibitor/ARB	↑↑	↓	↓
	Dihydropyridine CCB	↑	↓	↓
	Diuretic[a]	↑↑	↑	↓
	Mineralocorticoid receptor antagonist	↑↑	↑	↓
	SSRI		↑	↓

ARB = angiotensin receptor antagonist; CCB = calcium channel blocker; PAC = plasma aldosterone concentration; PRA = plasma renin activity; SSRI = selective serotonin reuptake inhibitor.

[a]Both potassium-sparing (amiloride) and potassium-wasting (hydrochlorothiazide) diuretics.

- Laparoscopic adrenalectomy for unilateral disease results in reduction of plasma aldosterone; medical therapy with an aldosterone receptor antagonist (spironolactone or eplerenone) is the treatment of choice for primary aldosteronism due to idiopathic hyperaldosteronism, or when patients with aldosterone-producing adenoma are not candidates for, or do not wish to undergo, surgery.

Pheochromocytoma and Paraganglioma

Pheochromocytomas and paragangliomas are catecholamine-secreting tumors that arise from chromaffin cells of the adrenal medulla (80%) and extra-adrenal (mostly abdominal) sympathetic ganglia, respectively. Tumors can also arise from parasympathetic ganglia in the head and neck, but these rarely secrete catecholamines.

At least one-third of pheochromocytomas/paragangliomas are associated with a germline mutation. Pheochromocytomas may occur in familial syndromes including multiple endocrine neoplasia type 2, von Hippel-Lindau syndrome, and neurofibromatosis type 2 (**Table 26**). All patients with catecholamine-secreting tumors should, therefore, be offered genetic counseling.

Hypertension associated with pheochromocytoma/paraganglioma can show a sustained pattern, with or without paroxysms, or occur as paroxysms only. Some patients (10% to 15%) remain normotensive. The classic triad of palpitations, headache, and diaphoresis is seen in fewer than 50% of patients with pheochromocytoma. Multiple symptoms related to catecholamine excess can occur including abdominal pain, skin pallor, blurred vision, or polyuria. Rarely, patients can present with acute myocardial infarction, cardiomyopathy, or stroke.

Indications for testing for pheochromocytoma are shown in Table 24. Initial tests for pheochromocytoma include

measurement of plasma-free metanephrine collected in a supine position or 24-hour urine fractionated metanephrine and catecholamine levels. Elevation in catecholamines can occur in patients under psychological or physical stress. Medications can affect results (**Table 27**) and should be discontinued at least 2 weeks prior to testing. Accurate diagnosis is further confounded by the fact that patients with or without hypertension may have adrenergic-type spells in the absence of a catecholamine-secreting tumor. Interpretation of the test results must consider the extent of metanephrine elevation rather than whether the result is normal or abnormal. Mild elevations may require repeat testing. Levels more than four times the upper limit of normal, in the absence of acute stress or illness, are consistent with a catecholamine-secreting tumor. The plasma-free metanephrine is highly sensitive (96% to 100%). The specificity is 85% to 89%. Urine fractionated metanephrine and catecholamines have higher specificity (98%) and high sensitivity (up to 97%). Neither test is superior, so clinicians can use an estimate of pretest probability to select the initial test. When there is a high index of suspicion, plasma-free metanephrine is chosen, and when suspicion is low, urine fractionated metanephrine and catecholamines may be a better option.

The search for a tumor should begin when a biochemical diagnosis of pheochromocytoma/paraganglioma is supported by laboratory results, to avoid misdiagnosing an incidental nonfunctioning adrenal mass as a pheochromocytoma. It is difficult to determine clinical relevance of significantly elevated metanephrine levels in hospitalized patients. The imaging modality of choice is an abdominal and pelvic contrast-enhanced CT as 85% of catecholamine-secreting tumors are intra-adrenal (and 95% reside in the abdomen or pelvis). Typical imaging features of pheochromocytomas are shown in **Table 28**. The average size of a symptomatic pheochromocytoma at diagnosis is 4 cm. If the CT is negative, reconsidering the diagnosis is the first step; however, if suspicion of a catecholamine-secreting tumor is high, the

TABLE 26.	Multiple Endocrine Neoplasm Syndromes		
Type	Mutation	Most Common Feature	Associated Features
1	*MEN1* (inheritance of one mutated allele with somatic mutation in other allele leads to neoplasia)	Parathyroid adenoma (often multiple)	Pancreatic islet cell and enteric tumors (gastrinoma, insulinoma most common)
			Pituitary adenoma
			Other (carcinoid tumors, adrenocortical adenoma)
2A	*RET* (exon 11, codon 634[a])	Medullary thyroid carcinoma	Pheochromocytoma (often multifocal)
			Parathyroid hyperplasia
2B	*RET* (exon 16, codon 918[a])	Medullary thyroid carcinoma	Pheochromocytoma (often multifocal)
			Mucosal neuroma
			Gastrointestinal ganglioneuroma
			Marfanoid body habitus

[a]Most common mutation observed.

TABLE 27. Substances Associated with False-Positive Biochemical Testing for Pheochromocytoma

Drug Class	Medication/Substance
Analgesics	Acetaminophen
Antiemetics	Prochlorperazine
Antihypertensives	Phenoxybenzamine[a]
Psychiatric medications	Antipsychotics
	Buspirone
	Monoamine oxidase inhibitors
	Serotonin norepinephrine reuptake inhibitors (SNRIs)
	Tricyclic antidepressants[a]
Stimulants	Amphetamines
	Methylphenidate
	Cocaine
	Caffeine
Other agents	Levodopa
	Decongestants (pseudoephedrine)
	Reserpine
Withdrawal	Clonidine
	Ethanol
	Illicit drugs

[a]Most likely to cause false-positive results.

next step is iodine 123 (^{123}I)-metaiodobenzylguanidine scanning. This test may also be indicated in patients with very large pheochromocytomas (>10 cm) to detect metastatic disease or paragangliomas to detect multiple tumors. Fludeoxyglucose-position emission tomography is more sensitive for detection of metastatic disease, but its use is generally reserved for those patients with established malignant tumors.

The definitive treatment for pheochromocytoma/paraganglioma is surgical resection. Preoperative β-receptor blockade with phenoxybenzamine for 10 to 14 days before surgery is essential to prevent hypertensive crises during surgery. The dose is progressively increased to achieve a blood pressure of 130/80 mm Hg or less and pulse of 60 to 70/min seated, and systolic pressure of 90 mm Hg or higher with pulse of 70 to 80/min standing. Side effects include dizziness, nasal congestion, and fatigue. To facilitate dose escalation and mitigate the volume contraction effects of α-receptor blockade, patients are instructed to liberalize their salt and fluid intake. A β-blocker is added once α-blockade is achieved to manage reflex tachycardia, but it should never be started prior to adequate α-blockade because unopposed α-adrenergic vasoconstriction can result in a hypertensive crisis.

For large pheochromocytomas with a high hormone secretion rate, other agents such as a calcium channel blocker and/or metyrosine are added to the treatment regimen. Calcium channel blockers can also be used in patients who develop significant hypotension on small doses of α-blocker. Selective α-1 receptor blockers such as doxazosin can be used as an alternative to phenoxybenzamine if availability or lack of insurance coverage of the latter is a problem. Postoperatively, patients can have significant hypotension, and most require fluid and vasopressor support at least briefly in the

TABLE 28. Typical Imaging Characteristics of Adrenal Masses

Adrenal Mass	Overall	CT	MRI Signal Intensity[a]
Adrenal adenoma	Diameter <4 cm Homogeneous enhancement[b] Round, clear margins	Density <10 HU Contrast washout >50% (10 min)	Isointense on T2-weighted images
Adrenocortical carcinoma	Usually >4 cm Heterogeneous enhancement[b] Irregular margins Calcifications, necrosis	Density >10 HU Contrast washout <50% (10 min)	Hyperintense on T2-weighted images
Pheochromocytoma	Variable size Heterogeneous enhancement[b], cystic areas Round, clear margins Can be bilateral	Density >10 HU Contrast washout <50% (10 min)	Hyperintense on T2-weighted images
Metastases	Variable margins Can be bilateral	Density >10 HU Contrast washout <50% (10 min)	Hyperintense on T2-weighted images

HU = Hounsfield units (measure of radiodensity compared with water).

[a]Signal intensity as compared with liver.

[b]Enhancement following intravenous contrast administration.

CONT.

postoperative period. Patients with pheochromocytoma may have impaired fasting glucose or type 2 diabetes related to insulin resistance induced by catecholamine excess. This can improve or reverse following adrenalectomy. H

Approximately 83% of pheochromocytomas/paragangliomas are benign. Pathologic findings do not predict which tumors will become malignant and develop metastases. Since metastases can occur decades after the initial diagnosis, patients should undergo long-term annual biochemical screening, typically with plasma-free metanephrine.

KEY POINTS

- Initial tests for pheochromocytoma include measurement of plasma free metanephrine levels or 24-hour urine fractionated metanephrine and catecholamine levels; certain medications can affect results and need to be discontinued at least 2 weeks prior to testing.

- The search for a tumor should begin when a biochemical diagnosis of pheochromocytoma/paraganglioma is clear in laboratory results, to avoid misdiagnosing an incidental nonfunctioning adrenal mass as a pheochromocytoma.

- The definitive treatment for pheochromocytoma/paraganglioma is surgical resection; preoperative α-blockade with phenoxybenzamine is essential to prevent hypertensive crises during surgery.

HVC
- Selective α-1 receptor blockers such as doxazosin can be used as an alternative to phenoxybenzamine if availability or lack of insurance coverage of the latter is a problem.

Androgen-Producing Adrenal Tumors

Androgen-producing adrenal tumors are rare and lead to menstrual irregularities and virilization in women including hirsutism, voice-deepening, increased muscle mass, increased libido, and clitoromegaly. Tumors secrete DHEA/DHEAS and androstenedione, which are subsequently converted to testosterone in the periphery. DHEAS-secreting tumors of the adrenal gland are readily visible on CT imaging, and adrenal vein sampling to localize the tumor is rarely required. Approximately 50% are benign, and the treatment of choice is resection.

Adrenal Hormone Deficiency

Primary Adrenal Insufficiency

Causes and Clinical Features

Primary adrenal insufficiency (AI) is a life-threatening disorder that often presents with insidious onset of symptoms making diagnosis a challenge (**Table 29**). It may also present as adrenal crisis, often precipitated by an acute illness or the initiation of thyroid hormone replacement in a patient with unrecognized chronic AI. Although skin hyperpigmentation from stimulation of melanocytes by high ACTH levels is considered a hallmark of primary adrenal insufficiency, it is not present in approximately 5% patients. The most common cause of primary adrenal insufficiency is autoimmune destruction of all layers of the adrenal cortex leading to progressive mineralocorticoid, glucocorticoid, and adrenal androgen deficiency. Most patients have positive 21-hydroxylase antibodies, and approximately 50% will develop another autoimmune

TABLE 29.	Clinical and Laboratory Manifestations of Primary Adrenal Failure		
Hormone Deficiency	**Symptoms**	**Signs**	**Laboratory Findings**
Cortisol	Fatigue	Hyperpigmentation[b] (palmar creases, extensor surfaces, buccal mucosa)	↓ Serum cortisol
	Weakness		↑ Plasma ACTH
	Low-grade fever	Decrease in BP	↓ Serum sodium[c]
	Weight loss		↓ Plasma glucose[d]
	Anorexia		
	Nausea/vomiting		
	Abdominal pain		
	Arthralgia		
	Myalgia		
Aldosterone	Salt craving	Orthostasis	↑ PRA
	Dizziness	Hypotension	↓ Serum sodium
			↑ Serum potassium
DHEAS	Reduced libido[a]	Decreased axillary or pubic hair[a]	↓ Serum DHEAS

ACTH = adrenocorticotropic hormone; BP = blood pressure; DHEAS = dehydroepiandrosterone sulfate; PRA = plasma renin activity.

[a]Women only.

[b]Occurs exclusively in primary adrenal failure.

[c]Cortisol inhibits the secretion of antidiuretic hormone (ADH), so hypocortisolemia will lead to increased secretion of ADH and hyponatremia.

[d]Rare in adults.

endocrine disorder in their lifetime (primary hypothyroidism, primary ovarian insufficiency, celiac disease, hypoparathyroidism, or type 1 diabetes mellitus).

Primary adrenal insufficiency can also be caused by infiltrative disorders such as infection (tuberculosis, fungal infections), sarcoidosis, and lymphoma, which result in bilateral adrenal gland enlargement. Metastatic disease involving the adrenals, most commonly from lung cancer, renal cell carcinoma, and melanoma rarely leads to adrenal insufficiency even if both adrenal glands are involved.

Bilateral adrenal hemorrhage can present as acute adrenal insufficiency and should be considered if unexpected hypotension develops. Risk factors for bilateral adrenal hemorrhage include protein C deficiency, anticoagulation, disseminated intravascular coagulopathy, and sepsis.

Diagnosis

An algorithm for the diagnosis of adrenal insufficiency is outlined in **Figure 5**. Initial evaluation includes the measurement of morning serum total cortisol and ACTH levels. Primary adrenal insufficiency is confirmed by the combination of low serum cortisol and elevated serum ACTH levels. Important considerations in the interpretation of the results are shown in Figure 5 and often require referral to an endocrinologist. Additional evaluation may include measurement of 21-hydroxylase antibodies; positive 21-hydroxylase antibodies are found in approximately 90% of autoimmune adrenalitis cases. If negative, CT scan of the adrenal glands should be obtained.

Treatment

Both glucocorticoid and mineralocorticoid therapy is required for treatment of primary AI. The preferred glucocorticoid is hydrocortisone taken 2 or 3 times daily. Adherence to multiple daily doses can be challenging so prednisone can be used as an alternative (**Table 30**). The principle of replacement is to administer a higher dose in the morning and to avoid replacement in the evening. Despite this attempt to mimic diurnal variation, patients with primary AI report a decrease in health-related quality of life. It is imperative to avoid overreplacement with glucocorticoid, to avoid iatrogenic Cushing syndrome with its risk of obesity, type 2 diabetes mellitus, hypertension, hyperlipidemia, bone loss, and cardiovascular disease. Some patients "feel better" at higher than physiologic replacement doses, but the risks outweigh the benefits of supraphysiologic doses. Mineralocorticoid replacement is achieved with daily fludrocortisone. DHEAS replacement is controversial in women due to lack of robust data for benefit and concerns regarding the safety and quality of U.S. preparations, which are supplements and not regulated as drugs.

Patients cannot mount an appropriate increase in cortisol with illness, and therefore, instruction in "sick day" rules is essential to prevent adrenal crisis (**Table 31**). For minor physiologic stress states such as respiratory infection, fever, or minor surgery under local anesthesia, patients should double or triple their baseline glucocorticoid dose for 2 to 3 days. Higher doses of glucocorticoid are required during moderate or major physiologic stress. Patients who present with adrenal

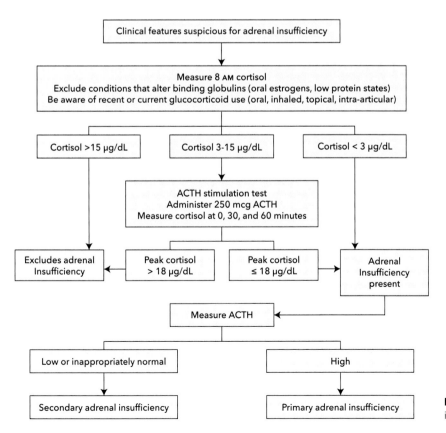

FIGURE 5. Algorithm for the diagnosis of adrenal insufficiency. ACTH = adrenocorticotropic hormone.

TABLE 30. Dose Equivalence and Relative Potencies of Common Synthetic Oral Glucocorticoids

Synthetic Glucocorticoid	Equivalent Dose (mg)	Biologic Half-Life (hours)	Relative Anti-Inflammatory Potency[a]	Relative Mineralocorticoid Potency[b]
Hydrocortisone	20	8-12	1	1/125
Prednisolone/ prednisone	5	18-36	4	1/150
Methylprednisolone	4	18-36	5	0
Dexamethasone	0.75	36-54	25-50	0

[a]Anti-inflammatory potency relative to hydrocortisone.

[b]Mineralocorticoid potency relative to fludrocortisone.

TABLE 31. Chronic Medical Treatment of Primary Adrenal Failure

Medication	Basal Dose	Considerations
Glucocorticoid[a]		*"Sick day rules"*:
Hydrocortisone	Usually 15-25 mg/d, divided into 2-3 doses over the day	Patient follows at home.
Prednisone	Prednisone 5 mg once daily *How to dose:* Titrate to clinical response with goal of no signs or symptoms of cortisol deficiency or excess (increase dose if symptoms of cortisol deficiency remain; decrease if CS signs and symptoms are present)	*For minor physiologic stress (upper respiratory infection, fever, minor surgery under local anesthesia):* 2-3 times basal dose for 2-3 days *Stress dosing*: Health care providers follow while patient is in the hospital. *For moderate physiologic stress (minor or moderate surgery with general anesthesia):* Hydrocortisone 25-75 mg/d orally or IV for 1-2 days *For major physiologic stress (major surgery, trauma, critical illness, or childbirth):* Hydrocortisone 100 mg IV followed by 50 mg every 6 h IV; rapid tapering and switch to oral regimen depending on clinical state
Mineralocorticoid		
Fludrocortisone	0.05-0.2 mg once daily in the morning *How to dose:* Titrate to: 1. Normal BP 2. Normal serum Na, K	Fludrocortisone is not required if hydrocortisone dose is >40 mg/d.
Adrenal androgen		
DHEA	25-50 mg once daily	Consider DHEA for women with impaired mood or sense of well-being when glucocorticoid replacement has been optimized.

BP = blood pressure; CS = Cushing syndrome; DHEA = dehydroepiandrosterone; IV = intravenous; Na = sodium; K = potassium.

[a]Shorter-acting glucocorticoids are preferred over longer-acting agents due to lower risk of glucocorticoid excess. Longer-acting preparations have the advantage of once-daily dosing.

crisis should receive fluid resuscitation and an initial immediate dose of intravenous hydrocortisone (100 mg), followed by intravenous hydrocortisone (100 mg) every 8 hours for the next 24 hours, with subsequent dosing governed by clinical status. Patients with concomitant untreated adrenal insufficiency and hypothyroidism should always receive glucocorticoid replacement therapy first to prevent precipitation of adrenal crisis by thyroid hormone replacement. Patients should also be counselled to wear a medic-alert identification at all times. No increase in mineralocorticoid dose is necessary with illness. **H**

The term "adrenal fatigue" is used by some alternative medicine providers to represent a constellation of symptoms purported to occur in patients who experience chronic emotional or physical stress that are claimed to be caused by simultaneous hyper- and hypocortisolism. There is no scientific evidence to support such a condition. Patients may undergo salivary cortisol testing, but interpretation of the results is often unreliable. Some patients labeled with "adrenal fatigue" are given hydrocortisone therapy or animal-derived adrenal gland extract that may contain active glucocorticoid, leading to exogenous suppression of ACTH production and iatrogenic Cushing syndrome. Sudden discontinuation of these products can lead to acute adrenal insufficiency. Patients with "adrenal fatigue" should be carefully tapered off any glucocorticoid therapy and other potential causes for their symptoms explored.

KEY POINTS

- The most common cause of primary adrenal insufficiency is autoimmune destruction of all layers of the adrenal cortex leading to progressive mineralocorticoid, glucocorticoid, and adrenal androgen deficiency.

- Both glucocorticoid and mineralocorticoid therapy is required for treatment of primary adrenal insufficiency.

- Patients cannot mount an appropriate increase in cortisol with illness, and therefore, instruction in "sick day" rules regarding glucocorticoid dosing is essential to prevent adrenal crisis.

Adrenal Function During Critical Illness

During times of physiologic stress, the hypothalamic-pituitary-adrenal axis is stimulated to produce increased levels of cortisol. In some patients, the increase in cortisol secretion is thought to be suboptimal and termed "relative AI." There is debate, however, as to whether the entity of relative adrenal insufficiency is a true disease. Cortisol-binding globulin and albumin decrease in critical illness, lowering the measured total cortisol. There is no agreement on a set of diagnostic criteria for relative AI despite the ability to measure free cortisol, calculated free cortisol, and basal and ACTH-stimulated total cortisol level in critically ill patients. Studies to date do not show improved survival in patients with relative AI treated with high-dose glucocorticoid therapy. Reversal of shock, however, may be improved, and hence it is currently recommended that stress-dose hydrocortisone be administered to patients with shock that is resistant to standard fluid and vasopressor therapy. **H**

Adrenal Mass

Incidentally Noted Adrenal Masses

An adrenal incidentaloma is defined as an adrenal mass greater than 1 cm in diameter that is detected on imaging performed for purposes other than suspicion of adrenal disease. The prevalence of adrenal incidentaloma increases with age and is estimated to be approximately 10% in those 70 years of age or older. Most lesions are benign, nonfunctioning adenomas, and approximately 10% to 15% secrete excess hormones. Other causes include metastases (probability increases if known

primary malignancy), myelolipoma, cysts, and adrenocortical carcinoma.

The finding of an incidental adrenal mass prompts two main questions: (1) Is it secreting excess hormone (aldosterone, cortisol, or catecholamines)? and (2) Is it benign or malignant? Patients with hypertension or with hypokalemia require testing for primary aldosteronism. Biochemical testing for pheochromocytoma, such as a 24-hour urine total metanephrine measurement, should be undertaken in all patients, even in the absence of typical symptoms or hypertension.

All patients should also be evaluated for subclinical Cushing syndrome, a condition characterized by ACTH-independent cortisol secretion that may result in metabolic (hyperglycemia and hypertension) and bone (osteoporosis) effects of hypercortisolism, but not the more specific clinical features of Cushing syndrome, such as supraclavicular fat pads, wide violaceous striae, facial plethora, and proximal muscle weakness. Initial testing for subclinical Cushing syndrome is achieved with a 1-mg overnight dexamethasone suppression test, with a cortisol level greater than 5 µg/dL (138 nmol/L) considered a positive test. Following a positive result, further tests are required to confirm cortisol autonomy and may include measurement of ACTH (suppressed), DHEAS (low), 24-hour urine free cortisol, and an 8-mg overnight dexamethasone suppression test; referral to an endocrinologist is recommended at this point. The decision whether to proceed to adrenalectomy should take into account the risks versus benefits of surgery. Studies to date have not been robust enough to show clear postoperative improvement in clinically important outcomes but suggest improved glucose, lipid, blood pressure, and bone density measurements.

Imaging findings can help differentiate between a benign and a malignant adrenal mass (see Table 28). Most adrenocortical carcinomas measure more than 4 cm at the time of discovery. Approximately 75% of benign adrenal masses, however, are also in this size range. Approximately 66% of benign adenomas are lipid-rich and exhibit low attenuation (<10 HU) on CT imaging. Benign adrenal adenomas also exhibit rapid washout (>50%) of contrast material compared to non-benign lesions. Adrenal biopsy has a limited role in evaluation of incidentalomas and is reserved for lesions suspicious for metastases or an infiltrative process such as lymphoma or infection. Pheochromocytomas should be ruled out prior to biopsy to avoid the possibility of a hypertensive crisis. Biopsy should not be performed when there is suspicion for primary adrenocortical carcinoma because, without review of the whole specimen, pathology cannot reliably distinguish this from a benign cortical adenoma, and tumor seeding is possible. If the former is suspected, the diagnosis should be established by adrenalectomy.

An algorithm for management of adrenal incidentaloma, including monitoring of lesions that do not require adrenalectomy, is shown in **Figure 6**.

- All patients with adrenal incidentaloma should be evaluated for pheochromocytoma; those with hypertension or hypokalemia should also be evaluated for primary aldosteronism, and all patients should be evaluated for subclinical Cushing syndrome.
- Imaging findings can help differentiate between a benign and malignant adrenal mass.

Adrenocortical Carcinoma

Adrenocortical carcinoma (ACC) is a rare, aggressive tumor that often secretes excess cortisol and/or androgens. Patients may present with rapid onset of Cushing syndrome, with or without virilization and/or symptoms from mass effect, such as increased abdominal girth and lower extremity edema. Fifty percent of ACCs secrete cortisol; 20% secrete multiple hormones, including cortisol and aldosterone precursors; and less than 10% secrete aldosterone. Some ACCs are discovered as an incidental adrenal mass that is either indeterminate or suspicious for ACC (see Table 28). Lesions are often large (>4 cm), and disease is at an advanced stage at the time of diagnosis. For localized disease, first-line therapy includes open resection. Debulking surgery, radiation therapy, and/or chemotherapy may also be options for palliation in advanced ACC.

Mitotane is an adrenolytic agent commonly used as adjuvant therapy that has been shown to be associated with longer recurrence-free survival. Mitotane causes primary AI, and daily glucocorticoid replacement therapy is required, often in supraphysiologic doses, due to mitotane-induced accelerated metabolism of glucocorticoids. Some patients also develop aldosterone deficiency manifested by hyponatremia, hyperkalemia, elevated renin levels, and postural hypotension, requiring fludrocortisone replacement. Five-year survival rates range from 62% to 82% for those with disease confined to the adrenal gland and 13% for tumors associated with distant metastases.

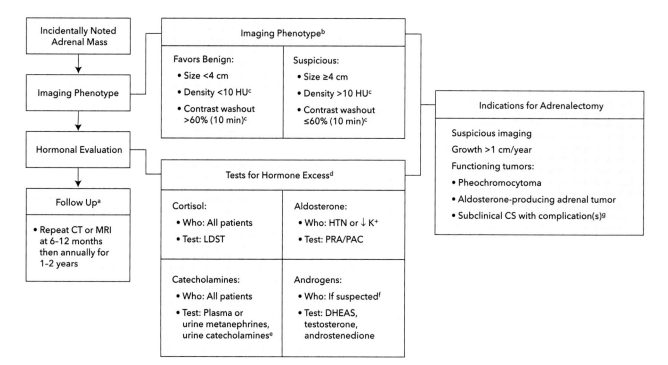

FIGURE 6. Algorithm for the initial diagnostic evaluation and follow up of an incidentally noted adrenal mass. CS = Cushing syndrome; DHEAS = dehydroepiandrosterone sulfate; HTN = hypertension; HU = Hounsfield units; K = potassium; LDST = low-dose (1-mg) dexamethasone suppression test; PAC = plasma aldosterone concentration; PRA = plasma renin activity.

[a]Repeat imaging is indicated for adrenal masses not meeting criteria for surgery at initial diagnosis.

[b]Refer to Table 28 for more CT and MRI findings. If imaging is suspicious in a patient with known malignancy, biopsy should be considered to confirm adrenal metastasis after screening for pheochromocytoma is completed.

[c]CT scan findings.

[d]Positive screening tests usually require further biochemical evaluation to confirm the diagnosis (see text).

[e]Measure plasma metanephrines if radiographic appearance is typical for a pheochromocytoma; otherwise measure 24-hour urine metanephrines and catecholamines.

[f]Hormonal evaluation for an androgen-producing adrenal tumor is indicated only if clinically suspected based on the presence of hirsutism, virilization, or menstrual irregularities in women.

[g]Adrenalectomy is considered for confirmed cases of subclinical CS associated with recent onset of diabetes, hypertension, obesity, or low bone mass.

KEY POINTS

- Adrenocortical carcinoma is a rare, aggressive tumor that often secretes excess cortisol and/or androgens and hormonal precursors causing hypertension and Cushing syndrome; patients may present with rapid onset of Cushing syndrome with or without virilization and/or symptoms from mass effect, such as increased abdominal girth and lower extremity edema.

- For localized disease, first-line therapy includes open resection; debulking surgery, radiation therapy, and/or chemotherapy may also be options for palliation in advanced adrenocortical carcinoma.

- Mitotane is an adrenolytic agent, commonly used as adjuvant therapy, that has been associated with longer recurrence-free survival.

Disorders of the Thyroid Gland

Thyroid Anatomy and Physiology

The thyroid gland is the largest dedicated endocrine organ. The usual anatomic location of the isthmus is just anterior to the second to fourth tracheal rings. The parathyroid glands are often located posterior to the superior and middle portions of each thyroid lobe. The recurrent laryngeal nerves, which innervate most of the intrinsic muscles of the larynx, course behind the thyroid gland. Thyroid pathology may cause compressive symptoms including shortness of breath, cough, dysphagia, and voice changes due to the close proximity of the thyroid to the trachea, esophagus, and recurrent laryngeal nerves.

The thyroid gland contains thyroid follicular cells and parafollicular cells (c-cells). Calcitonin is produced by the parafollicular cells and inhibits bone resorption; however, it plays a minor role in bone physiology. Follicular cells produce the thyroid hormones, thyroxine (T_4) and triiodothyronine (T_3). The synthesis and secretion of thyroid hormones is tightly regulated by the hypothalamic-pituitary-thyroid axis. Thyrotropin-releasing hormone (TRH) from the hypothalamus triggers the pulsatile release of thyroid-stimulating hormone (TSH) from thyrotrope cells in the anterior pituitary gland. TSH, through activation of the TSH-receptor, stimulates thyroid cell growth, iodide metabolism, and thyroid hormone synthesis and secretion. T_4 and T_3 exert negative feedback on the hypothalamus and pituitary gland to moderate further hormone synthesis.

Iodine is an essential dietary micronutrient and a key structural component of T_4 and T_3.

The thyroid gland is the exclusive source of T_4, whereas approximately 80% of T_3 is the result of removing one iodine molecule from T_4, through deiodinase activity in peripheral tissues. This occurs primarily in the liver and kidney. Most of T_4 (99.96%) and T_3 (99.6%) are bound to proteins in serum. Approximately 70% of T_4 and T_3 are bound to thyroxine-binding globulin. Albumin, transthyretin, and lipoproteins carry a smaller proportion. Only the tiny amount of free T_4 and T_3 is biologically active. While T_4 largely serves as a pro-hormone, T_3 binds with high affinity to thyroid hormone nuclear receptors affecting gene transcription in target tissues and mediating its physiologic effects. It has positive inotropic and chronotropic effects in the heart and enhances myocardial adrenergic sensitivity. It also increases the rate of myocardial diastolic relaxation, augments intravascular volume, and lowers peripheral vascular resistance. It increases gastrointestinal motility, bone turnover, and regulates heat generation and energy expenditure.

Thyroid Examination

The thyroid gland is located in the neck midway between the sternal notch and thyroid cartilage. It attaches to the trachea posteriorly and elevates with swallowing. Examination involves both visualization and palpation while the patient swallows liquid. It can be palpated with the examiner behind the patient with circumferential hand positioning to allow focus on palpation or with the examiner facing the patient, which allows the examiner to see the thyroid during palpation. The anterior approach is preferred with necks of larger diameter.

Structural Disorders of the Thyroid Gland

Thyroid Nodules

Thyroid nodules are discrete structural lesions, distinct from the background gland parenchyma on ultrasound. They are most commonly detected as incidental findings on imaging studies performed for other reasons. The prevalence of nodules palpated on examination is 5% in women and 1% in men. They are detected on ultrasound in 40% of the U.S. population and are more common with increasing age. Thyroid nodules can result from multiple pathologic processes, ranging from benign cysts and inflammatory nodules, to malignancies including primary thyroid, lymphoma, or metastatic lesions. Non-thyroidal lesions, such as parathyroid adenomas, can also present as nodules. Primary thyroid neoplasms are clonal in origin and include follicular adenomas and thyroid cancer.

The initial evaluation of a thyroid nodule begins with measuring serum TSH (**Figure 7**). TSH suppression may indicate the presence of autonomously functioning or "hot" nodules, which account for 5% to 10% of palpable thyroid nodules. Autonomous nodules may cause hyperthyroidism and are associated with a very low risk of malignancy. They do not require fine-needle aspiration biopsy (FNAB). Patients with thyroid nodules and a suppressed TSH are evaluated with thyroid scintigraphy. A radioactive isotope, preferably iodine

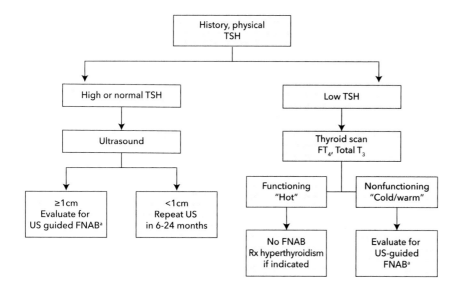

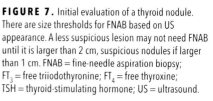

FIGURE 7. Initial evaluation of a thyroid nodule. There are size thresholds for FNAB based on US appearance. A less suspicious lesion may not need FNAB until it is larger than 2 cm, suspicious nodules if larger than 1 cm. FNAB = fine-needle aspiration biopsy; FT_3 = free triiodothyronine; FT_4 = free thyroxine; TSH = thyroid-stimulating hormone; US = ultrasound.

[a]Need for US-guided FNAB depends on clinical risk factors for thyroid cancer, nodule size, and US appearance.

123 (^{123}I), is administered, the percentage taken up by the thyroid is calculated (radioactive iodine uptake [RAIU]), and an image is obtained (thyroid scan). Hot nodules concentrate radioactive iodine to a greater extent than normal thyroid tissue.

Thyroid/neck ultrasound is performed in patients with a normal or elevated TSH to confirm the presence of thyroid nodules. The management of nonfunctioning thyroid nodules is determined by the ultrasound results and presence of symptoms. The 2015 American Thyroid Association guidelines classify thyroid nodules into five sonographic patterns based on echogenicity, whether they are solid, cystic, or both, and features of malignancy (**Table 32**). Hyperechoic nodules are brighter, isoechoic nodules are equally bright, and hypoechoic nodules are darker than the background parenchyma. Ultrasound can determine the size of the nodule. FNAB is not recommended for subcentimeter nodules unless associated with symptoms, pathologic lymphadenopathy, or extrathyroidal extension.

Thyroid nodule FNAB should be performed under ultrasound guidance when possible because of improved accuracy compared with palpation biopsy. Thyroid cytopathology is usually interpreted and classified according to criteria developed at the National Cancer Institute Thyroid Fine Needle Aspiration State of the Science Conference (Bethesda Conference). The Bethesda classification system is summarized in **Table 33**. Thyroid FNAB cytology can be nondiagnostic in up to 5% to 10% of specimens. Approximately 60% to 70% of biopsied nodules have benign cytology, 20% are indeterminate, and 5% to 10% have evidence of malignancy.

The management of cytologically indeterminate thyroid nodules (Bethesda III-V) can be challenging, and referral to an endocrinologist is recommended. Clinical monitoring is indicated for all thyroid nodules and should include measurement of serum TSH, as structurally abnormal thyroid glands are at increased risk for thyroid dysfunction (see Disorders of Thyroid Function). American Thyroid Association sonographic

pattern and clinical context guide the timing of initial ultrasound follow up for benign nodules and those not evaluated with FNAB. Repeat ultrasound should be performed in 6 to 12 months for all high suspicion nodules, 12 to 24 months for intermediate and low suspicion nodules, and 24 months or longer for very low suspicion nodules. Repeat FNAB is indicated for all high suspicion nodules, nodules with concerning new sonographic findings, and intermediate or low suspicion nodules that increase significantly in size, which is defined as a 20% increase in at least two dimensions or an increase in nodule volume of more than 50%. Repeat FNAB is not recommended for nodules that have had two negative biopsies.

KEY POINTS

- The initial evaluation of a thyroid nodule begins with measuring serum thyroid-stimulating hormone.

- Patients with a suppressed thyroid-stimulating hormone level are evaluated with thyroid scintigraphy; those patients with normal or elevated thyroid-stimulating hormone are evaluated with ultrasonography.

- Patients with nodules 1 cm or larger should be evaluated with fine-needle aspiration biopsy.

- Fine-needle aspiration biopsy is not recommended for subcentimeter nodules unless associated with symptoms, pathologic lymphadenopathy, or extrathyroidal extension. **HVC**

Goiters

The term "goiter" denotes an enlarged thyroid gland. Goiters can be seen in the setting of normal thyroid function, hypothyroidism, or hyperthyroidism. The most common cause worldwide is endemic goiter due to severe iodine deficiency. Patients presenting with goiter should be questioned about iodine intake, rate of change in size, and risk factors for thyroid cancer (see Thyroid Cancer). Clinical history should focus on

TABLE 32. Summary of 2015 American Thyroid Association Guidelines: Sonographic Patterns and Recommendations for Fine-Needle Aspiration Biopsy

Sonographic Pattern	Representative Image	Description	Estimated Risk of Malignancy	Size Threshold for Fine-Needle Aspiration Biopsy
Benign		Pure cyst (anechoic with no internal blood flow)	<1%	Fine-needle aspiration biopsy not recommended
Very low suspicion		Some mixed cystic and solid nodules (spongiform nodules)[a]	<3%	2 cm[c]
Low suspicion		Isoechoic/hyperechoic solid nodules; some mixed cystic and solid nodules	5%-10%	1.5 cm
Intermediate suspicion		Hypoechoic solid nodules	10%-20%	1 cm
High suspicion		Hypoechoic solid nodules with one or more suspicious feature[b]	>70%-90%	1 cm

[a]Microcystic spaces occupying more than 50% of the nodule volume is highly correlated with benign cytology.

[b]Microcalcifications, shape taller than wide in the transverse plane, irregular margins, extrathyroidal extension or pathologic lymph nodes (image shows hypoechoic solid nodule with irregular margins).

[c]Clinical observation is an acceptable alternative.

Reprinted and adapted from: Haugen Bryan R., Alexander Erik K., Bible Keith C., Doherty Gerard M., Mandel Susan J., Nikiforov Yuri E., Pacini Furio, Randolph Gregory W., Sawka Anna M., Schlumberger Martin, Schuff Kathryn G., Sherman Steven I., Sosa Julie Ann, Steward David L., Tuttle R. Michael, and Wartofsky Leonard. Thyroid. Jan 2016. ahead of print http://doi.org/10.1089/thy.2015.0020 Published in Volume: 26 Issue 1: January 12, 2016; Online Ahead of Editing: October 14, 2015.

symptoms suggestive of thyroid hormone excess or deficiency and compression. Compressive symptoms include shortness of breath, cough, dysphagia, and voice changes and are evident in 10% to 20% of patients with goiter, most of whom also have clinically apparent thyromegaly. On examination tracheal deviation should be assessed and the size, symmetry, and consistency of the thyroid and presence of nodules should be noted. Possible venous obstruction should be assessed by having the patient raise the arms above the head. The findings of jugular venous distension, facial plethora, and flushing indicate possible thoracic outlet obstruction with reduced venous return (Pemberton sign) (**Figure 8**). Serum TSH level should be assessed in patients with goiter. If low, free T_4 and total T_3 should be measured and thyroid scintigraphy performed. If normal or elevated, thyroid/neck ultrasound is indicated in patients with risk factors for thyroid cancer, palpable thyroid nodules, gland asymmetry, large goiters, rapid growth pattern, or compressive symptoms. Patients with signs or symptoms of compression require additional testing as outlined below, and surgery may be needed for symptomatic

TABLE 33. Diagnoses Obtained by Fine-Needle Aspiration Biopsy of Thyroid Nodules and Risk for Malignancy

Fine-Needle Aspiration Biopsy Diagnosis	Risk for Malignancy[a]	Management
Benign	0%-3%	Repeat ultrasound in 6-24 months[b]
Atypia of uncertain significance/follicular lesion of uncertain significance	10%-30%	Repeat FNAB in 3 months[c]
Suspicious for follicular neoplasm	25%-40%	Lobectomy[b]
Suspicious for malignancy	50%-70%	Lobectomy or total thyroidectomy
Malignant	97%-99%	Lobectomy or total thyroidectomy
Nondiagnostic	5%-10%	Repeat FNAB If two nondiagnostic FNABs, surgery

FNAB = fine-needle aspiration biopsy.

[a]Risk for malignancy by cytology diagnosis includes noninvasive follicular thyroid neoplasm with papillary-like nuclear features (NIFTP), a "pre-cancerous" lesion. If counted as benign, the risk of malignancy is reduced for all Bethesda categories except nondiagnostic and benign readings. Data from Cibas ES, Ali SZ. The 2017 Bethesda System for reporting thyroid cytopathology. Thyroid. 2017 Nov;27(11):1341-1346. doi: 10.1089/thy.2017.0500. PubMed PMID: 29091573.

[b]If American Thyroid Association "high suspicion" pattern, repeat ultrasound and FNAB in 6 to 12 months.

[c]Supplementary management strategies include molecular genetic testing of the nodule and selective use of thyroid scintigraphy (when serum thyroid-stimulation hormone level is low-normal).

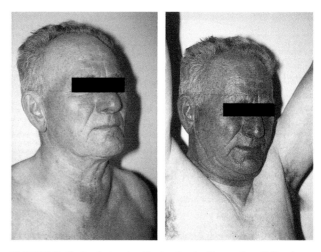

FIGURE 8. The Pemberton sign. Head and neck with arms down (*left*) and arms elevated (*right*).

management. Treatment of hypothyroid and hyperthyroid conditions in the setting of goiter is discussed below.

KEY POINTS

- The most common worldwide cause of goiter is severe iodine deficiency.

- Patients with goiter should be questioned about iodine intake, rate of change in size, assessed for signs and symptoms of compression, and evaluated for clinical manifestations of thyroid hormone excess or deficiency.

- Serum thyroid-stimulating hormone should be assessed in patients with goiter; if low, free thyroxine (T_4) and total triiodothyronine (T_3) should be measured and thyroid scintigraphy performed; if T_4 and T_3 are normal or elevated, a thyroid/neck ultrasound is indicated in the presence of risk factors for thyroid cancer, palpable thyroid nodules, gland asymmetry, large goiters, rapid growth pattern, or compressive symptoms.

Multinodular Goiter

Multinodular goiter is the most common cause of goiter in older adults in the United States. Evaluation includes measurement of serum TSH and, when TSH is not suppressed, thyroid/

neck ultrasound should be performed and discrete nodules evaluated as discussed previously (see Thyroid Nodules). The frequency of thyroid malignancy in patients with multinodular goiter is similar to those with solitary thyroid nodules. Signs and symptoms of compression or suspected substernal extension require additional testing. CT or MRI of the neck and chest (when substernal goiter is suspected) can define anatomic relationships and assess for tracheal narrowing. The administration of iodinated contrast should be avoided when possible to avoid precipitating iodine-induced hyperthyroidism (Jod-Basedow phenomenon). A flow-volume loop study is indicated in patients with symptoms of airway compression or when the tracheal lumen measures less than 1 cm in diameter on CT or MR (see MKSAP 18 Pulmonary and Critical Care Medicine). Endoscopy or a swallowing study can assess for extrinsic compression of the esophagus in patients with cervical dysphagia. Consultation with an otolaryngologist is indicated to confirm clinically suspected vocal cord paralysis. Surgery is indicated for significant compression or suspected malignancy.

Diffuse Goiter

The most common cause of diffuse goiter is autoimmune thyroid disease associated with thyroid dysfunction (Hashimoto thyroiditis and Graves disease). Infiltrative disorders, such as Riedel (IgG4-related) thyroiditis, are rare causes of diffuse goiter. Diffuse goiter may also occur in euthyroid patients in the absence of predisposing inflammatory or neoplastic processes. Genetic predisposition, iodine insufficiency, and cigarette smoking are contributing factors. Thyroid/neck ultrasound is indicated in euthyroid patients with diffuse goiter. It is recommended for patients with Graves disease or Hashimoto thyroiditis when there is thyroid gland asymmetry or nodules on examination. As discussed previously, additional testing is indicated if compressive signs or symptoms are present. Thyroid surgery is considered in the setting of significant compression.

Thyroid Cancer

Thyroid cancer is diagnosed in 13.9 per 100,000 people per year in the United States. The incidence of thyroid cancer has increased over the last four decades and now is the fifth most common cancer in women. Much of this change is attributable to a rise in the diagnosis of small noninvasive cancers, initially detected incidentally on imaging done for other reasons (carotid Doppler studies, neck/chest CT, PET scan). Mortality rates have remained stable with an overall 5-year survival rate of 98.1%. Papillary thyroid carcinoma and follicular thyroid carcinoma, collectively known as differentiated thyroid cancer, account for the most thyroid cancer diagnoses in the United States. Papillary thyroid carcinoma commonly spreads to cervical lymph nodes but is associated with a low risk of distant metastases; whereas lymph node metastases are rare in follicular thyroid carcinoma, metastases to lung, bone, and other sites can be seen. The types and frequency of thyroid cancer are shown in **Figure 9**.

Thyroid cancer is often identified incidentally; however, it may be detected on neck examination. Risk factors for thyroid cancer include a personal history of ionizing radiation exposure with a higher prevalence of papillary thyroid carcinoma in persons exposed to ionizing radiation (>10 rads), with the highest risk seen following childhood exposures, such as with nuclear accidents (Chernobyl), and a personal or family history of thyroid malignancy. Additional risk factors for thyroid cancer include extremes of age (younger than 30 or older than 60) and male gender. Findings suggestive of malignancy include rapid nodule growth, a hard fixed nodule, dysphagia, vocal cord paralysis (hoarseness), and cervical lymphadenopathy. The diagnosis is confirmed by fine-needle aspiration biopsy.

Surgery is the mainstay of thyroid cancer treatment. Either total thyroidectomy or hemithyroidectomy is acceptable for unilateral differentiated thyroid cancers measuring 1 to 4 cm, as long as locoregional spread is not suspected. Total thyroidectomy is otherwise indicated. Unique risks of

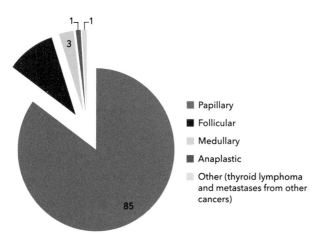

FIGURE 9. Relative frequency of the types of thyroid cancer.

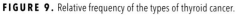

Data from Hundahl SA, Fleming ID, Fremgen AM, Menck HR. A National Cancer Data Base report on 53,856 cases of thyroid carcinoma treated in the U.S., 1985-1995. Cancer. 1998 Dec 15;83(12):2638-48. [PMID: 9874472]

thyroid surgery include hypocalcemia as a result of removal or devascularization of the parathyroid glands and difficulty breathing or voice changes from recurrent laryngeal nerve injury. Referral to a high-volume thyroid surgeon (>90 cases per year) is preferred due to a lower risk of postoperative complications.

Postoperative radioactive iodine (^{131}I) should be considered for the dual purposes of thyroid remnant ablation and adjuvant therapy for patients with differentiated thyroid cancer and an intermediate to high risk of recurrence, such as with extrathyroidal extension, lymphovascular invasion, poorly differentiated/more aggressive histology, or metastatic disease. TSH stimulation, achieved either by withdrawal of thyroid hormone (levothyroxine) replacement or administration of recombinant human TSH (rhTSH), is required to promote ^{131}I uptake by thyroid follicular cells. Following ^{131}I therapy, patients undergo whole-body scanning to identify areas of ^{131}I uptake corresponding to metastatic disease. Uptake is expected in the postsurgical thyroid bed but not elsewhere. ^{131}I therapy is also used to treat thyroid cancer recurrences not amenable to surgical resection.

After initial cancer treatment, serum thyroglobulin (Tg), a sensitive marker for the detection of persistent or recurrent disease, and thyroglobulin antibody (TgAb) titers are monitored. When TgAb is present, Tg levels are uninterpretable because TgAb can falsely lower Tg measurement. In this case, the TgAb level serves as a surrogate marker. A falling TgAb titer over time correlates with a favorable prognosis, whereas a rising titer is suspicious for persistent or recurrent disease.

Neck ultrasound is regularly performed in routine thyroid cancer surveillance, usually 6 to 12 months after the initial cancer treatment. In patients at high risk of recurrent disease, diagnostic radioactive iodine (^{123}I or ^{131}I) whole-body scanning with TSH-stimulated Tg measurement can be performed. If residual or recurrent thyroid cancer is suspected, such as when serum Tg is persistently elevated or rising over time but not identified by neck ultrasound or radioactive iodine whole-body scanning, adjunctive imaging tests including CT, MRI, bone scan, or PET/CT can be useful in disease localization.

Treatment of intermediate to high-risk differentiated thyroid cancer includes TSH suppression with daily levothyroxine. Thyroid follicular cells are TSH responsive, as are most well-differentiated thyroid cancers. To reduce cancer recurrence, a sufficient dose of levothyroxine is administered to suppress the serum TSH below normal with the specific goal individualized. A serum TSH level less than or equal to 2 but at or above the lower limit of the reference range can be targeted in patients with low risk thyroid cancer. Monitoring and dose adjustment by internists is appropriate in conjunction with the endocrinologist. Metastatic thyroid cancer is managed with active surveillance, additional surgery, or ^{131}I therapy, followed by external beam radiation therapy and/or chemotherapy (tyrosine kinase inhibitors).

Anaplastic thyroid cancer is a rare but aggressive thyroid malignancy that can occur in patients with preexisting differentiated thyroid cancer or de novo. It carries a dismal prognosis with median survival of 5 months. Anaplastic thyroid cancer presents with a rapidly enlarging neck mass and may be unresectable at the time of diagnosis. Treatment is palliative in most cases with surgery, external beam radiation therapy, and chemotherapy.

Medullary thyroid cancer arises from parafollicular cells. Germline *RET* oncogene mutations occur with familial medullary thyroid cancer and multiple endocrine neoplasia (MEN) 2A and 2B. MEN should be ruled out with genetic testing prior to surgery, given its association with pheochromocytoma. Medullary thyroid cancer is treated with total thyroidectomy and central neck lymph node dissection. Levothyroxine is indicated to treat postoperative hypothyroidism in patients with medullary thyroid cancer with a goal serum TSH level within the reference range. Serum calcitonin, serum carcinoembryonic antigen levels, and neck ultrasound are part of routine cancer surveillance.

Low-risk papillary thyroid cancer, confined to the thyroid gland, that has been completely resected, has not metastasized, and does not demonstrate aggressive pathologic features (lymphovascular invasion or tall cell variant), requires no additional treatment. The risk of disease-related death is less than 1%, and the risk of structural disease recurrence is 1% to 2% for low-risk unifocal papillary microcarcinomas. Patients receiving either lobectomy or thyroidectomy have similarly excellent outcomes.

KEY POINTS

- Thyroid cancer is often detected incidentally but can be detected when a thyroid nodule or abnormal lymph node is noted on neck examination.

- Surgery is the mainstay of thyroid cancer treatment; either hemithyroidectomy or total thyroidectomy is acceptable for unilateral differentiated thyroid cancers measuring 1 to 4 cm, as long as locoregional spread is not suspected, while total thyroidectomy is preferred in all other cases.

- In addition to surgery, patients with differentiated thyroid cancer and an intermediate to high risk of recurrence are treated with radioactive iodine therapy (^{131}I) and thyroid-stimulating hormone suppression with levothyroxine.

Evaluation of Thyroid Function

Serum TSH is the most sensitive and recommended initial test of thyroid function. It is used to determine euthyroidism, hypothyroidism or hyperthyroidism. If TSH is suppressed, free T_4 and total T_3 should be assessed to detect overt or subclinical hyperthyroidism, and if TSH is elevated, free T_4 should be assessed to detect overt or subclinical hypothyroidism.

Measuring serum TSH alone is sufficient except in certain circumstances, such as suspected central hypothyroidism, where free T_4 measurement is also indicated (see Disorders of the Pituitary Gland).

Total and free T_4 and total T_3 concentrations can be assessed with a variety of assays and can be accurately measured in most patients with overt thyroid dysfunction. Commercially available free T_3 assays are less reliable. Perturbations in thyroxine-binding globulin and other binding proteins can occur with physiologic changes (pregnancy), certain disease states (nephrotic syndrome), and as a result of medications (oral estrogen therapy). Levels of total T_4 and T_3 will vary based on increasing or decreasing binding proteins and do not reflect actual thyroid function. Measurement of free T_4, the unbound fraction of T_4 in serum, is most commonly determined using widely available immunometric assays. These tests are accurate in most clinical settings, including in patients with mild binding protein derangements; however, they can be inaccurate with more significant perturbations (familial dysalbuminemic hyperthyroxinemia). Measuring free T_4 by equilibrium dialysis is highly accurate, but expensive, not widely available, and rarely necessary.

Patients taking more than 5 to 10 mg/day of biotin should be counseled to discontinue ingestion for 2 days prior to the laboratory assessment of thyroid function. Biotin is a water-soluble vitamin that is commonly found in over-the-counter dietary supplements. High circulating levels of biotin have been shown to interfere with laboratory assays that utilize streptavidin–biotin as an immobilizing system. Biotin interference causes falsely high results with competitive immunoassays used to measure small molecules (free T_4, free T_3, total T_4, and total T_3) and causes falsely low results with sandwich assays used to measure large molecules (TSH).

Measurement of T_3 is recommended in three settings: (1) in the evaluation of thyrotoxicosis to identify isolated T_3 toxicosis, (2) to assess the severity of hyperthyroidism and response to therapy, and (3) potentially, to differentiate hyperthyroidism from destructive thyroiditis. In T_3 toxicosis, the T_3:T_4 ratio is often greater than 20 due to preferential secretion of T_3. Multiple drugs can affect thyroid function and replacement (**Table 34**).

Measurement of T_3 in the setting of hypothyroidism is not necessary or recommended; normal levels are maintained unless hypothyroidism is severe. TSH will become elevated in hypothyroidism first, followed by abnormalities in T_4 level.

There is no clinical indication to assess reverse T_3 levels, and thus it is not recommended.

KEY POINT

- Measurement of triiodothyronine in the setting of hypothyroidism is not necessary or recommended; normal levels are maintained unless hypothyroidism is severe.

HVC

TABLE 34. Medications that Affect Thyroid Function or Replacement

Mechanism of Action	Drugs	Comments
Decreased absorption or enterohepatic circulation of levothyroxine	Calcium Proton pump inhibitors Iron Cholestyramine Aluminum hydroxide Soybean oil Sucralfate Psyllium	Recommend that levothyroxine administration be separated from these medications by several hours
Increased metabolism of levothyroxine	Phenytoin Carbamazepine Rifampin Phenobarbital Sertraline	Higher levothyroxine doses may be required to maintain TSH in the normal range
Thyroiditis	Amiodarone Lithium Interferon alfa Interleukin-2 Tyrosine kinase inhibitors Immune checkpoint inhibitors	May cause hypo- or hyperthyroidism Sunitinib Nivolumab, pembrolizumab
De novo development of antithyroid antibodies	Interferon alfa	May develop Hashimoto thyroiditis, Graves disease, or painless thyroiditis
Inhibition of TSH synthesis or release	Glucocorticoids Dopamine Dobutamine Octreotide	Leads to TSH suppression; TSH should be rechecked 6-8 weeks after these medications are stopped to assess for return to normal.
Increased thyroxine-binding globulin	Estrogen Tamoxifen Methadone	False elevation of total T_3 and T_4 levels; free T_3 and T_4 are a more accurate reflection of hormone levels
Decreased thyroxine-binding globulin	Androgen therapy Glucocorticoids Niacin	False lowering of total T_3 and T_4 levels; free T_3 and T_4 are a more accurate reflection of hormone levels

T_3 = triiodothyronine; T_4 = thyroxine; TSH = thyroid-stimulating hormone.

Disorders of Thyroid Function

Thyroid Hormone Excess (Hyperthyroidism and Thyrotoxicosis)

The term *thyrotoxicosis* describes the exposure of tissues to high levels of circulating thyroid hormones (T_4 and/or T_3) from any cause. Hyperthyroidism is thyrotoxicosis caused by excessive endogenous production of thyroid hormones. The overall prevalence of hyperthyroidism in the United States is 1.3%. In primary hyperthyroidism, the thyroid gland is the anatomic site of dysfunction. Increased secretion of TSH is a rare secondary cause of hyperthyroidism.

Clinical Features and Diagnosis

Table 35 lists signs and symptoms of thyroid hormone excess. In elderly patients hyperthyroidism may be apathetic instead of presenting with classic symptoms. Lid lag (eyelid retraction) can be seen in thyrotoxicosis of any cause and results from increased adrenergic tone. The diagnosis of hyperthyroidism is based on biochemical testing demonstrating a low-serum TSH level and elevated concentrations of free T_4 and/or total T_3. Thyroid scintigraphy with radioactive iodine uptake (RAIU) can verify the cause. RAIU is high (above 30%) or inappropriately normal in hyperthyroidism and low (less than 10%) in other causes of thyrotoxicosis.

TABLE 35. Clinical Manifestations of Thyrotoxicosis and Thyroid Hormone Deficiency[a]

Sign or Symptom	Thyrotoxicosis	Thyroid Hormone Deficiency
General	Fatigue, weight loss,[b] heat intolerance	Fatigue, weight gain, cold intolerance
Neuropsychiatric	Decreased concentration, anxiety, irritability, insomnia	Decreased concentration, depression, psychomotor retardation, hypersomnolence
	Hyperreflexia, tremor, lid lag	Delayed relaxation of DTRs
Cardiovascular	Palpitations, tachycardia, systolic hypertension, high output heart failure	Bradycardia, diastolic hypertension
Gastrointestinal	Hyperphagia, increased frequency of bowel movements, loose stools, diarrhea	Constipation
Genitourinary	Menstrual disturbance (oligomenorrhea, amenorrhea)	Menstrual disturbance (menorrhagia)
Musculoskeletal	Muscle weakness	Myalgia, arthralgia
Cutaneous	Hair loss, increased sweating, increased oil production/acne; periorbital edema	Hair loss, dry skin, brittle nails, periorbital edema, lateral truncation of the eyebrows, myxedematous skin changes

DTRs = deep tendon reflexes.

[a]Goiter may be present in thyrotoxicosis or thyroid hormone deficiency. See text for physical findings characteristic of Graves disease.

[b]Mild weight gain can occur with subclinical hyperthyroidism (thyroid-stimulating hormone suppression without T_4 or T_3 elevation) due to appetite stimulation.

Additional testing can be done when the clinical diagnosis is not clear; when RAIU is unavailable or unreliable (patients on amiodarone, lithium, or exposed to recent iodinated contrast material); or when scintigraphy is contraindicated (pregnancy and lactation). Tests include measurement of thyroid-stimulating immunoglobulin (TSI) or thyrotropin (TSH) receptor antibodies (TRAb) if Graves disease is suspected but the diagnosis remains clinically unclear, and thyroid ultrasound to assess for patterns of vascularity.

KEY POINTS

- The diagnosis of hyperthyroidism is based on biochemical testing demonstrating a low serum thyroid-stimulating hormone level and elevated concentrations of free thyroxine and/or total triiodothyronine.

- Thyroid scintigraphy with determination of radioactive iodine uptake can verify the cause of hyperthyroidism.

Causes

Causes of thyrotoxicosis are listed in **Table 36**. Graves disease, toxic multinodular goiter, and toxic adenoma are the most common causes of hyperthyroidism.

Graves Disease

Graves disease is a multisystem disease and can affect the thyroid, ocular muscles, and skin. It causes 80% of hyperthyroidism in iodine-sufficient areas. It is an autoimmune thyroid disorder predominantly affecting women with a peak incidence among patients aged 30 to 60 years. Graves disease is also more common in patients with other autoimmune disorders or a family history of thyroid autoimmunity. T lymphocytes become sensitized to thyroid antigens and

TABLE 36. Causes of Thyrotoxicosis

Disorder	Comments
Graves disease	Common; TRAb mediated activation of TSHR
Toxic multinodular goiter	Common; autonomously functioning thyroid tissue
Toxic adenoma	Common; autonomously functioning thyroid tissue
Thyroiditis (acute, subacute, painless)	Common; thyroid inflammation resulting in release of stored thyroid hormones
Medication induced	Common; amiodarone, lithium, interferon alfa, interleukin-2, tyrosine kinase inhibitors, immune checkpoint inhibitors
Thyrotoxicosis factitia	Common; administration of exogenous thyroid hormone; ingestion of contaminated pork or beef products
HCG-mediated (Pregnancy, trophoblastic disease, germ cell tumor)	Common in pregnancy, other forms rare; indiscriminant binding of HCG to TSHR due to common alpha subunit shared by TSH and HCG.
Struma ovarii	Rare; autonomously functioning thyroid tissue in an ovarian teratoma accounting for >50% of the tumor
Follicular thyroid cancer metastases	Rare; autonomously functioning follicular thyroid carcinoma metastases
Thyrotrope adenoma	Rare; TSH-secreting pituitary adenoma

HCG = human chorionic growth hormone; TSH = thyroid-stimulating hormone; TRAb = thyrotropin (TSH) receptor antibodies; TSHR = TSH receptor.

stimulate B lymphocytes to produce antibodies against the TSH receptor (TSI or TRAb). The thyroid is diffusely enlarged, may have a bruit, and has a firm, smooth texture on examination; cervical lymphadenopathy can occur. Systolic hypertension, tachycardia, hyperreflexia, and warm moist skin are often present.

Graves ophthalmopathy affects 25% of patients. Cigarette smoking is a risk factor. Clinical manifestations include periorbital edema, chemosis (conjunctival edema), proptosis (protrusion of the globe), diplopia (due to oculomotor paresis), and vision loss. Graves ophthalmopathy does not respond to the treatment of hyperthyroidism and often requires glucocorticoids or surgery.

Pretibial myxedema is a rare infiltrative dermopathy of Graves disease that affects 2% to 3% of patients; it is a nonpitting edema that is indurated, with a peau d'orange appearance, typically on the shins (see MKSAP 18 Dermatology).

KEY POINTS

- In Graves disease, the thyroid is diffusely enlarged, may have a bruit, and has a firm, smooth texture on examination; cervical lymphadenopathy can also occur.

- Graves ophthalmopathy does not respond to the treatment of hyperthyroidism and often requires glucocorticoids or surgery.

Toxic Adenoma and Multinodular Goiter

Toxic adenoma and multinodular goiter typically affect older adults as the prevalence of thyroid nodules increases with age. Thyroid nodules synthesize and secrete thyroid hormones independent of TSH stimulation. Exposure to iodinated contrast can precipitate conversion from nontoxic to toxic adenoma(s), such as with contrasted CT scanning and cardiac catheterization.

Destructive Thyroiditis

Thyrotoxicosis occurs in destructive thyroiditis as a result of unregulated release of preformed thyroid hormone from thyroid follicles damaged by inflammation. Causes are listed in **Table 37**. Thyroiditis typically has three phases: thyrotoxic, hypothyroid, and return to euthyroidism. The first two phases can last up to 3 months each. A person has increased risk of additional bouts of thyroiditis once the initial thyroiditis has resolved.

Management

Most thyrotoxic patients benefit from β-blockers (atenolol, metoprolol, propranolol) to reduce adrenergic symptoms rapidly. Propranolol decreases the peripheral conversion of T_4 to T_3, but is non-cardioselective and requires twice or three times daily dosing. Atenolol and metoprolol are preferred owing to once-daily dosing that increases adherence and their cardioselective nature that decreases central nervous system side effects.

There are three treatment modalities for hyperthyroidism: thioamides (methimazole and propylthiouracil [PTU]),

TABLE 37.	Causes of Destructive Thyroiditis
Disorder	**Comments**
Painless (silent) thyroiditis	Seen with underlying autoimmune thyroid disease (Hashimoto thyroiditis)
Postpartum thyroiditis	Painless thyroiditis occurring postpartum; permanent hypothyroidism occurs in 20%
Medication-induced thyroiditis	Painless thyroiditis; amiodarone, lithium, interferon alfa, interleukin-2, tyrosine kinase inhibitors, immune checkpoint inhibitors
Subacute thyroiditis (de Quervain or subacute granulomatous)	Painful thyroiditis; follows a viral upper respiratory tract infection
Infectious (suppurative)	Painful thyroiditis; *Staphylococcus* or *Streptococcus* species infection usually seen in immunocompromised patients
Radiation-induced thyroiditis	Painful thyroiditis; occurs after radioactive iodine therapy or neck external beam radiation therapy

radioactive iodine (^{131}I) ablative therapy, and thyroidectomy. The choice of treatment is predicated on the cause of the hyperthyroidism and patient preference. Short-term use of methimazole to normalize thyroid function prior to ^{131}I therapy or thyroidectomy is recommended for patients 65 years of age or older or who have prevalent cardiovascular disease or multiple comorbidities. Referral to an endocrinologist is recommended.

Graves Disease

Antithyroid drugs (thionamides) are often used in the initial treatment of Graves hyperthyroidism because up to 50% will have spontaneous remission of hyperthyroidism within 24 months, especially if the goiter is small and only low doses of thioamide are required to achieve euthyroidism. Recurrent hyperthyroidism is likely if TRAb levels remain elevated at the time of drug discontinuation. If Graves hyperthyroidism recurs, definitive treatment is recommended.

Agranulocytosis and liver dysfunction are two rare but serious side effects of thioamides. Prior to treatment, baseline CBC with differential and liver profile should be assessed. Agranulocytosis should be suspected and the patient's neutrophil count assessed in the setting of fever or pharyngitis. Liver function should be assessed in any patient with symptoms or signs of hepatic dysfunction (jaundice, icterus). Methimazole is the antithyroid drug of choice, except in the first trimester of pregnancy, because PTU has been associated with fatal hepatonecrosis.

The goal of ^{131}I ablative therapy in Graves disease is to render the patient hypothyroid. Women receiving ^{131}I therapy must avoid pregnancy for 6 to 12 months after treatment. In patients with Graves ophthalmopathy, there is an acute escalation of thyroid autoantibody titers following radioiodine therapy that may exacerbate ocular symptoms. Pretreatment of

Graves ophthalmopathy or selection of alternative treatments depends on the severity of the eye disease.

Thyroidectomy in Graves hyperthyroidism is most appropriate when there is a large goiter with compressive symptoms, moderate to severe Graves ophthalmopathy, and/or with coexistent thyroid cancer or primary hyperparathyroidism.

Other Causes

First-line therapy for a toxic adenoma or toxic multinodular goiter is either ^{131}I therapy or thyroid surgery. Choice is determined by patient preference, presence of compressive symptoms, and access to a high-volume thyroid surgeon.

Destructive thyroiditis is managed expectantly with β-blockers to control adrenergic symptoms and NSAIDs, followed by high-dose glucocorticoid therapy, for pain control in painful thyroiditis.

KEY POINTS

- Most thyrotoxic patients benefit from β-blockers to reduce adrenergic symptoms.

- The three treatment modalities for hyperthyroidism are thionamides (methimazole and propylthiouracil), radioactive iodine (^{131}I) ablative therapy, and thyroidectomy; the choice of treatment is predicated on the cause of the hyperthyroidism and patient preference.

- Antithyroid drugs (thionamides) are associated with up to a 50% spontaneous remission rate within 24 months; agranulocytosis and liver dysfunction are two rare but serious side effects.

Subclinical Hyperthyroidism

Subclinical hyperthyroidism diagnosis is based on suppression of the serum TSH, with normal T_4 and T_3 levels. Subclinical hyperthyroidism affects 0.7% of the U.S. population. Approximately 0.5% to 7% progress to overt hyperthyroidism per year and 5% to 12% revert to normal thyroid function. The most common cause is toxic multinodular goiter.

Subclinical hyperthyroidism has been associated with an increased risk of atrial fibrillation and cardiovascular events. A recent large prospective cohort study demonstrated higher rates of hip fracture with subclinical hyperthyroidism (7% in subclinical hyperthyroidism vs. 4.5% in euthyroid patients); however, it is unknown whether treatment reduces fracture risk.

The TSH will normalize at 6 weeks in more than 25% of patients with subclinical hyperthyroidism. Therefore, observation and rechecking thyroid function prior to the initiation of treatment is reasonable unless the risk of complications is high, such as in patients with cardiac disease. Higher risk of cardiovascular and skeletal complications is seen with serum TSH level under 0.1 µU/mL (0.1 mU/L). Treatment of subclinical hyperthyroidism is recommended for patients with serum TSH levels below 0.1 µU/mL (0.1 mU/L) and with symptoms, cardiac risk factors, heart disease, or osteoporosis, as well as

for postmenopausal women not taking estrogen therapy or bisphosphonates.

KEY POINTS

- Subclinical hyperthyroidism is diagnosed based on suppression of the serum thyroid-stimulating hormone, but normal thyroxine and triiodothyronine levels.

- Treatment of subclinical hyperthyroidism is recommended for patients with serum thyroid-stimulating levels below 0.1 µU/mL (0.1 mU/L) and symptoms, cardiac risk factors, heart disease, or osteoporosis, as well as for postmenopausal women not taking estrogen therapy or bisphosphonates.

Thyroid Hormone Deficiency

Thyroid hormone deficiency affects more than 10 million Americans. It is 10 times more common in women than men.

Clinical Features and Diagnosis

Signs and symptoms of thyroid hormone deficiency are listed in Table 35. Thyroid hormone deficiency is also associated with laboratory abnormalities including anemia, elevated LDL cholesterol, and hyponatremia.

The diagnosis of primary hypothyroidism is made by measuring serum TSH, and if elevated, measuring free T_4, which can be added on in most laboratories. Serum TSH is elevated in both overt and subclinical hypothyroidism, but free T_4 is normal when subclinical and low in overt hypothyroidism. Thyroid autoantibodies [thyroid peroxidase (TPO) antibodies] are present in most patients with Hashimoto thyroiditis; however, measurement of TPO antibody titer is not necessary unless the diagnosis is unclear. The diagnosis of hypothyroidism is discussed elsewhere (see Disorders of the Pituitary Gland).

KEY POINTS

- The diagnosis of hypothyroidism is made by measuring serum thyroid-stimulating hormone, and if elevated, then measuring free thyroxine.

- Serum thyroid-stimulating hormone is elevated in both overt and subclinical hypothyroidism, but free thyroxine is normal in subclinical hypothyroidism and low in overt hypothyroidism.

- Thyroid autoantibodies [thyroid peroxidase (TPO) antibodies] are present in most patients with Hashimoto thyroiditis; however, measurement of TPO antibody titer is not necessary unless the diagnosis is unclear. **HVC**

Causes

Causes of hypothyroidism are listed in **Table 38**. The most common cause in the United States is autoimmune thyroid gland failure (due to Hashimoto thyroiditis), while iodine deficiency, which affects 2 billion people worldwide, is the most common cause globally. Iodide deficiency is uncommon in the

TABLE 38. Causes of Thyroid Hormone Deficiency

Disorder	Comments
Hashimoto thyroiditis	Autoimmune thyroid disorder associated with anti-TPO antibodies
Post-thyroidectomy	Treatment of Graves disease, goiter, thyroid nodules, or thyroid cancer
Post-radioactive iodine therapy	Treatment of Graves disease or toxic adenoma/multinodular goiter
External beam radiation to the neck	Treatment of Hodgkin lymphoma and head/neck malignancies
Thyroiditis (acute, subacute, suppurative)	Typically a transient hypothyroidism prior to recovery of euthyroid state
Central hypothyroidism	TSH deficiency from hypothalamic or pituitary disease; TSH should not be used to assess for replacement dose adequacy; T_4 level should be used for dosing
Congenital hypothyroidism	Universal neonatal screening in the United States where the incidence is 1 in 3500
Iodide deficiency	Common worldwide in developing countries with severe iodine deficiency
Drug-induced	Amiodarone, lithium, interferon-alpha, interleukin-2, iodine, thionamides (methimazole), ethionamide, tyrosine kinase inhibitors (sunitinib), immune checkpoint inhibitors (ipilimumab)

Anti-TPO = anti-thyroid peroxidase; TSH = thyroid-stimulating hormone; T_4 = thyroxine.

United States as a result of efforts to fortify food (iodized salt). Central hypothyroidism is also uncommon.

Primary Hypothyroidism

Hashimoto thyroiditis (chronic lymphocytic thyroiditis) is an autoimmune thyroid disorder characterized by diffuse infiltration of the thyroid gland by lymphocytes and plasma cells with subsequent follicular atrophy and scarring. It is more common in patients with other autoimmune disorders or a family history of thyroid autoimmunity. Diffuse goiter can be seen most commonly in younger patients. Most patients (90%) have TPO antibodies, and the risk of developing hypothyroidism is four times higher in euthyroid patients with TPO antibodies.

Hypothyroidism occurs in all patients after thyroidectomy and 20% of patients after thyroid lobectomy. Postablative hypothyroidism occurs after ^{131}I therapy in 90% of patients with Graves disease within 1 year of radioactive iodine therapy, and in 60% of patients with toxic multinodular goiter, although onset of hypothyroidism may be delayed for many years in the latter case. External beam radiation to the neck also can cause hypothyroidism, as with Hodgkin lymphoma and head/neck malignancies.

Drug-induced hypothyroidism is another cause of primary hypothyroidism (see Table 38).

KEY POINTS

- The most common cause of primary hypothyroidism is autoimmune thyroid gland failure due to Hashimoto thyroiditis, typically associated with thyroid perioxidase antibodies.
- In addition to Hashimoto thyroiditis, common causes of hypothyroidism include thyroid surgery and postablative hypothyroidism following ^{131}I therapy for treatment of Graves disease or toxic multinodular goiter.

Subclinical Hypothyroidism

Subclinical hypothyroidism is typically asymptomatic and diagnosed by a serum TSH level above the upper limit of the reference range and a normal free T_4 level. It affects 5% to 10% of the general population. Transient elevation of serum TSH should be ruled out by repeating the measurement in 6 to 8 weeks. The rate of progression from subclinical to overt hypothyroidism is 2% to 4% per year, while one-third of patients spontaneously revert to normal thyroid function. The normal range for TSH increases with age, and a TSH level of up to 10 µU/mL (10 mU/L) is within the normal range for persons 80 years of age and older.

Subclinical hypothyroidism with TSH above 10 µU/mL (10 mU/L) may be a risk factor for coronary artery disease and heart failure. There is no evidence that treating subclinical hypothyroidism improves quality of life, cognitive function, blood pressure, or weight, but in patients with elevated LDL cholesterol, normalization of the TSH will lower LDL cholesterol.

Management

Thyroid hormone replacement with levothyroxine is the treatment of choice for thyroid hormone deficiency. Goals of treatment are to normalize serum TSH (in primary hypothyroidism) or free T_4 (in central hypothyroidism) and to resolve signs and symptoms of hypothyroidism. Beginning a full replacement dose (1.6 µg/kg lean body weight) is appropriate for most patients with overt hypothyroidism, except in older adults and patients with cardiovascular disease for whom lower initial doses (25-50 µg/day) are recommended. Assessment of the adequacy of treatment should be done with a repeat serum TSH level at least 6 weeks after initiation or change in dose with a goal of a normal TSH.

T_3-containing compounds are not recommended in the treatment of hypothyroidism due to its short half-life, which results in spikes in T_3 levels. Studies have failed to show that T_3 alone or in combination with T_4 has clear benefit in treatment of hypothyroidism.

Subclinical hypothyroidism with a serum TSH value above 10 µU/mL (10 mU/L) should be treated. Initial treatment is 25 to 50 µg of levothyroxine per day. There is unclear benefit and potential for harm in treating mild subclinical hypothyroidism

(TSH > 5-10 µU/mL [5-10 mU/L]). Overtreatment is seen in more than one-third of patients over 65, which may increase risk for dysrhythmia and bone loss.

Oral levothyroxine is absorbed in the jejunum and ileum. Ideally it should be taken on an empty stomach (60 minutes before breakfast or coffee are consumed). If the patient is having difficulty adhering to morning adminis-tration, then it can be taken before bed. Missed doses can be taken the following day in younger patients struggling with daily adherence. The absorption of an orally administered dose is 70% to 80% under optimum fasting conditions. Gastrointestinal disorders (such as celiac disease) may impact absorption and result in higher than expected levo-thyroxine dose requirements. Medications can also interfere with the absorption or metabolism of levothyroxine (see Table 34).

KEY POINTS

- Levothyroxine is the treatment of choice for thyroid hormone deficiency; it should be taken on an empty stomach 60 minutes before eating breakfast or consum-ing coffee.

HVC
- Triiodothyronine-containing compounds are not rec-ommended in the treatment of hypothyroidism due to its short half-life, which results in spikes in triiodothy-ronine levels.

HVC
- Overtreatment of subclinical hypothyroidism is com-mon, especially in patients older than 65 years of age, and should be avoided.

Drug-Induced Thyroid Dysfunction

Many medications can affect thyroid function and are listed in Table 34.

Amiodarone is an antiarrhythmic medication with high iodine content (37%) and prolonged half-life of approximately 60 days. Thyroid dysfunction occurs in approximately 25% of ami-odarone-treated patients and can present as hypothyroidism, hyperthyroidism, painless thyroiditis, or goiter. Hypothyroidism, seen in 20% of affected patients, is usually seen in the setting of Hashimoto thyroiditis. All patients can have a transient rise in TSH levels in the first few months of amiodarone therapy due to the Wolff-Chaikoff effect (temporary decrease in thyroid pro-duction due to iodine load), but most regain normal thyroid function.

Thyrotoxicosis affects 5% of patients treated with ami-odarone. Type 1 (hyperthyroidism) amiodarone-induced thy-rotoxicosis occurs in patients with Graves disease or thyroid nodules. It is a form of iodine-induced hyperthyroidism (Jod-Basedow phenomenon). It is treated with thioamides, typically methimazole. Type 2 (destructive thyroiditis) amiodarone-induced thyrotoxicosis is more common and occurs in patients without underlying thyroid disease. It is usually self-limiting but sometimes requires treatment with moderate- to high-dose glucocorticoids. The decision to discontinue amiodarone

depends on the patient's cardiac condition and type of thyro-toxicosis (type 1 or 2).

KEY POINT

- Thyroid dysfunction occurs in approximately 25% of patients taking amiodarone and can present as hypo-thyroidism, hyperthyroidism, painless thyroiditis, or goiter.

Thyroid Function and Dysfunction in Pregnancy

Thyroid hormones are essential for normal fetal development. The size of the maternal thyroid gland can increase up to 40% during pregnancy. Production of T_4 and T_3 increases up to 50% to compensate for the increased thyroxine-binding globulin production associated with pregnancy-related increase in estrogen. Iodine requirements also increase up to 50%. Pregnant and lactating women should therefore be counseled to supplement their dietary iodine intake with a daily oral supplement containing 150 µg of iodine, which is included in some but not all over-the-counter and prescription prenatal vitamins. Universal screening of TSH in pregnant women is not recommended. However, those at increased risk of thy-roid dysfunction should be screened, which includes those 30 years of age and older; with known hypothyroidism and/or a strong family history of thyroid dysfunction; prior head/neck irradiation; prior neck surgery; positive TPO, TSI, or TRAb status; or other autoimmune disorders.

Changes in thyroid function tests are depicted in **Figure 10**. Placental human chorionic gonadotropin (hCG) stimulates

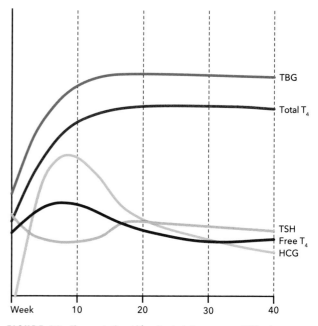

FIGURE 10. Changes in thyroid function tests in pregnancy. HCG = human chorionic gonadotropin; T_4 = thyroxine; TBG = thyroid-binding globulin; TSH = thyroid-stimulating hormone.

thyroid hormone secretion and TSH may be mildly suppressed as a result. In the late first trimester (weeks 7-12) the lower limit of the TSH reference range decreases by 0.4 µU/mL (0.4 mU/L) and upper limit by 0.5 µU/mL (0.5 mU/L). Serum TSH gradually returns to the nonpregnant reference range in the second and third trimester.

Measured total T_4 concentrations increase linearly during pregnancy. After week 16, the upper limit of the total T_4 reference range can be estimated by multiplying the nonpregnant upper limit by 1.5. Free T_4 measured by indirect analogue immunoassays are inaccurate in pregnancy unless method and trimester-specific reference ranges are applied.

Consultation with an endocrinologist is indicated for management of thyrotoxicosis during pregnancy. Gestational thyrotoxicosis from high human chorionic gonadotropin levels is the most common cause of transient TSH suppression. If serum total or free T_4 remains within the trimester-specific reference range, treatment is not needed. Women with moderate to severe hyperthyroidism in early pregnancy should be treated with PTU because potential teratogenic effects are less severe than with methimazole. After the first trimester, women can be transitioned to methimazole. Thyroid function should be followed closely and the serum total or free T_4 should be maintained at or just above the trimester-specific reference range to avoid fetal hypothyroidism.

Graves disease affects 0.2% of pregnant women and can be confirmed by classic physical findings or elevated TSI or TRAb. Women with Graves disease are considered high-risk pregnancies and should be followed by maternal fetal specialists throughout the pregnancy.

Hypothyroidism in pregnancy is associated with increases in miscarriage, premature birth, low birth weight, and decreased infant neurocognitive function. Levothyroxine is the treatment of choice.

For women with preexisting hypothyroidism, levothyroxine dosing can be empirically increased by 30% when pregnancy is confirmed. In treatment-naïve pregnant women with positive TPO antibodies, levothyroxine is started if TSH level is ≥2.5 µU/mL (2.5 mU/L). Treatment is indicated for TPO-negative pregnant women if TSH is above the pregnancy-specific reference range. TSH should be measured every 4 weeks for the first half of pregnancy and around 30 weeks in all hypothyroid women and in those at risk for hypothyroidism (antibody positive or history of hemithyroidectomy or ^{131}I therapy). A TSH level less than 2.5 µU/mL (2.5 mU/L) should be targeted in treated hypothyroid women both preconception and during pregnancy.

Thyroid nodules detected in pregnant women should be evaluated as in nonpregnant patients. The timing of FNAB, whether during or after pregnancy, is determined by the likelihood of cancer and patient preference. Consultation with an endocrinologist is indicated for management of thyroid cancer

detected during pregnancy. Pregnant women with a history of thyroid cancer should be managed as when not pregnant.

KEY POINTS

- For women with preexisting hypothyroidism, levothyroxine dosing can be empirically increased by 30% when pregnancy is confirmed.

- In treatment-naïve pregnant women with positive thyroid peroxidase (TPO) antibodies, levothyroxine is started if thyroid-stimulating hormone level is 2.5 µU/mL (2.5 mU/L) or higher; and treatment is indicated for TPO-negative pregnant women if the thyroid-stimulating hormone level is above the pregnancy-specific reference range.

Nonthyroidal Illness Syndrome (Euthyroid Sick Syndrome)

Nonthyroidal illness syndrome (NTIS) commonly occurs in patients who are hospitalized and critically ill. Up to 75% of hospitalized patients have thyroid function test abnormalities. Nonthyroidal illness suppresses thyrotropin-releasing hormone, which typically results in suppressed but detectable TSH. An undetectable TSH is not consistent with NTIS. Infrequently, TSH can be mildly elevated in NTIS, but a TSH level of 20 µU/mL (20 mU/L) or greater is not consistent with NTIS. T_4 is typically normal, but due to decreased deiodinase activity in T_4 metabolism, T_3 decreases and reverse T_3 increases (biologically inactive). Thyroid-binding globulin decreases in illness, lowering the total T_4 and T_3 levels. NTIS can be interpreted as an adaptive response to systemic illness and macronutrient restriction.

Treatment of NTIS is not recommended due to lack of significant clinical benefit. In general, thyroid function should not be assessed in hospitalized patients unless there is a strong clinical suspicion of thyroid dysfunction. If NTIS is diagnosed, TSH should be rechecked approximately 6 weeks after the patient has recovered from their nonthyroidal illness to assess for return to normal.

KEY POINTS

- Treatment of nonthyroidal illness syndrome is not recommended due to lack of significant clinical benefit. **HVC**

- Thyroid function should not be assessed in hospitalized patients unless there is a strong clinical suspicion of thyroid dysfunction. **HVC**

Thyroid Emergencies

Thyroid Storm

Thyroid storm is a rare disorder with high mortality (up to 30%) characterized by severe thyrotoxicosis (suppressed TSH, elevated free T_4 and/or total T_3) and systemic hemodynamic decompensation (shock). Serum thyroid hormone concentrations do not differentiate thyroid storm from severe thyrotoxicosis. It is the presence of shock that makes the diagnosis of thyroid storm.

Presentation often follows discontinuation of antithyroid drug therapy, systemic illness, labor and delivery, surgery, or trauma. Patients with Graves disease are at higher risk. Clinical manifestations include high fever, tachycardia, altered mental status, and cardiac and hepatic dysfunction. A scoring system, such as the Burch and Wartofsky Point Scale (**Table 39**), can support the diagnosis, but thyroid storm is diagnosed clinically.

Management includes ICU-level care, treatment of any precipitant illness, thyrotoxicosis-directed therapy, and supportive measures. Thyrotoxicosis is treated with intravenous β-blockers (esmolol infusion), thioamide (typically PTU, transitioning to methimazole when more stable), intravenous high-dose glucocorticoids, and potassium iodide. Iodide should be administered more than 1 hour after antithyroid drugs to avoid providing substrate to the gland. Glucocorticoid therapy is a potent inhibitor of peripheral T_4 to T_3 conversion. Bile acid sequestrants can be used to decrease T_4 and T_3 levels, especially in patients unable to take thioamides. Plasmapheresis or emergent thyroidectomy is used in patients who respond poorly to medical therapy. Definitive treatment with thyroidectomy or ^{131}I therapy is indicated in patients who survive thyroid storm.

KEY POINTS

- Thyroid storm is a rare disorder with high mortality (up to 30%) characterized by severe thyrotoxicosis and systemic hemodynamic decompensation.

- Thyroid storm often occurs with discontinuation of antithyroid drug therapy, systemic illness, labor and delivery, surgery, or trauma.

- ICU-level care; treating any precipitating illness; and the use of intravenous β-blockers, thioamide, intravenous high-dose glucocorticoids, and potassium iodide are all used to manage thyroid storm.

Myxedema Coma

Myxedema coma is a life-threatening presentation of severe hypothyroidism with hemodynamic compromise that affects 0.22 people per million per year. Mortality is high (up to 40%), and ICU-level care is required. Risk factors for myxedema coma are female gender, advanced age, cold exposure, or a precipitant event in patients with undiagnosed hypothyroidism, such as myocardial infarction, sepsis, trauma, or stroke. Mental status changes ranging from lethargy to coma to psychosis, coupled with hypothermia (temperature below 34.4 °C (94.0 °F) are the most common clinical manifestations. Bradycardia, hypotension, or decreased respiration rate with resultant hypoxia and hypercapnia are also frequently present. Careful examination of the neck for thyroidectomy scar is critical. Free T_4 is low in myxedema coma. TSH is typically elevated, but without an overtly low free T_4, myxedema coma

TABLE 39. Burch and Wartofsky Point Scale to Support the Diagnosis of Thyroid Storm[a]

Criteria	Points
Thermoregulatory Dysfunction	
Temperature °F (°C)	
99-99.9 (37.2-37.7)	5
100-100.9 (37.8-38.2)	10
101-101.9 (38.3-38.8)	15
102-102.9 (38.9-39.3)	20
103-103.9 (39.4-39.9)	25
≥104 (40)	30
Cardiovascular	
Tachycardia (bpm)	
100-109	5
110-119	10
120-129	15
130-139	20
≥140	25
Atrial fibrillation	
Absent	0
Present	10
Congestive heart failure	
Absent	0
Mild	5
Moderate	10
Severe	20
Gastrointestinal-Hepatic Dysfunction	
Absent	0
Moderate (diarrhea, abdominal pain, nausea, vomiting)	10
Severe (jaundice)	20
Central Nervous System Disturbance	
Absent	0
Mild (agitation)	10
Moderate (delirium, psychosis, extreme lethargy)	20
Severe (seizure, coma)	30
Precipitant History	
Absent	0
Present	10
Scores Totaled	
<25	Thyroid storm is unlikely
25-45	Impending thyroid storm
>45	Thyroid storm is likely

[a]Thyroid storm is diagnosed clinically in the presence of hemodynamic compromise.

From Burch HB, Wartofsky L. Life-threatening thyrotoxicosis: thyroid storm. Endocrinol Metab Clin North Am. 1993 Jun;22(2):263-77. Review. PMID: 8325286.

is unlikely regardless of how high the TSH. Other metabolic derangements include hyponatremia and hypoglycemia. Cortisol should be drawn with initial laboratory studies to assess for concomitant cortisol deficiency.

Aggressive supportive measures include fluids, vasopressors if necessary, ventilator support, and passive warming rather than active warming to avoid vasodilation, which can worsen hypotension. Stress-dose glucocorticoids (100 mg intravenous hydrocortisone every 8 hours) are administered empirically before thyroid hormone is initiated to treat possible concomitant adrenal insufficiency. If random cortisol level is above 18 mg/dL (496.8 nmol/L), hydrocortisone can be discontinued. Replacement of thyroid hormone requires consideration of the need to normalize the thyroid hormone level rapidly and the risk of a fatal cardiac event caused by thyroid hormone administration. Initial treatment is intravenous levothyroxine with loading dose of 200 to 400 μg, followed by a daily oral dose of 1.6 μg/kg. The dose should be reduced to 75% if administered intravenously. Lower levothyroxine doses are recommended with advanced age and/or cardiac disease. Goals of treatment are improved mental status, metabolic parameters, and cardiopulmonary function. When the patient is stable, transition to oral levothyroxine is the goal. **H**

KEY POINTS

- Myxedema coma is a life-threatening presentation of severe hypothyroidism with hemodynamic compromise; it most often occurs when a systemic illness is superimposed on previously undiagnosed hypothyroidism.

- In addition to aggressive supportive measures, stress-dose glucocorticoids (100 mg intravenous hydrocortisone every 8 hours) are administered empirically before thyroid hormone is initiated to treat possible concomitant adrenal insufficiency.

Reproductive Disorders
Physiology of Female Reproduction

Coordinated actions of the hypothalamus, pituitary gland, and ovaries (known as the hypothalamic-pituitary-ovarian axis) give rise to ovulatory cycles in women. The pulsatile release of gonadotropin-releasing hormone (GnRH) drives the anterior pituitary cells to secrete follicle-stimulating hormone (FSH) and luteinizing hormone (LH) (**Figure 11**). FSH regulates estradiol production and follicle growth in the follicular phase of the menstrual cycle. A sudden rise in LH levels causes release of an ovum midcycle, signaling the start of the luteal phase, which is a constant 14 days. Endometrial sloughing follows decreased estrogen or progesterone levels if a fertilized embryo does not implant. Menses occur every 25 to 35 days; menstrual cycles shorter than 25 days or longer than 35 days in women

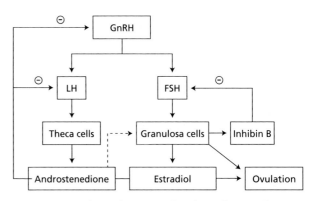

FIGURE 11. Female reproductive axis. Pulses of GnRH drive LH and FSH production. LH acts on theca cells to stimulate androgen (principally androstenedione) production. Androstenedione is metabolized to estradiol in granulosa cells. FSH acts on granulosa cells to enhance follicle maturation. Granulosa cells produce inhibin B as a feedback regulator of FSH production. FSH = follicle-stimulating hormone; GnRH = gonadotropin-releasing hormone; LH = luteinizing hormone; − (circled) = negative feedback.

younger than age 40 years are likely anovulatory, resulting in abnormal uterine bleeding or oligomenorrhea. Before puberty, ovaries are quiescent due to immaturity of the hypothalamus. After menopause, all reproductive function and most endocrine function of the ovaries ceases.

KEY POINT

- In women younger than age 40 years, menstrual cycles shorter than 25 days or longer than 35 days are likely anovulatory.

Amenorrhea

Amenorrhea, the absence of menses, can be intermittent or permanent. It may result from hypothalamic, pituitary, ovarian, uterine, or outflow tract disorders.

Clinical Features
Primary Amenorrhea

Primary amenorrhea is defined as absence of menses at age 15 years in the presence of normal growth and secondary sexual characteristics. Primary amenorrhea is most commonly caused by a genetic (50%) or anatomic (15%) abnormality. Most causes of secondary amenorrhea can also present as primary amenorrhea.

The most common cause of primary amenorrhea is gonadal dysgenesis, most commonly with Turner syndrome (45,X0). Turner syndrome is caused by loss of part or all of an X chromosome. It occurs in 1 in 2500 live female births. It is associated with short stature and primary ovarian insufficiency (POI); primary amenorrhea is seen in approximately 90% of patients with Turner syndrome.

Anatomic abnormalities that can cause primary amenorrhea include an intact hymen, transverse vaginal septum, and vaginal agenesis. Vaginal agenesis (also known as müllerian agenesis or Mayer-Rokitansky-Küster-Hauser syndrome) is the second most common cause of primary amenorrhea, with an incidence of 1 in 5000 live female births. Women with vaginal agenesis have a normal female karyotype and ovarian function, and thus, normal external genitalia and secondary sexual characteristics.

Secondary Amenorrhea

Secondary amenorrhea is defined as absence of menses for more than 3 months in women who previously had regular menstrual cycles or for 6 months in women who have irregular menses. In women with oligomenorrhea, defined as fewer than nine menstrual cycles per year or cycle length longer than 35 days, the evaluation is the same as for secondary amenorrhea.

Functional hypothalamic amenorrhea (FHA) is caused by a disruption of the hypothalamic-pituitary-ovarian axis and is the most common cause of secondary amenorrhea after pregnancy. Disruption of the pulsatile release of hypothalamic GnRH may occur due to stress, weight loss, or exercise. In many cases, all three factors are present. FHA is a diagnosis of exclusion; history and physical examination, biochemical testing, and, imaging, when appropriate, should be undertaken to rule out other causes of secondary amenorrhea including intracranial tumor, infiltrative or destructive disorders such as lymphocytic hypophysitis, histiocytosis X, sarcoidosis, Sheehan syndrome, and acute or chronic systemic illness.

Premenopausal women with hyperprolactinemia present more often with oligomenorrhea or amenorrhea than galactorrhea. Hyperprolactinemia accounts for 10% to 20% of non-pregnancy-mediated amenorrhea. Menstrual dysfunction in hyperprolactinemia results from inhibition of GnRH.

Menstrual dysfunction is common in women with thyroid disorders; while heavy bleeding is typical with hypothyroidism, secondary amenorrhea can also occur.

Hyperandrogenic disorders are associated with amenorrhea, with polycystic ovary syndrome by far the most common hyperandrogenic cause.

Spontaneous primary ovarian insufficiency (POI) can be diagnosed in women younger than age 40 years with menstrual dysfunction in association with two serum FSH levels in the menopausal range. POI affects 1 in 100 women. In addition to disordered menses, affected women may develop symptoms related to estrogen deficiency, such as vasomotor symptoms, sleep disturbance, and dyspareunia related to vaginal dryness. Most cases are sporadic, but a first-degree relative with POI suggests a familial etiology, whereas a personal history of autoimmune disorders can suggest an autoimmune polyglandular syndrome. Women with POI have increased risk for development of autoimmune adrenal insufficiency.

Intrauterine adhesions are the only uterine cause of secondary amenorrhea. Amenorrhea results from the development of scar tissue within the uterine cavity preventing build up and shedding of endometrial cells. Adhesions develop following uterine instrumentation, most commonly associated with uterine curettage for pregnancy complications (Asherman syndrome).

Evaluation of Amenorrhea

A thorough history and physical examination is the first step in evaluating amenorrhea. Important data include medication and illicit drug exposure, changes in weight, exercise history, psychosocial stressors, and family history related to menarche. Symptoms can include headaches or visual changes suggesting pituitary pathology, symptoms of thyroid excess or deficiency, galactorrhea suggesting hyperprolactinemia, or vasomotor symptoms associated with estrogen deficiency.

Physical examination should include a pelvic examination to evaluate the vagina, cervix, and uterus for abnormalities. Imaging may be necessary to confirm a normal uterus. Physical examination should also include evaluation for features of Turner syndrome, such as a low hairline, webbed neck, shield chest, and widely spaced nipples.

In patients with primary or secondary amenorrhea, measurement of height, weight, and BMI is important. A low BMI (<18.5) may suggest FHA due to an eating disorder, excessive exercise, or systemic illness. A high BMI (≥30) is frequently seen in women with polycystic ovary syndrome (PCOS). Additional physical examination findings suggestive of PCOS include acne and hirsutism. Hypercortisolism is associated with acne and hirsutism, as well as abnormal fat pad distribution, centripetal obesity, facial plethora, proximal muscle weakness, and wide (>1 cm) violaceous striae. Vitiligo or other signs of autoimmune disease increase the likelihood of autoimmune POI. Breast examination should include assessment for expressible galactorrhea. Vulvovaginal atrophy suggests estrogen deficiency.

After ruling out pregnancy, initial laboratory testing in both primary and secondary amenorrhea should include measurement of FSH, thyroid-stimulating hormone (TSH), free thyroxine, and prolactin levels. Next steps are guided by these laboratory results (**Figure 12**).

If the TSH level is abnormal, evaluation and management of thyroid dysfunction should occur (see Disorders of the Thyroid Gland).

If the prolactin level is elevated, repeat prolactin testing is needed to confirm the diagnosis. A careful review of medications is essential because many drugs can cause hyperprolactinemia. Kidney and liver function testing is also required (see Disorders of the Pituitary Gland).

If the FSH level is elevated, testing should be repeated in 1 month with simultaneous serum estradiol testing. If the FSH

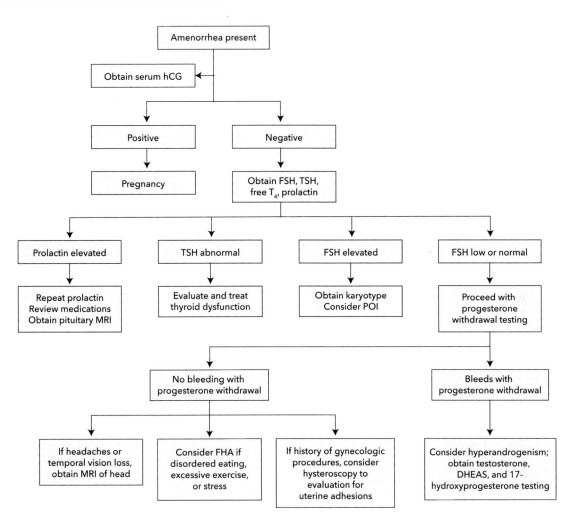

FIGURE 12. Algorithm for evaluating amenorrhea. FHA = functional hypothalamic amenorrhea; FSH = follicle-stimulating hormone; DHEAS = dehydroepiandrosterone sulfate; hCG = human chorionic gonadotropin; POI = primary ovarian insufficiency; T₄ = thyroxine; TSH = thyroid-stimulating hormone.

level is elevated on repeat testing and estradiol level is low, karyotype analysis is indicated to evaluate for Turner syndrome. POI and menopause also cause elevated FSH levels.

In women with normal or low FSH levels, the history and physical examination findings determine next steps. Further assessment of estrogen status can be determined by a progestin withdrawal test. If a normal estrogen state is confirmed (bleeding within a week of stopping progesterone), hyperandrogenism should be considered. Laboratory evaluation for hyperandrogenism includes measurement of total testosterone and sex hormone-binding globulin (SHBG) levels. PCOS is the most likely cause of menstrual dysfunction in women with hyperandrogenism; however, other hyperandrogenic disorders must be excluded before diagnosing PCOS. If no bleeding occurs, a low-estrogen state due to hypothalamic hypogonadism is most likely.

Imaging studies that can be utilized in the evaluation of amenorrhea include MRI of the sellar region (to evaluate for structural integrity of the pituitary), pelvic ultrasound (to assess for anatomic abnormalities of uterus, vagina, and ovaries), hysterosalpingogram and hysteroscopy (to assess for

uterine outflow obstructions). Choice of imaging study, as well as necessity of imaging at all, is predicated on prior biochemical test results indicating the cause of the amenorrhea.

KEY POINT

- After ruling out pregnancy, initial laboratory testing in both primary and secondary amenorrhea should include measurement of follicle-stimulating hormone, thyroid-stimulating hormone, free thyroxine, and prolactin.

Treatment of Amenorrhea

Almost all women with Turner syndrome will need exogenous estrogen therapy with cyclic progestin to prevent endometrial hyperplasia. Estrogen-progestin therapy is continued until age 51 years, the average age of menopause.

Treatment for FHA includes less-restrictive eating patterns, weight gain, or a reduction in strenuous exercise to restore menses. Additionally, it is important to treat conditions associated with FHA, including low bone mass, eating disorders, anxiety, and other mood disorders.

Amenorrhea due to hyperprolactinemia with a lactotroph adenoma is managed with dopamine agonist therapy if fertility is desired, or with estrogen/progestin if not, to prevent bone loss. If hyperprolactinemia-induced amenorrhea is related to medications that cannot be stopped (such as antipsychotic agents), estrogen/progestin therapy is indicated.

Treatment of POI includes estrogen/progestin therapy until approximately age 51 years. Psychosocial support is important due to higher scores on depression, anxiety, and negative affect scales in patients with POI; subspecialty consultation to discuss fertility options is also indicated.

Treatment of vaginal agenesis includes nonsurgical vaginal dilation; surgical options can be considered if nonsurgical therapy fails.

Hyperandrogenism Syndromes

Hirsutism and Polycystic Ovary Syndrome

Elevated serum concentrations of androgens in women most commonly manifest with hirsutism and may also present with acne, androgenetic alopecia, and/or virilization. Hirsutism is the presence of excessive terminal hair in male-pattern growth distribution; it affects approximately 10% of women. Virilization (voice deepening, clitoromegaly, male pattern baldness, severe acne) occurs only in severe hyperandrogenism and raises concern for ovarian hyperthecosis or an androgen-producing ovarian or adrenal tumor. Onset of hirsutism in a woman older than age 30 years also raises concern for an androgen-producing tumor. Although androgen-secreting ovarian tumors are rare, they should be considered in patients with abrupt, rapidly progressive hirsutism or severe hyperandrogenism as well as in women with marked hyperandrogenemia (total testosterone >150 ng/dL [5.2 nmol/L]).

Women with chronic hirsutism and menstrual cycles every 25 to 35 days most likely have idiopathic hirsutism or PCOS. Fifteen to 40% of women with hyperandrogenism and menses every 21 to 35 days have ovulatory dysfunction. PCOS is the most common cause of hirsutism, accounting for 95% of cases.

PCOS is a disorder characterized by hyperandrogenism and ovulatory dysfunction. PCOS affects 6% to 10% of women and is the most common cause of anovulatory infertility in women. It is associated with rapid GnRH pulses, an excess of LH, and insufficient FSH secretion, resulting in excessive ovarian androgen production and ovulatory dysfunction. It is accompanied by insulin resistance. Elevated insulin levels in PCOS further enhance ovarian and adrenal androgen production, as well as increase bioavailability of androgens related to a reduction in SHBG. PCOS is associated with increased incidence of metabolic syndrome, prediabetes, type 2 diabetes mellitus, hypercholesterolemia, and obesity.

There are a variety of diagnostic criteria for PCOS (**Table 40**). It is important to remember that PCOS is a diagnosis of exclusion; other causes of oligo-/anovulation must be considered including thyroid dysfunction, nonclassical congenital adrenal hyperplasia, hyperprolactinemia, and androgen-secreting tumors.

KEY POINTS

- Polycystic ovary syndrome is a disorder characterized by hyperandrogenism and ovulatory dysfunction affecting 6% to 10% of women.

- Polycystic ovary syndrome is a diagnosis of exclusion; other causes of oligo-/anovulation must be considered including thyroid dysfunction, nonclassical congenital adrenal hyperplasia, hyperprolactinemia, and androgen-secreting tumors.

Evaluation of Hyperandrogenism

The history and physical examination should include details about the onset of hirsutism and other symptoms/signs of hyperandrogenism, menstrual history, family history of hyperandrogenism, signs of insulin resistance (obesity, acanthosis nigricans, skin tags), distribution of terminal hair growth, and hair loss. Exposure to exogenous testosterone (topical, oral, or injected) should be assessed as a possible cause of hyperandrogenism and virilization.

Women with hirsutism should have total testosterone with SHBG measured, as well as morning 17-hydroxyprogesterone to screen for congenital adrenal hyperplasia. Laboratory evaluation for oligomenorrhea or amenorrhea (human chorionic gonadotropin [hCG], prolactin, FSH, TSH, free thyroxine) is also indicated. Serum dehydroepiandrosterone sulfate (DHEAS) measurement should be obtained in cases of recent onset of rapidly progressive hirsutism and/or virilization.

Markedly high DHEAS and/or testosterone levels are not consistent with PCOS. Patients with total testosterone levels

TABLE 40. Diagnostic Criteria for Polycystic Ovary Syndrome		
NIH Consensus Criteria 1990 (All Required)	**Rotterdam Criteria 2003 (Two of Three Required)**	**Androgen Excess and Polycystic Ovary Syndrome Society Criteria (All Required)**
Menstrual irregularity due to oligo-/anovulation	Oligo-/anovulation	Clinical and/or biochemical signs of hyperandrogenism
Clinical and/or biochemical signs of hyperandrogenism	Clinical and/or biochemical signs of hyperandrogenism	Ovarian dysfunction - oligo-/anovulation and/or polycystic ovaries on ultrasound
Exclusion of other disorders	Polycystic ovaries on ultrasound	Exclusion of other androgen excess or ovulatory disorders

greater than 200 ng/dL (6.9 nmol/L) or DHEAS values greater than 7.0 µg/mL (18.9 µmol/L) require imaging to assess for adrenal tumor (adrenal CT or MRI) or ovarian tumor (transvaginal ultrasound).

Management of Hyperandrogenism

Mechanical hair removal (threading, depilatories, electrolysis, laser) may be adequate for cosmesis in women with idiopathic hirsutism. First-line pharmacologic management of hirsutism is combined hormonal (estrogen-progestin) oral contraceptive agents; these agents suppress gonadotropin secretion and ovarian androgen production, as well as increase SHBG levels. Antiandrogen therapy (spironolactone) can be added for a better cosmetic response; concomitant contraception is mandatory with this therapy due to teratogenesis in male fetuses. Topical eflornithine is also approved for treatment of unwanted hair growth.

In PCOS, weight loss is a first-line intervention in patients with BMI of 25 or greater. Sustained weight loss of 5% to 10% improves androgen levels, menstrual function, and possibly fertility. Oral contraceptive agents are first-line pharmacologic therapy for hirsutism and menstrual dysfunction unless fertility is desired. An antiandrogen agent is added after 6 months if cosmesis is suboptimal with oral contraceptive agents. If fertility is desired, clomiphene citrate or letrozole can be used to correct oligo-/anovulation. Metformin reduces hyperinsulinemia and androgen levels but has minimal impact on hirsutism and ovulation.

Patients with PCOS should be screened for prediabetes/diabetes mellitus, hypercholesterolemia, obesity, hypertension, and obstructive sleep apnea due to increased risk for these conditions. Metformin is indicated when impaired glucose tolerance, prediabetes, or type 2 diabetes mellitus does not respond adequately to lifestyle modification.

KEY POINTS

- Oral contraceptive agents are first-line drug therapy for hirsutism and menstrual dysfunction; an antiandrogen agent may be added for better cosmetic response.
- Patients with polycystic ovary syndrome should be screened for prediabetes/diabetes mellitus, hypercholesterolemia, obesity, hypertension, and obstructive sleep apnea.

Female Infertility

Infertility evaluation is appropriate after 1 year of unprotected intercourse, on average twice weekly, in women younger than age 35 years and after 6 months in women age 35 years or older. Treatment of infertility is typically managed by a reproductive endocrinologist. Both partners should be evaluated concurrently; often, multiple factors are present (see Male Infertility).

History and physical examination findings may suggest the cause of infertility. Key factors include menstrual history (to determine ovulatory status) and assessment for thyroid dysfunction, galactorrhea, hirsutism, pelvic pain, dysmenorrhea, and dyspareunia. History of previous pregnancies, cancer therapy, substance use disorder, sexually transmitted infections, pelvic inflammatory disease, and gynecologic procedures should be explored. Frequency of coitus is important information. Physical examination should include BMI and assessment for signs of hyperandrogenism, estrogen deficiency, hyperprolactinemia, and thyroid dysfunction.

Assessment of ovulatory function is the first step in evaluation. Women with menses approximately every 28 days with molimina symptoms (breast tenderness, abdominal bloating, ovulatory pain) are likely ovulatory. In women without such cycles, assessment of ovulatory status is assessed with a midluteal phase serum progesterone level (obtained 1 week before the expected menses); a progesterone level greater than 3 ng/mL (9.5 nmol/L) is evidence of recent ovulation. If anovulatory cycles are suspected, the initial evaluation includes prolactin, TSH, and FSH measurements, with subsequent assessment for PCOS.

Hysterosalpingogram is used to assess for tubal occlusion and to evaluate the uterine cavity. Exploratory laparoscopy may be used if endometriosis or pelvic adhesions are suspected. If no abnormalities are found, fertility treatments will be offered under the direction of a reproductive endocrinologist, possibly including ovarian stimulation with clomiphene citrate or letrozole, intrauterine insemination, and in vitro fertilization, which may be offered to women age 40 years or older as first-line therapy.

KEY POINTS

- Infertility evaluation is appropriate after 1 year of unprotected intercourse in women younger than age 35 years and after 6 months in women age 35 years or older.
- Both partners should be evaluated concurrently; often, **HVC** multiple factors are present.
- Assessment of ovulatory function is the first step in evaluation for female infertility.

Physiology of Male Reproduction

The testes contain two anatomical units: the spermatogenic tubules composed of germ cells and Sertoli cells, and the interstitium containing Leydig cells. The three steroids of primary importance in male reproduction are testosterone, dihydrotestosterone, and estradiol. It is the pulsatile secretion of gonadotropin-releasing hormone (GnRH) by the hypothalamus that elicits pulsatile secretion of luteinizing hormone (LH) and follicle-stimulating hormone (FSH) by the gonadotroph cells of the anterior pituitary.

LH regulates testosterone synthesis in Leydig cells in a diurnal pattern; LH secretion is regulated by negative feedback of testosterone and estradiol. FSH regulates Sertoli cell spermatogenesis. Inhibin B is an important peptide inhibitor of pituitary FSH secretion (**Figure 13**). The hypothalamic-pituitary-testicular axis is sensitive to stressors, including acute and chronic illness, fasting, and strenuous exercise, all of which can lower testosterone levels.

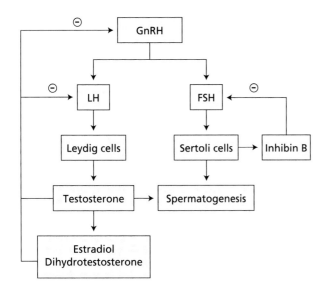

FIGURE 13. Male reproductive axis. Pulses of GnRH elicit pulses of LH and FSH. FSH acts on Sertoli cells, which assist sperm maturation and produce inhibin B, the major negative regulator of basal FSH production. The Leydig cells produce testosterone, which feeds back to inhibit GnRH and LH release. Some testosterone is irreversibly converted to dihydrotestosterone or estradiol, which are both more potent than testosterone in suppressing GnRH and LH. FSH = follicle-stimulating hormone; GnRH = gonadotropin-releasing hormone; LH = luteinizing hormone; − (circled) = negative feedback.

Hypogonadism

Causes

Male hypogonadism is a clinical syndrome that results from failure of the testes to produce physiologic levels of testosterone and a normal number of spermatozoa due to disruption of the hypothalamic-pituitary-testicular axis.

Primary hypogonadism is caused by testicular abnormalities. Common causes of acquired primary hypogonadism in adults include mumps orchitis, sequelae of radiation treatment, antineoplastic agents or toxins, testicular trauma or torsion, and acute and chronic systemic illnesses. Klinefelter syndrome (47,XXY) is the most common congenital cause of primary hypogonadism and is associated with tall stature, small testes, developmental delay, and socialization difficulties.

Secondary hypogonadism reflects a hypothalamic (GnRH) and/or pituitary (LH/FSH) deficiency. There are rare congenital causes, such as Kallmann syndrome, which are associated with anosmia. Common causes of acquired hypogonadotrophic hypogonadism are hyperprolactinemia, medications, critical illness, untreated sleep disorders, obesity, liver and kidney disease, alcoholism, marijuana use, and disordered eating. Tumors, trauma, thalassemias, and infiltrative diseases that cause disruption of gonadotropin production (such as sarcoidosis and hemochromatosis) are uncommon causes.

KEY POINT

- Primary hypogonadism is caused by testicular abnormalities; secondary hypogonadism reflects hypothalamic and/or pituitary dysfunction.

Clinical Features

Specific symptoms of hypogonadism in the adult male include decreased morning and spontaneous erections, decreased libido, mastodynia, gynecomastia, decreased need for shaving, and/or decreased axillary and genital hair. Hot flashes, decreased bone mass, and low-trauma fractures are associated with profound and/or longstanding testosterone deficiency. Nonspecific symptoms include decreased mood, energy, concentration, muscle strength and bulk, and stamina, as well as poor sleep and memory. Infertility is more likely to occur with primary than secondary hypogonadism.

Men who develop hypogonadism before puberty have small testes and phallus and lack secondary sexual characteristics. With onset after puberty, there may be some regression of secondary sexual characteristics. A decrease in testes and/or phallus size and development of gynecomastia in adults is more likely due to a primary cause.

Evaluation

Screening men with nonspecific symptoms of hypogonadism is not recommended. In men with specific signs and symptoms, measuring an 8 AM total testosterone level is indicated. If the testosterone level is low, a second 8 AM testosterone level is measured. The diagnosis is made with two low serum testosterone measurements. Measurement of free testosterone is appropriate in obese men because obesity lowers SHBG, leading to a falsely low measured total testosterone level. If testosterone is low, a serum LH measurement is indicated.

An elevated LH level reflects primary hypogonadism and further evaluation should be directed toward identifying the cause.

A low or normal LH level with simultaneous low testosterone reflects secondary hypogonadism. Medications including GnRH analogues (prostate therapy treatment), gonadal steroids (such as anabolic steroid use or megestrol for appetite stimulation), high-dose glucocorticoid treatment, and chronic opiate use can all suppress gonadotropins, resulting in secondary hypogonadism. Additional evaluation includes measurement of serum prolactin and screening for hemochromatosis. Assessment for other pituitary hormone deficiencies is indicated if signs or symptoms are present. Dedicated pituitary MRI should be performed if hyperprolactinemia is present, other pituitary hormone abnormalities are identified, testosterone level is less than 150 mg/dL (5.2 nmol/L), or if there are signs or symptoms of mass effect (**Figure 14**).

KEY POINTS

- Screening men with nonspecific symptoms of hypogonadism is not recommended.   **HVC**
- The diagnosis of male hypogonadism is made with two 8 AM low serum total testosterone measurements.

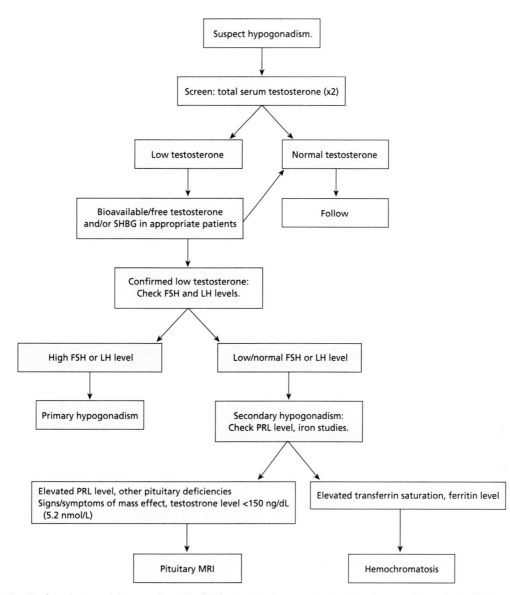

FIGURE 14. Algorithm for evaluating male hypogonadism. FSH = follicle-stimulating hormone; LH = luteinizing hormone; PRL = prolactin; SHBG = sex hormone-binding globulin; ×2 = two separate measurements.

Management

In men with biochemically proven hypogonadism, testosterone therapy can be initiated, after the etiology is determined. There are a variety of testosterone replacement preparations available (**Table 41**). The goal is to replace testosterone so that the measured total testosterone value is in the mid-normal range.

Clinical benefits of testosterone therapy include an increase in libido, lean muscle mass, fat free mass, bone density, and secondary sexual characteristics. Potential adverse effects include acne, impact on prostate tissue, obstructive sleep apnea, thrombophilia, and erythrocytosis (**Table 42**).

Testosterone therapy is only indicated for treatment of testosterone deficiency; it is not used for impaired spermatogenesis, and in fact further impairs spermatogenesis by suppressing pituitary FSH secretion. Patients should be counselled on the decreased fertility associated with exogenous testosterone therapy.

KEY POINTS

- After the etiology of hypogonadism is determined, testosterone therapy should be initiated with a goal of achieving a mid-normal range total testosterone measurement.
- Testosterone therapy is only indicated for treatment of testosterone deficiency; it is not used for impaired spermatogenesis.

HVC

TABLE 41. Recommended Testosterone Replacement Therapy

Route of Administration	Preparation	Typical Dosing Pattern	Timing of Initial Monitoring	Advantages; *Disadvantages*
Intramuscular injection	Testosterone cypionate	100-200 mg every 2 weeks	Testosterone midway between injections	Low cost; *fluctuation in testosterone level*
Intramuscular injection	Testosterone enanthate	100-200 mg every 2 weeks	Testosterone midway between injections	Low cost; *fluctuation in testosterone level*
Transdermal patch	Testosterone transdermal 24-hour patch	2-6 mg/day	Morning testosterone ~14 days after starting therapy	Stable levels; *skin rash/ poor adherence to skin*
Transdermal gel	AndroGel 1%	50-100 mg daily	Morning testosterone ~14 days after starting therapy	Stable levels; *potential for skin transfer to others*
Transdermal gel	AndroGel 1.62%	20.25-81 mg daily	Morning testosterone 14-28 days after starting therapy	Stable levels; *potential for skin transfer to others*
Transdermal gel	Fortesta	10-70 mg daily	2 hours after application ~14 days after starting therapy	Stable levels; *potential for skin transfer to others*
Transdermal gel	Testim	50-100 mg daily	Morning testosterone ~14 days after starting therapy	Stable levels; *potential for skin transfer to others*
Transdermal gel	Vogelxo	50-100 mg daily	Morning testosterone ~14 days after starting therapy, prior to application	Stable levels; *potential for skin transfer to others*
Transdermal solution	Axiron	30-120 mg daily	2-8 hours after application ~14 days after starting therapy	Stable levels; *potential for skin transfer to others*
Subcutaneous implants	Testosterone implant pellets	150-450 mg every 3-6 months	Measure at the end of the dosing interval	Infrequent dosing/Incision required for insertion; *risk of recurrent symptomatic hypogonadism as the duration of action is widely variable*

TABLE 42. Endocrine Society Clinical Guidelines for Monitoring Adverse Effects of Testosterone Replacement Therapy

Parameter	Recommended Screening Schedule	Alerts
Hematocrit	Value obtained at baseline and then at 3 months and 6 months after therapy initiation, followed by yearly measurements.	Value >54%
PSA level	For patients >40 years of age with a baseline value >0.6 ng/mL (0.6 µg/L), DRE and PSA level (determined at 3 and 6 months after therapy initiation followed by regular screening).	Increase >1.4 ng/ mL (1.4 µg/L) in 1 year or >0.4 ng/mL (0.4 µg/L) after 6 months of use; abnormal results on DRE; AUA prostate symptoms score/ IPSS >19

AUA = American Urological Association; DRE = digital rectal examination; IPSS = International Prostate Symptom Score; PSA = prostate-specific antigen.

Data from Bhasin S, Cunningham GR, Hayes FJ, Matsumoto AM, Snyder PJ, Swerdloff RS, et al; Task Force, Endocrine Society. Testosterone therapy in men with androgen deficiency syndromes: an Endocrine Society clinical practice guideline. J Clin Endocrinol Metab. 2010;95:2536-59. [PMID: 20525905]

Anabolic Steroid Abuse in Men

Abuse of anabolic steroids is a serious public health concern that goes beyond the professional athlete. The prevalence of anabolic steroids use in men approaches 7%. Steroids are often purchased on the internet and dosing patterns vary. Labile mood, acne, excessive muscle bulk, and small testes may indicate anabolic steroid abuse. Reproductive side effects of anabolic steroid abuse include gynecomastia (due to peripheral conversion of testosterone to estradiol), testicular atrophy, diminished spermatogenesis and fertility, and iatrogenic hypogonadotropic hypogonadism, which may be permanent. Laboratory evidence suggestive of anabolic steroid abuse includes elevated hematocrit, undetectable or low LH level, low SHBG level, and low total testosterone level with elevated testosterone precursor(s), such as androstenedione.

KEY POINTS

- Labile mood, acne, excessive muscle bulk, and small testes may indicate anabolic steroid abuse.

- Side effects of anabolic steroid abuse include gynecomastia, testicular atrophy, diminished spermatogenesis and fertility, and iatrogenic hypogonadotropic hypogonadism, which may be permanent.

Testosterone Changes in the Aging Man

With aging, total testosterone and free testosterone levels in men decline and SHBG increases, which results from testicular and hypothalamic-pituitary dysfunction. While serum testosterone levels decline 1% to 2% per year, most men do not become hypogonadal. Sperm production does not change significantly with age. The consequences of "andropause" are not fully elucidated, but adverse effects may include a negative impact on sexual function, muscle mass, erythropoiesis, and bone health.

The Endocrine Society supports treating older men with biochemically confirmed testosterone deficiency. The goal is replacement to a low-normal range of testosterone. Prior to initiation of treatment, some recommend shared decision making with the patient and discussion of the uncertainty of harms and benefits of testosterone therapy. This strategy is controversial.

Testosterone therapy in men without biochemical evidence of deficiency has not been shown to be beneficial, and studies have shown increased risk for cardiovascular disease and death, venous thromboembolism, and prostate cancer with use of testosterone therapy.

KEY POINTS

- Testosterone changes in men associated with aging do not result in symptomatic hypogonadism in most men.

HVC
- Testosterone therapy in men without biochemical evidence of deficiency has not been shown to be beneficial, and studies have shown increased risk for cardiovascular disease and death, venous thromboembolism, and prostate cancer with use of testosterone therapy.

Male Infertility

In couples with infertility, assessment of male infertility should be undertaken concurrently with female assessment. A comprehensive history should focus on potential causes of infertility: developmental history, chronic illness, infection, surgery, drugs and environmental exposures, sexual history, and prior fertility. Physical examination should focus on evidence of androgen deficiency, with careful examination of the external genitals. If testicular examination is abnormal, consider referral to a urologist. Semen analysis is the initial laboratory assessment; collection should occur after 2 to 3 days of sexual abstinence, but no longer to avoid decreased sperm motility. If semen analysis is abnormal, it should be repeated at least 2 weeks later, and if results are abnormal, referral to a reproductive endocrinologist is recommended.

KEY POINT

- Semen analysis is the initial laboratory assessment for male infertility; if results are abnormal, testing should be repeated at least 2 weeks later, with referral to a reproductive endocrinologist if results are abnormal again.

Gynecomastia

Gynecomastia, a benign proliferation of breast glandular tissue due to an increased action of estrogen relative to androgens, occurs in one- to two-thirds of older men. A thorough history and careful review of medications is necessary. Antiandrogen agents, such as spironolactone, cimetidine, and protease inhibitors, have a clear association with gynecomastia. Other identified causes include substance use disorder, malnutrition, cirrhosis, hypogonadism, testicular germ cell tumors, hyperthyroidism, and chronic kidney disease.

On physical examination, gynecomastia presents as a rubbery, concentric, subareolar mass. It is typically bilateral and may be tender if early in its course of development. Unilateral, nontender, and/or fixed breast masses should prompt an evaluation for breast cancer with a mammogram. Pseudogynecomastia is characterized by increased subareolar fat without glandular enlargement.

In a male presenting with painful gynecomastia, measurement of human chorionic gonadotropin, LH, morning total testosterone, and estradiol levels should be obtained if no clear cause is identified on history and physical examination.

Treatment of a specific cause of gynecomastia during the active proliferative phase may result in regression. If gynecomastia is longstanding, regression (spontaneously or with medical therapy) is unlikely due to fibrotic changes. In this scenario, plastic surgery referral may be the best option for cosmetic improvement.

KEY POINT

- Treatment of a specific cause of gynecomastia during the active proliferative phase may result in regression; if gynecomastia is longstanding, regression is unlikely due to fibrotic changes.

Transgender Hormone Therapy Management

Transgender medicine involves the care of persons whose gender identity differs from their sexual assignment at birth. Gender incongruence is persistent incongruence between gender identity and external sexual anatomy at birth not arising from a confounding mental disorder; gender dysphoria is discomfort arising from incongruence between a person's gender identity and their external sexual anatomy at birth. A transgender man is someone with a male gender identity and a female birth-assigned sex; a transgender woman is someone with a female gender identity and a male birth-assigned sex.

Transgender people may avoid health care because of discriminatory or disrespectful interactions in prior health care encounters. Providing a safe environment is critical to ensure that transgender people establish and continue primary and gendering-affirming care. It is important for providers to understand basic terminology used by the trans community, which varies regionally.

Psychological and medical care must be provided in an environment that avoids preconceptions, and proper environmental signage, terminology, and staff training is essential (see WPATH Standards of Care). Accurate collection of gender identity information is also important; many organizations use a "two-step" method to collect these data: (1) gender identity and (2) sex listed on the original birth certificate, thus avoiding invisibility of transgender status.

Prior to a physical examination, history taking is necessary to understand an individual's anatomic changes associated with gender-affirming hormone therapy (GAHT) and surgical intervention. Secondary sex characteristics present on a wide spectrum of development in transgender patients. Providers should offer appropriate health maintenance and cancer screening based on an individual's anatomy.

GAHT is the most common medical intervention sought by transgender people and does not require subspecialty care. Primary care providers, gynecologists, and endocrinologists may prescribe this therapy. Treatment includes medications for hirsutism (spironolactone), contraception (estradiol/progestin), abnormal uterine bleeding (estradiol/progestins), menopause (estradiol/progestin), testosterone deficiency (testosterone), and benign prostatic hyperplasia (5-α reductase inhibitors).

GAHT must be patient-centered and individualized to the patient's goals. A discussion of the risks/benefits associated with treatment and informed consent are essential before beginning treatment. Criteria to consider before initiating GAHT include persistent, well-documented gender dysphoria, capacity to make a fully informed decision, age of majority in a given country, and if present, control of significant medical or psychological conditions. GAHT limits fertility, thus reproductive options should be discussed with patients prior to initiation of GAHT. Endocrine Society Clinical Practice Guidelines for GAHT are available. With GAHT, most physical changes occur over the course of 2 years, but the exact timeline of change is highly variable.

Feminizing hormone therapy is typically estradiol in combination with an androgen blocker. Goals are breast development; fat redistribution; and reductions in muscle mass, body hair, erectile function, sperm count, and testicular size. Estrogen therapy increases risk of deep venous thrombosis (DVT) and, to a lesser extent based on cohort study results, ischemic stroke and myocardial infarction; contraindications to estrogen therapy include a history of DVT, estrogen-sensitive neoplasm, and end-stage liver disease. Tobacco cessation should be encouraged prior to initiation of estrogen therapy due to increased risk of DVT. Anti-androgen therapy, such as spironolactone, diminishes secondary male sex characteristics and minimizes the estrogen dose needed, thus reducing risks associated with high-dose exogenous estrogen therapy.

Monitoring testosterone and estradiol levels for adequate response to therapy is necessary for the first year.

Masculinizing hormone therapy is achieved using topical or injected testosterone with a goal of cessation of menses, facial hair growth, voice deepening, fat redistribution, increased muscle mass and body hair, and clitoral growth. Contraindications to testosterone therapy include pregnancy, unstable coronary artery disease, and polycythemia. Monitoring testosterone and estradiol levels for adequate response to therapy should occur for the first year. Hemoglobin also should be monitored.

Gender confirmation surgery is often the last intervention in transgender persons. Many transgender persons do not pursue surgery, but it is essential for alleviation of gender dysphoria in others. For transgender women, surgical procedures may include augmentation mammoplasty, genital surgery (penectomy, orchiectomy, vaginoplasty, clitoroplasty, vulvoplasty), and non-genital, non-breast surgery (facial feminization, voice surgery, thyroid cartilage reduction). For transgender men, surgical procedures may include mastectomy, hysterectomy with oophorectomy, phalloplasty, vaginectomy, scrotoplasty, and implantation of penile and/or testicular prostheses.

Stringent criteria must be met prior to undergoing irreversible gender reassignment surgery.

KEY POINTS

- Gender-affirming hormone therapy is the most common medical intervention sought by transgender people and does not require subspecialty care; criteria for gender-affirming hormone therapy include persistent, well-documented gender dysphoria, capacity to make a fully informed decision, age of majority in a given country, and if present, control of significant medical or psychological conditions.

- Screening and preventive medicine in transgender patients should be based on the individual's anatomy.

Calcium and Bone Disorders

Calcium Homeostasis and Bone Physiology

Regulation of serum calcium level is complex and dependent on the actions of vitamin D and parathyroid hormone (PTH). The primary effect of vitamin D is to enhance the absorption of calcium within the intestinal tract, whereas the effects of PTH are primarily mediated through regulation of calcium retention and excretion in the kidney (**Figure 15**). Measured calcium levels depend on the amount bound to albumin, which can be affected by nutrition and acid-base status. Hypoalbuminemia of any cause, such as cirrhosis or

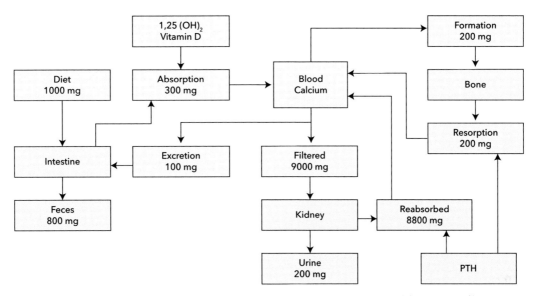

FIGURE 15. Neutral flux of calcium between bone and blood in adults is coordinated by parathyroid hormone (PTH). While most calcium filtered into urine is reabsorbed independent of PTH, PTH further increases retention of calcium from the urine. PTH indirectly augments calcium absorption in the gut by increasing production of 1,25 (OH)$_2$ vitamin D. Both effects of PTH are increasingly important at lower intakes of calcium and as blood levels of calcium decline. Amounts of calcium shown illustrate relative contribution of each organ to calcium homeostasis in a healthy adult.

malignancy-related cachexia, will cause low total calcium levels. When albumin concentration is low, measurement of ionized calcium or calculation of corrected total calcium is required to accurately assess calcium levels.

The level of vitamin D is determined by both production in the skin in response to sunlight and by ingestion, either from food or supplements. While vitamin D$_2$ (ergocalciferol) and vitamin D$_3$ (cholecalciferol) are available as supplements, the latter may be more efficacious due to greater potency, longer half-life, and being identical to that formed from ultraviolet light exposure. Activation of vitamins D$_2$ and D$_3$ requires hydroxylation initially by the liver and subsequently by the kidney, resulting in the active form of vitamin D, 1,25-dihydroxyvitamin D, calcitriol. 25-Hydroxyvitamin D is the storage form of vitamin D in the body, and measurement of 25-hydroxyvitamin D is the most appropriate test for assessing vitamin stores.

The initial response to a decline in serum calcium is an increase in PTH secretion, which decreases renal calcium excretion and increases calcium resorption from the bones to raise the serum calcium level. PTH also induces increased renal conversion of 25-hydroxyvitamin D to the active metabolite 1,25-dihydroxyvitamin D, which improves the efficiency of intestinal calcium absorption. Continued PTH-mediated mobilization of calcium from bone over months to years in response to chronic negative calcium balance can lead to metabolic bone disease. In contrast, the skeleton, gut, and vitamin D metabolism do not significantly contribute to the correction of hypercalcemia. Instead, an increased filtered load and suppression of PTH secretion leads to robust excretion of calcium by the kidneys provided that effective circulating volume is adequate.

In addition to its role in mineral metabolism, the adult skeleton provides a reservoir of calcium, structural support for mobility, muscle attachment, and protection of vital organs. Bone remodeling allows for continuous skeletal adaptation and repair. Osteocytes coordinate bone remodeling, which is initiated by osteoclastic resorption then followed by much slower osteoblastic bone formation and mineralization of a collagen/protein matrix. The entire skeleton is remodeled approximately every 10 years.

KEY POINTS

- The primary effect of vitamin D is to enhance the absorption of calcium within the intestinal tract, whereas the effects of parathyroid hormone are primarily mediated through regulation of calcium retention and excretion in the kidney.

- Measurement of 25-hydroxyvitamin D is the most appropriate test for vitamin D deficiency.

Hypercalcemia
Clinical Features of Hypercalcemia

Hypercalcemia is diagnosed when the calcium level exceeds normal levels, typically 10.5 mg/dL (2.6 mmol/L). Incidental finding of asymptomatic hypercalcemia on routine or screening blood tests is common.

Classic symptoms of hypercalcemia include polyuria, polydipsia, and nocturia. Additional symptoms may include anorexia, nausea, abdominal pain, constipation, and mental status changes. At higher levels, patients may become obtunded. Symptoms do not correlate linearly with serum calcium or PTH levels.

Severe hypercalcemia and hypercalciuria can lead to volume depletion and acute kidney injury, nephrolithiasis, or nephrocalcinosis. Skeletal manifestations reflect the underlying cause of hypercalcemia. Primary hyperparathyroidism may present as osteoporosis with fragility fractures and low bone density. Severe hyperparathyroidism from parathyroid carcinoma or secondary hyperparathyroidism due to kidney disease may be associated with bone pain and osteitis fibrosa cystica (a radiographic diagnosis). Hypercalcemia associated with lytic bone lesions is often the result of multiple myeloma or breast cancer.

KEY POINT

- Symptoms of hypercalcemia are variable but may include polyuria, polydipsia, nocturia, anorexia, nausea, abdominal pain, constipation, and mental status changes, and they may be associated with acute kidney injury, nephrolithiasis, nephrocalcinosis, and skeletal changes.

Causes and Diagnosis of Hypercalcemia

Clues to the underlying cause of hypercalcemia include the severity, acuity of illness, and patient factors including concurrent illnesses. Hypercalcemia is categorized as mild (<12 mg/dL [3 mmol/L]), moderate (12-14 mg/dL [3–3.5 mmol/L]), or (severe >14 mg/dL [3.5 mmol/L]). When hypercalcemia is incidentally noted, repeat measurement is indicated. If hypercalcemia is confirmed, simultaneous measurement of serum calcium and PTH is a critical first step in diagnosing the cause and categorizing PTH-mediated and non–PTH-mediated hypercalcemia. Ionized calcium measurement is not helpful when the serum albumin level is normal or when there are no acute acid-base disorders. A thorough history and physical examination, as well as careful review of all medications including supplements, should be done in all patients with hypercalcemia.

KEY POINT

- Initial diagnostic testing for hypercalcemia requires simultaneous measurement of serum calcium and parathyroid hormone (PTH), which allows classification as PTH-related and non–PTH-related disease.

Medications Causing Hypercalcemia

Thiazide diuretics may cause mild hypercalcemia, especially in the setting of previously unrecognized, mild primary hyperparathyroidism. Hypercalcemia associated with lithium therapy is due to altered PTH secretion and may occur years after initiation of therapy. If possible, stopping the medication and rechecking calcium levels is a reasonable first step in management. If the calcium returns to normal, this suggests the medication was responsible.

Parathyroid Hormone–Mediated Hypercalcemia

PTH secretion decreases abruptly in response to a rise in serum calcium concentration. Therefore, an elevated or inappropriately normal (usually in the upper half of the reference range) PTH level in a patient with hypercalcemia is diagnostic of PTH-mediated hypercalcemia (**Figure 16**). Patients with an elevated PTH level but normal levels of calcium and vitamin D (normocalcemic primary hyperparathyroidism) may be managed similarly to those with asymptomatic primary hyperparathyroidism.

Primary Hyperparathyroidism

Primary hyperparathyroidism is typically caused by a solitary parathyroid adenoma. Women are more often affected than men, with a peak incidence in the seventh decade of life. Hypercalcemia is usually mild (within 1 mg/dL [0.25 mmol/L] of the upper limits of normal) and may be intermittently normal. Hypercalciuria is present in up to 30% of patients. Since

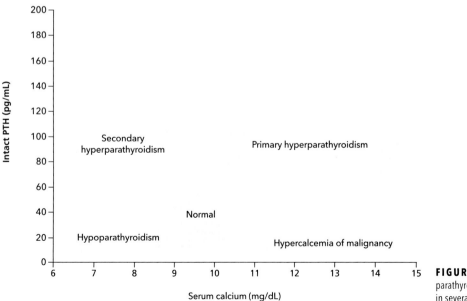

FIGURE 16. Relationship of calcium and parathyroid hormone (PTH) in normal conditions and in several diseases.

PTH enhances kidney phosphate excretion, low or low-normal serum phosphorus concentrations support the diagnosis. Assessment of bone mineral density (BMD) with dual-energy x-ray absorptiometry (DEXA) should include the nondominant forearm, which can be particularly affected in patients with hyperparathyroidism. Although parathyroid imaging with sestamibi or neck ultrasound may localize an adenoma, the presence of an adenoma does not influence the decision to proceed with surgery in the setting of primary hyperparathyroidism. Imaging may be beneficial to the surgeon for planning surgical intervention. In the absence of a history of calcium nephrolithiasis, kidney imaging may be indicated to exclude occult stones if this finding would change management.

Dietary calcium intake should be approximately 1000 mg/d to avoid further increases in urine calcium excretion and PTH secretion. Measurement of 25-hydroxyvitamin D and cautious correction of vitamin D deficiency is important. Repletion is recommended in patients whose levels are below 30 ng/dL (75 nmol/L) with careful attention to urine calcium excretion and serum calcium once vitamin D values are greater than 30 ng/dL (75 nmol/L).

Changes in specific endpoints during monitoring that lead to a recommendation for parathyroid surgery are outlined in **Table 43**. Surgery results in a 95% cure rate and less than 1% rate of complications with an experienced surgeon using minimally invasive techniques. Preoperative correction of vitamin D deficiency is important to avoid postoperative hypocalcemia, which is the result of relative hypoparathyroidism and reduced PTH-mediated production of 1,25-dihydroxyvitamin D culminating in a rapid flux of calcium into bone (hungry bone syndrome). Patients with mild primary hyperparathyroidism commonly require calcium supplementation for up to

1 week after parathyroidectomy until residual parathyroid tissue normalizes serum calcium concentrations. Reassessment of BMD 1 year after parathyroidectomy may show improvement in BMD, especially at the spine.

Approximately one in three patients with asymptomatic primary hyperparathyroidism who initially defer surgery will develop indications for surgery during 10 to 15 years of observation. In those not deemed eligible or who elect not to undergo surgery, evaluation should include annual measurement of serum calcium, creatinine, and glomerular filtration rate (GFR). If kidney stones are suspected, imaging and 24-hour urine collection for biochemical stone profile should be considered. BMD should be obtained every 2 years, and spine imaging should be considered if the patient has significant loss of height or back pain in the setting of a normal BMD.

KEY POINT

- Measurement of 25-hydroxyvitamin D and cautious correction of vitamin D deficiency is important in patients with primary hyperparathyroidism.

Parathyroid Carcinoma

Parathyroid carcinoma is very rare, but may present with symptoms of severe hypercalcemia, with serum levels greater than 14 mg/dL (3.5 mmol/L) and markedly high PTH concentrations. Imaging is not useful and fine-needle aspiration is not recommended due to concerns of tumor seeding. The primary treatment is surgical resection. Unfortunately, 50% of patients may have residual or recurrent disease. Severe hypercalcemia in parathyroid carcinoma that is not amenable to surgery can be treated chronically with cinacalcet. Medical management options are limited, and patients are most likely to die from complications of hypercalcemia.

Tertiary Hyperparathyroidism

In patients with end-stage kidney disease, multigland hyperplasia results from chronic stimulus of PTH (a sequela of long-standing secondary hyperparathyroidism) due to poorly controlled hypocalcemia and hyperphosphatemia. In some cases of secondary hyperparathyroidism, the serum calcium can normalize if the hyperplasia and associated PTH secretion is robust. Chronic stimulation of the parathyroid glands can lead to autonomous production of PTH by all four glands, resulting in hypercalcemia. Tertiary hyperparathyroidism is most commonly recognized after kidney transplantation. Although historically treated with subtotal multigland parathyroidectomy, the hypercalcemia can be resolved in most patients by treatment with paricalcitol or cinacalcet.

Genetic Causes of Hypercalcemia

Familial Hypocalciuric Hypercalcemia

Familial hypocalciuric hypercalcemia (FHH) is an autosomal dominant condition and the most common type of familial hypercalcemia. Patients are asymptomatic. The parathyroid glands and kidney detect serum calcium concentrations

TABLE 43.	Indications for Parathyroid Surgery During Monitoring
Assessment	**Indication[a]**
Serum calcium (>upper limit of normal)	>1 mg/dL (>0.25 mmol/L)
Skeletal	T-score <−2.5 at lumbar spine, total hip, femoral neck, or distal 1/3 radius; or a significant reduction in BMD[a]
	Vertebral fracture by x-ray, CT, MRI, or VFA
Renal	CrCl <60 mL/min
	Clinical development of a kidney stone or by imaging (x-ray, ultrasound, or CT)

CrCl = creatinine clearance; MRI = magnetic resonance imaging; VFA = vertebral fracture assessment.

[a]A significant change is defined by a reduction that is greater than the least significant change as defined by the International Society for Clinical Densitometry.

From Bilezikian JP, Brandi ML, Eastell R, Silverberg SJ, Udelsman R, Marcocci C, et al. Guidelines for the Management of Asymptomatic Primary Hyperparathyroidism: Summary Statement from the Fourth International Workshop. J Clin Endocrinol Metab. 2014;99:3561-9. [PMID: 25162665] through the calcium-sensing receptor (CaSR). In FHH, inactivating mutation of the CaSR gene causes the parathyroid gland to perceive serum calcium concentrations as low, resulting in increased PTH secretion and a higher serum calcium level. Simultaneously, the mutated CaSR in the kidney increases kidney reabsorption of calcium, leading to paradoxical hypocalciuria in the setting of hypercalcemia.

Although these patients appear to have primary hyperparathyroidism, FHH is a benign condition that is not treated with parathyroidectomy. Hypercalcemia will not resolve with surgery. Patients do not have sequelae of hypercalcemia, such as stones or osteoporosis. Signs suggestive of FHH include: mild hypercalcemia since childhood; low 24-hour urine calcium excretion, especially if calcium-creatinine clearance ratio is below 0.01; and/or family history of parathyroidectomy without resolution of hypercalcemia. If clinically ambiguous, the diagnosis can be confirmed by CaSR genetic testing.

KEY POINT

- The distinction between primary hyperparathyroidism and familial hypocalciuric hypercalcemia can be made by a 24-hour urine collection for calcium and creatinine, which will establish the amount of kidney calcium excretion and will allow evaluation of the calcium-creatinine clearance ratio.

Multiple Endocrine Neoplasia Syndrome

Primary hyperparathyroidism in adolescents and young adults may be the first sign of multiple endocrine neoplasia syndrome (MEN). Primary hyperparathyroidism is associated with MEN1 and MEN2A syndromes. If the family history reveals primary hyperparathyroidism, pituitary tumor, Zollinger-Ellison syndrome, early death from pancreatic neoplasm, pheochromocytoma, or medullary thyroid cancer, MEN is more likely and screening should be considered. In contrast to sporadic primary hyperparathyroidism, MEN syndromes have recurrence of hyperparathyroidism due to ongoing hyperplasia in the remaining parathyroid tissue after parathyroidectomy. MEN1 is associated with mutation of the tumor suppressor *MEN1* gene, and MEN2A is associated with mutation of the *RET* gene. This is best managed in conjunction with or by an endocrinologist.

Non–Parathyroid Hormone-Mediated Hypercalcemia

The differential diagnosis of hypercalcemia with suppressed PTH is broad. In patients with severe hypercalcemia, the history, symptoms, and findings may suggest the underlying cause. Treatment should commence without delay while awaiting results of laboratory testing. In PTH-independent hypercalcemic states, hypercalciuria can be severe and may precede hypercalcemia. PTH is usually undetectable but may be very low (<20 pg/mL [20 ng/L]) if hypercalcemia is mild.

Malignancy-Associated Hypercalcemia

The most common cause of non–parathyroid hormone-mediated hypercalcemia is malignancy, and it is typically severe (>14 mg/dL [3.5 mmol/L]). It is often the result of tumor-produced PTH-related protein (PTHrP) leading to extensive resorption of bone. Renal cell carcinoma, breast cancer, and squamous cell cancers are associated with PTHrP-related hypercalcemia. Rarely, locally mediated osteolysis from extensive skeletal metastases, typically in multiple myeloma and breast cancer, may cause efflux of calcium from bone resulting in significant hypercalcemia. For more information, see MKSAP 18 Hematology and Oncology.

Vitamin D–Dependent Hypercalcemia

Vitamin D–dependent hypercalcemia is associated with normal to elevated serum phosphorus levels because vitamin D enhances intestinal absorption of phosphorus and suppressed PTH secretion reduces kidney phosphorus excretion.

Unregulated conversion of 25-hydroxyvitamin D to 1,25-dihydroxyvitamin D may occur in granulomatous tissue associated with fungal infection, tuberculosis, sarcoidosis, and lymphoma, leading to increased intestinal absorption of calcium. These conditions are associated with an inappropriately normal or frankly elevated 1,25-dihydroxyvitamin D level and suppressed PTH. Decreased serum and urine calcium after intake of calcium and vitamin D is restricted or a rapid decrease in calcium after glucocorticoid therapy (which inhibits the hydroxylation of 25-hydroxyvitamin D) is consistent with these disorders.

Vitamin D intoxication from chronic high-dose ingestion of vitamin D (typically >50,000 units daily in patients without malabsorptive conditions) and increased storage in fat causes protracted hypercalciuria, nephrolithiasis, impaired kidney function, and elevated 25-hydroxyvitamin D levels.

Other Causes

Ingestion of large amounts of calcium typically from antacid use (for example, calcium carbonate), especially with coexistent chronic kidney disease, causes milk-alkali syndrome.

Glucocorticoid and mineralocorticoid replacement and volume repletion resolve the mild hypercalcemia sometimes associated with Addisonian crisis.

Severe thyrotoxicosis occasionally causes hypercalcemia or hypercalciuria by increasing bone resorption.

Acute prolonged immobilization, as seen in spinal cord injuries, can cause large efflux of calcium from the skeleton through uncoupled bone remodeling with decreased osteoblastic activity despite increased osteoclastic activity. Patients with primary hyperparathyroidism or skeletal metastases are predisposed to hypercalcemia due to immobilization as are young patients where increased bone remodeling is normal.

Management of Hypercalcemia

Management is dependent on the severity of the hypercalcemia. If mild (<12 mg/dL [3 mmol/L]), treatment of the underlying disorder (for example, parathyroidectomy in primary hyperparathyroidism) is sufficient. Hospitalization may be needed in patients with acute kidney injury, mental status changes, or calcium levels above 12 mg/dL (3 mmol/L). Initial treatment of severe hypercalcemia is aggressive hydration to replete volume loss and increase kidney excretion of calcium. Loop diuretics are not recommended unless kidney failure or heart failure is present, in which case volume expansion should precede the administration of loop diuretics to avoid hypotension and further kidney injury. For the acutely symptomatic patient, subcutaneous calcitonin can be used; however, the drug effect wanes after 48 hours. Long-term management of hypercalcemia may require intravenous bisphosphonate therapy to prevent mobilization of calcium from the skeleton, but requires adequate kidney function. Glucocorticoids and restriction of calcium and vitamin D intake are uniquely beneficial in vitamin D–dependent hypercalcemia. Hemodialysis is reserved for the treatment of severe hypercalcemia in oliguric patients. **H**

KEY POINT

- Initial treatment of moderate to severe hypercalcemia is aggressive hydration to replete volume loss and increase kidney excretion of calcium; loop diuretics are not recommended unless kidney failure or heart failure is present, in which case volume expansion should precede the administration of loop diuretics to avoid hypotension and further kidney injury.

Hypocalcemia

Clinical Features of Hypocalcemia

Signs and symptoms of hypocalcemia reflect its severity and acuity. Hypocalcemic disorders in outpatients are typically detected on screening blood tests and are mild, with serum calcium 7.5 to 8.9 mg/dL (1.9-2.2 mmol/L). It may also be detected during evaluation for low-intensity traumatic fractures or low bone mass. Most patients will be asymptomatic or report symptoms of intermittent paresthesia of the hands and feet or perioral numbness. Hypocalcemia due to chronic hypoparathyroidism can also be associated with cataract formation, basal ganglia calcification, papilledema, and dental enamel hypoplasia.

Patients with severe hypocalcemia may present with neuromuscular symptoms and signs. Carpopedal spasm with characteristic hand posture (flexion at metacarpophalangeal joints and extension at interphalangeal joints) may be spontaneous or triggered by transient distal limb ischemia during blood pressure assessment (Trousseau sign). Facial nerve hyperirritability and muscle spasm can be demonstrated by percussion of the facial nerve just anterior to the ear (Chvostek sign). Importantly, laryngospasm, seizure, myocardial dysfunction, and QT-interval prolongation leading to sudden cardiac death due to severe hypocalcemia (<7.5 mg/dL [1.9 mmol/L]) can occur without prodromal paresthesia or muscle cramping. **H**

KEY POINT

- Laryngospasm, seizure, myocardial dysfunction, and QT-interval prolongation leading to sudden cardiac death due to severe hypocalcemia (<7.5 mg/dL [1.9 mmol/L]) can occur without prodromal paresthesia or muscle cramping.

Causes and Diagnosis of Hypocalcemia

Hypocalcemia should be confirmed with a second measurement, which requires assessment of and correction for serum albumin concentrations. Ionized calcium measurement is indicated in the setting of fluctuating acid/base status. Simultaneous measurement of serum calcium, phosphorus, creatinine, and PTH is the next step. PTH should be elevated in the setting of hypocalcemia (see Figure 16).

Hypoparathyroidism

Hypoparathyroidism is most commonly caused by inadvertent injury during anterior neck surgery (thyroidectomy, parathyroidectomy) or surgery to treat parathyroid gland hyperplasia, both of which present within a few hours of surgery. Depending on the extent of injury/resection, surgical hypoparathyroidism may last days to weeks. Permanent hypoparathyroidism may be partial or complete; the latter is associated with undetectable serum PTH levels and a higher prevalence of hyperphosphatemia. **H**

Inappropriately normal PTH levels with concurrent hypocalcemia represents the former. Other causes of hypocalcemia due to insufficient PTH secretion include infiltrative disorders (hemochromatosis or Wilson disease), radiation, autoimmunity, and congenital disorders (such as 22q11.2 deletion syndrome). Chronic hypocalcemia with inappropriately normal PTH occurring within a family may represent an activating mutation of the *CaSR* gene. Hypomagnesemia, seen in the settings of malnutrition, alcoholism, and with use of loop diuretics and chronic proton pump inhibitor therapy, causes functional, reversible parathyroid hypofunction and must be excluded before a low or inappropriately normal PTH level is attributed to hypoparathyroidism. PTH resistance (pseudohypoparathyroidism) is a rare genetic cause of hypocalcemia.

KEY POINT

- Hypomagnesemia causes functional, reversible parathyroid hypofunction and must be excluded before a low or inappropriately normal parathyroid hormone level is attributed to hypoparathyroidism.

Other Causes of Hypocalcemia

Malnutrition and/or malabsorption of either or both vitamin D and calcium may be suspected based on clinical history (bariatric surgery, celiac disease) and confirmed by low serum 25-hydroxyvitamin D level or low 24-hour urine calcium excretion (a proxy indicator of calcium intake and absorption). The most common cause of acquired hypocalcemia is chronic kidney failure due to impaired production of 1,25-dihydroxy-vitamin D and hyperphosphatemia. Hypercalciuria is most often idiopathic, but can also be due to chronic loop diuretic use. Rhabdomyolysis and tumor lysis syndrome increase serum phosphorus and calcium phosphate binding in the vascular space, causing low ionized calcium.

Hungry bone syndrome (rapid flux of calcium into bone after parathyroidectomy for severe primary hyperparathyroidism) and widespread osteoblastic metastases (prostate cancer, breast cancer) can cause hypocalcemia, as can saponification of calcium (and magnesium) in necrotic fat in acute pancreatitis.

Potent antiresorptive drugs, such as intravenous bisphosphonates and denosumab, can cause severe and protracted hypocalcemia by impairing physiologic efflux of calcium from the skeleton in patients with vitamin D deficiency. Therefore, it is important to assess vitamin D levels and correct deficiency before beginning treatment with an antiresorptive drug.

Management of Hypocalcemia

Because severe neuromuscular complications of hypocalcemia can occur in the absence of prodromal muscle tetany, severe hypocalcemia (<7.5 mg/dL [1.9 mmol/L]) requires urgent treatment with intravenous calcium. Slow administration through central intravenous access with electrocardiographic monitoring is preferred. Alternatively, teriparatide 20 µg twice per day rapidly eliminates hypocalcemic symptoms in acute postsurgical hypoparathyroidism (off-label indication).

Vitamin D supplementation 1000 to 4000 IU/d and oral calcium carbonate or calcium citrate at doses of 1 to 3 g/d in divided doses may normalize or sufficiently treat mild or chronic hypocalcemia. Calcitriol is needed in the setting of hypoparathyroidism with undetectable PTH and kidney failure because 1,25-dihydroxyvitamin D activation requires both PTH and sufficient kidney function.

In chronic hypoparathyroidism, goals of therapy are to eliminate symptoms while avoiding complications of therapy. A reasonable goal for most patients is a serum calcium concentration at or just below the reference range without hypercalciuria. Monitoring of urine calcium excretion is mandatory because hypercalciuria often limits therapy. Correction of coexisting hypomagnesemia is also required. Thiazide diuretics are commonly used because they decrease urine calcium excretion.

Initial treatment of hyperphosphatemia is reduction of dietary phosphorus but occasionally requires the addition of oral phosphate binders if serum phosphorus exceeds the normal range. Recombinant human PTH is available for patients who do not meet treatment goals with calcium and calcitriol therapy alone.

KEY POINT

- A reasonable goal for most patients with hypoparathyroidism is a serum calcium concentration at or just below the reference range without hypercalciuria.

Metabolic Bone Disease

Low Bone Mass and Osteoporosis

Bone mass, mineral content, and macro- and microarchitecture determine bone strength. Bone mineral density (BMD) reflects bone mass and mineral content and, in older adults, predicts deterioration of microarchitecture. This relationship and epidemiologic data underpin the use of BMD determined by dual-energy x-ray absorptiometry (DEXA) to diagnose low bone mass and refine fracture risk assessment in older adults. Fragility fractures (those occurring with minimal trauma, equivalent or less than a fall from a standing height) after age 50 indicate low bone strength and define clinical osteoporosis regardless of BMD. Skull, feet, and hand fractures cannot, by definition, be fragility fractures.

Pathophysiology

Low bone mass in adults may represent poor bone formation, bone loss, or both. Factors that can affect peak bone mass formation include genetic conditions, lifestyle factors, and poor health, especially in the second decade of life. Net loss of bone mass can occur in adults when osteoclastic bone remodeling is faster than osteoblastic bone formation. The list of risk factors for low bone mass and osteoporosis is extensive and is included in **Table 44** and **Table 45**. Some patients, however, have osteoporosis caused by secondary causes. Testing for secondary causes is summarized in **Table 46**.

Screening for Osteoporosis

Current guidelines recommend screening average risk postmenopausal women beginning at age 65. Guidelines vary in their recommendations for routine screening for osteoporosis in men. The American College of Rheumatology recommends BMD testing within 6 months of starting long-term glucocorticoid therapy in adults 40 years of age and older and in adults under 40 years of age with risk factors for osteoporosis or a history of fragility fractures.

Patients with risk factors for low bone mass or osteoporosis, fragility fractures of the femur, vertebra (**Figure 17**), pelvis, humerus or radius, height loss of 4 cm (1.6 in) or more, or kyphosis, should have BMD testing earlier than standard screening recommendations. BMD may also be indicated if the risk of fractures is elevated based on the results of risk assessment tools such as the Simple Calculated Osteoporosis Risk Estimate (SCORE), Osteoporosis Self-Assessment Tool (OST), the Osteoporosis Risk Assessment Instrument (ORAI), and Fracture Risk Assessment Tool (FRAX). **Table 47** lists recommendations for BMD testing and vertebral imaging.

Screening of younger women may be indicated if one or more risk factors for osteoporosis are present. In premenopausal women without risk factors, assessment of BMD for fracture risk is not advised or validated. However, if testing is done in an otherwise healthy person, results that are below age- and gender-matched averages (Z-score <0) generally do not require further evaluation or serial monitoring.

TABLE 44. Risk Factors for Low Bone Density and Osteoporosis

Lifestyle/Modifiable	Non-Modifiable	Medications/Supplements
Alcohol use	Race/Ethnicity	Anticonvulsants
Immobilization	Age	Antiretroviral therapy (tenofovir)
BMI <17	Gender	Aromatase inhibitors
Low calcium intake	First-degree relative with low BMD	Calcineurin inhibitors
Smoking	Genetic	Depo-medroxyprogesterone
Vitamin D deficiency	Cystic fibrosis	Glucocorticoids (≥5 mg/day prednisone or equivalent for ≥3 months)
Weight loss	Hypophosphatasia	Heparin
Recurrent falls	Ehlers-Danlos	GnRH agonists
	Osteogenesis imperfecta	Proton pump inhibitors
		Thiazolidinediones
		Lithium
		Androgen deprivation therapy

BMD = bone mineral density; GnRH = gonadotropin-releasing hormone.

TABLE 45. Conditions and Comorbidities Associated with Increased Risk for Low Bone Mass and Osteoporosis

Endocrine	Gastrointestinal	Hematologic	Rheumatologic	Neurologic	Other
Anorexia nervosa	Bariatric surgery	Amyloidosis	Ankylosing spondylitis	Multiple sclerosis	AIDS/HIV
Cushing syndrome	Celiac disease	Leukemia and lymphoma	Rheumatoid arthritis	Muscular dystrophy	Chronic obstructive lung disease
Diabetes mellitus	Inflammatory bowel disease	Monoclonal gammopathies	Systemic lupus	Spinal cord injury with paralysis	End-stage kidney disease
Hyperparathyroidism	Malabsorption	Multiple myeloma			Idiopathic hypercalciuria
Hypogonadism	Primary biliary	Amyloidosis			
Thyrotoxicosis					
Turner syndrome					

TABLE 46. Diagnostic Studies to Evaluate for Secondary Causes of Osteoporosis

Blood Testing
Complete blood count
Calcium, phosphorus, and magnesium
Kidney function tests
Liver function tests
Thyroid-stimulating hormone
25-hydroxyvitamin D
Total testosterone (younger men)
Tryptase
Urine Testing
24-h urinary calcium
Urinary free cortisol level

Extent of testing should be influenced by clinical suspicion and severity of osteoporosis.

KEY POINT

- Current guidelines recommend screening average risk postmenopausal women beginning at age 65; screening recommendations for men vary by organization.

Diagnosis

In postmenopausal women and men over 50 years of age, the diagnosis of osteopenia is determined by BMD testing (T-score between -1 and -2.5) alone, whereas osteoporosis can be diagnosed clinically based on the presence of fragility fractures, hip fracture, vertebral compression fracture, or by DEXA. Without secondary causes of low BMD or a fragility fracture, osteoporosis is diagnosed when the femur neck, total hip, nondominant radius, or composite (two or more consecutive diagnostic vertebrae) lumbar spine T-score is -2.5 or less, as defined by the World Health Organization. If hip or spine cannot be accurately measured by BMD, DEXA of the distal third of the radius can be used.

Diagnosis of osteoporosis in premenopausal women and men under 50 years can be made with diagnosis of a fragility fracture or low bone mass on DEXA defined by a Z-score less than -2, which indicates "low bone mass for age."

BMD assessment using quantitative calcaneal ultrasonography may be used to screen for osteoporosis, but abnormal results require confirmation by DEXA. Quantitative CT provides a DEXA equivalent T-score, is not hindered by degenerative changes in the lumbar spine, and is highly sensitive for detection of vertebral compression fractures, but its cost and

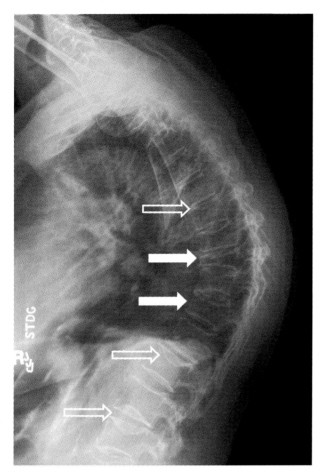

FIGURE 17. Asymptomatic vertebral compression fractures detected by spine radiograph in a patient with height loss and kyphosis. Depicted is vertebral endplate depression without loss of vertebral height in upper lumbar vertebrae (*empty arrows*) and severe wedging and height loss of multiple mid-thoracic vertebral bodies (*solid arrows*).

TABLE 47. Recommendations for Measurement of Bone Mineral Density and Vertebral Imaging
Bone Mineral Density Testing[a]
Women age 65 and older
For men, evidence is insufficient to assess the benefits/harms of screening for osteoporosis[b]
Postmenopausal women and men age 50 to 69, based on risk-factor profile
Those who have had a fracture, to determine degree of disease severity
Radiographic findings suggestive of osteoporosis or vertebral deformity
Glucocorticoid therapy for more than 3 months
Primary hyperparathyroidism
Vertebral Imaging[c]
Women ≥70 and men ≥80 if T-score at the spine, total hip, or femoral neck is ≤ −1.0
Women aged 65-69 and men aged 75-79 if T-score at the spine, total hip, or femoral neck is ≤1.5
In postmenopausal women age 50-64 and men aged 50-69 with the following risk factors:
Low-trauma fractures
Historic height loss of 1.5 in or more (4 cm)
Height loss of 0.8 inches or more (2 cm)
Recent or ongoing long-term glucocorticoid treatment

[a]BMD testing should be performed at DEXA facilities using accepted quality assurance measures.

[b]The National Osteoporosis Foundation recommends screening men 70 and older, and the Endocrine Society recommends screening men 70 and older and men aged 50-69 who have risk factors such as low body weight, prior fracture as an adult, or smoking.

[c]Vertebral imaging should be repeated when a new loss of height is noted or new back pain is reported.

radiation exposure are greater and is not recommended for osteoporosis screening.

KEY POINTS

- Osteoporosis can be diagnosed clinically based on fragility fractures, hip fracture, vertebral compression fracture, or a bone mineral density measurement of ≤-2.5.

HVC
- Quantitative CT provides a dual-energy x-ray absorptiometry equivalent T-score, is not hindered by degenerative changes in the lumbar spine, and is highly sensitive for detection of vertebral compression fractures, but its cost and radiation exposure are greater and is not recommended for osteoporosis screening.

Evaluation of Secondary Causes of Low Bone Mass

Non-modifiable factors are the most common cause of low bone mass, but there are many other causes (see Table 44 and Table 45). Low bone mass may be the presentation for conditions such as idiopathic hypercalciuria or celiac disease. All patients should have a thorough history and physical

examination and additional testing based on findings (see Table 46). Although BMD may not be required in all patients to make the diagnosis of osteoporosis, it may be helpful to determine if additional testing is needed and to guide treatment.

Osteomalacia

Osteomalacia is most commonly caused by severe and prolonged vitamin D deficiency, which results in inadequate concentrations of calcium and/or phosphate in the bone, which in turn prevents mineralization of newly formed bone matrix. Unlike osteoporosis, osteomalacia does not result in permanent loss of bone structure. A period of months to years of disordered mineralization is required before bone strength is compromised.

Symptoms of osteomalacia include diffuse bone pain, bone tenderness to palpation (tibial plateau and sternum), and proximal muscle weakness; however, early osteomalacia may present only with low bone mass on DEXA and can be indistinguishable from osteoporosis without further testing. Very low BMD (Z-score ≤-2), low or low-normal serum calcium and phosphorus levels, very low 25-hydroxyvitamin D (<10 ng/mL [25 nmol/L]) level, and secondary hyperparathyroidism distinguishes osteomalacia from osteoporosis. Elevated serum alkaline phosphatase level is particularly suggestive of osteomalacia, although mild elevation can be seen with recent osteoporotic fracture. Radiographs may display an unusual distribution of fractures in severe osteomalacia (**Figure 18**). When bone pain is not explained by conventional radiographic findings in the setting of suspected osteomalacia, imaging with radionuclide bone scan or MRI may reveal fractures.

The goal of treatment is to optimize conditions for bone mineralization using supplementation to normalize serum 25-hydroxyvitamin D (>30 ng/mL [75 nmol/L]), calcium, and phosphorus concentrations. The skeletal response to treatment is reflected by gradual normalization of alkaline phosphatase level and symptom relief. Resolution of osteomalacia may take as long as 12 months; subsequent BMD testing will show significant increases and/or normalization of BMD.

Other Causes

Low bone mass and fragility fractures in young and middle-aged adults may result from genetic disorders (see Table 45). Patients with mild (type 1) osteogenesis imperfecta may present with a history of childhood fractures that decrease in frequency as adults. Hypermobility raises suspicion for Ehlers-Danlos and related syndromes. Hypophosphatasia should be suspected in middle-aged patients with fractures and serum alkaline phosphatase levels well below the reference range.

Nonpharmacologic Management

Exercise involving weight-bearing, resistance, and balance is important for bone health and may reduce fracture risk at any age, but especially in patients over 65 years. Although the

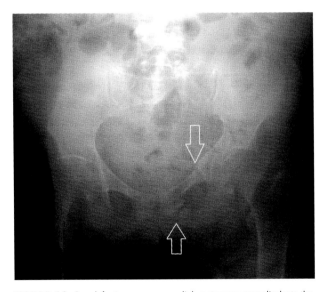

FIGURE 18. Pseudofractures appear as radiolucent areas perpendicular to the bone surface and are typically bilateral and/or symmetrical. The pubic rami (shown here), medial aspect of the proximal femur, proximal fibula, and metatarsals are common sites.

measurable treatment effect may be small, calcium and vitamin D were universally supplemented in osteoporosis pharmacotherapy trials; the National Academy of Medicine recommends calcium intake of 1000 to 1200 mg/d, ideally from dietary sources. A calcium supplement may be used for patients whose diets are insufficient, but should not be recommended independent of dietary assessment and intervention. As many osteoporosis clinical trials, including those testing pharmacotherapy, sought to achieve 25-hydroxyvitamin D levels of at least 30 ng/mL (75 nmol/L), a vitamin D supplement of 1000 to 2000 IU/d may be appropriate in the context of osteoporosis care.

Pharmacologic Management

The goal of treatment is reduce risk of fractures in patients with osteoporosis or those at increased risk of fracture (primary prevention). The U.S. National Osteoporosis Foundation recommends pharmacologic treatment for patients with osteoporosis-related hip or spine fractures, those with a BMD T-score of −2.5 or less, and those with a BMD T-score between −1 and −2.5 with a 10-year risk of 3% or greater for hip fracture or risk of 20% or greater for major osteoporosis-related fracture as estimated by the Fracture Risk Assessment Tool (FRAX). Some studies suggest that different thresholds for initiation of treatment should be considered in other at-risk populations. The American College of Rheumatology recommends treatment for glucocorticoid-induced osteoporosis based on age, gender, and fracture risk.

Pharmacotherapy may also be used to prevent loss of BMD in postmenopausal women at risk of osteoporosis and to prevent or treat glucocorticoid-induced osteoporosis. Although estrogen therapy may be considered for management of vasomotor symptoms in postmenopausal women, it is no longer considered first-line therapy for prevention of osteoporosis. The FDA has recently approved a combination pill, bazedoxifene and conjugated estrogen, for prevention of postmenopausal osteoporosis. FDA-approved drugs for treatment of osteoporosis and options for prevention are listed in **Table 48**.

Bisphosphonates

Oral bisphosphonates, alendronate and risedronate, are antiresorptive agents and are generally first-line treatment in postmenopausal women and men over 50 years of age. They have been shown to reduce the risk for spine, hip, and nonvertebral fractures. Another bisphosphonate, ibandronate, has only shown efficacy in reducing vertebral fractures. In glucocorticoid-induced osteoporosis with moderate to high fracture risk, oral bisphosphonates are recommended as first-line therapy in adult men and women regardless of age. Intravenous zoledronic acid once a year is an option if patients experience upper gastrointestinal symptoms or have difficulty taking the medication as directed. An acute-phase response reaction including pyrexia and myalgia may occur after first administration in as many as one in three patients, but does not occur typically with subsequent administrations. Bisphosphonates

TABLE 48. FDA-Approved Medications for Treatment and Prevention of Osteoporosis and Skeletal Sites of Proven Fracture Prevention When Used to Treat Osteoporosis

	Prevention		Documented Fracture Prevention			
	PMO	GIO	Recurrent	Hip	Vertebral	Non-Vertebral
Bisphosphonates						
Alendronate	√			√	√	√
Risedronate	√	√		√	√	√
Ibandronate	√				√	
Zoledronic acid (IV)	√	√	√	√	√	√
Denosumab				√	√	√
Raloxifene	√				√	
Anabolic						
Abaloparatide					√	√
Teriparatide					√	√

GIO = glucocorticoid-induced osteoporosis; PMO = postmenopausal osteoporosis.

are contraindicated in patients with reduced kidney function (glomerular filtration rate [GFR] <35 mL/min/1.73 m^2) and should not be given until vitamin D deficiency and hypocalcemia are treated, if present.

Rare side effects of antiresorptive agents are osteonecrosis of the jaw and atypical femur fracture. Osteonecrosis of the jaw may occur at any point in therapy; whereas the risk for atypical femur fracture appears to increase with duration of therapy. For most patients, the benefits in reduction of osteoporosis fractures far outweigh the risk of these uncommon side effects. A drug holiday can be considered in women who are not at high fracture risk after 3 years (intravenous) to 5 years (oral) of bisphosphonate treatment. In postmenopausal women at high risk due to a T-score -3.5 or below, previous osteoporotic fracture, or who sustain a fracture while on therapy, continuation of treatment for up to 10 years (oral) or 6 years (intravenous) should be considered. While there are no data to guide the duration of the drug holiday, factors taken into consideration include the bisphosphonate used and whether BMD is maintained on DEXA.

KEY POINTS

- Bisphosphonates are generally the first-line treatment of osteoporosis; only alendronate and risedronate reduce the risk for spine, hip, and nonvertebral fractures.

- A drug holiday can be considered in postmenopausal women who are not at high fracture risk after 3 years (intravenous) to 5 years (oral) of bisphosphonate treatment.

Receptor Activator of Nuclear Factor KB (RANK) Ligand Inhibitors

Denosumab is a monoclonal antibody that inhibits osteoclast activation. When administered subcutaneously twice yearly, denosumab suppresses bone resorption, increases bone density, and reduces the incidence of osteoporotic fractures in men and women. The effects of denosumab are not sustained when treatment is stopped. Denosumab may be preferred in patients with stage 4 chronic kidney disease and in those intolerant of or incompletely responding to bisphosphonate therapy. Adverse effects include hypocalcemia, especially in older patients with vitamin D deficiency, and an increased rate of cellulitis and bronchitis. Medication-related osteonecrosis of the jaw and atypical femur fracture have been reported with denosumab use as well.

Anabolic Agents

Teriparatide, rhPTH (1-34), is approved for use in postmenopausal women and men or women with glucocorticoid-induced osteoporosis who are at high risk of osteoporotic fracture. It is also used to improve bone mass in men with primary or hypogonadism-related osteoporosis at high risk of fracture. Abaloparatide, rhPTHrP (1-34), is approved for the treatment of postmenopausal women with osteoporosis at high risk for fracture. Both agents stimulate bone formation and require daily subcutaneous injection. Treatment should be limited to 2 years. Improvement in BMD is most evident at the spine. To prevent the loss of newly formed bone, sequential therapy with an antiresorptive agent must begin within 1 month of completing the course of anabolic treatment.

Follow-up of Patients with Low Bone Mass

Routine serial DEXA measurements of BMD are not indicated for follow-up of low-risk patients who do not have osteoporosis. Subsequent BMD testing depends on baseline BMD. Repeating after 15 years may be reasonable if the hip T-score is normal (>-1), while retesting at 2 years may be considered if the hip T-score is -2 to -2.4.

The primary reason for repeating BMD testing in patients taking antiresorptive agents is to detect treatment failure. Declining BMD, indicated by a statistically significant percent drop in g/cm² of bone (not declining T-scores in subsequent DEXA scans) or a fracture while on treatment, raises concern for an unrecognized secondary cause, nonadherence, or insufficient response that necessitates reevaluation. The American College of Physicians recommends against monitoring of bone mineral density during treatment because data from several studies showed that women treated with antiresorptive treatment benefited from reduced fractures even if BMD did not increase. Instead follow-up management should include review of indication for treatment, monitoring of adherence to treatment, and reinforcement of lifestyle measures to prevent fractures, minimize bone loss, and avoid frailty. Drug holiday from antiresorptive therapy usually involves measurement of BMD to establish a baseline and repeated measurement in 2 to 3 years. Although this approach would ostensibly inform subsequent treatment decisions, it has not been validated.

Vitamin D Deficiency

The most appropriate test to assess adequacy of vitamin D is measurement of serum 25-hydroxyvitamin D, which reflects dietary and skin-derived vitamin D. At least 20 ng/mL (50 nmol/L) is recommended to prevent metabolic bone disease in otherwise healthy populations and generally can be met with an intake of 600 to 800 IU/d.

Routine screening for vitamin D deficiency is not recommended in healthy populations; however, testing for deficiency is appropriate in groups at high risk or in patients presenting with low bone mass, fractures, hypocalcemia, or hyperparathyroidism. In patients with bone, parathyroid, or calcium disorders, to raise blood levels consistently above 30 ng/dL (75 nmol/L) may require 1000 to 2000 U/d. Patients with malabsorption, chronic lack of sun exposure, BMI greater than 40, advanced liver disease, and medications interfering with vitamin D metabolism, such as phenytoin and phenobarbital, may require 2000 to 4000 U/d for repletion and maintenance of vitamin D stores as guided by 25 hydroxyvitamin D levels obtained 3 months after initiation of treatment.

Loading doses using 50,000 U/d of either vitamin D_2 (ergocalciferol) or vitamin D_3 (cholecalciferol) once weekly for 8 weeks is appropriate in severe deficiency especially in the setting of malabsorption. Candidates for loading doses include: undetectable 25-hydroxyvitamin D, hypocalcemia, and osteomalacia due to vitamin D deficiency. Maintenance therapy of 1000 to 4000 U/d is recommended to maintain sufficiency after a loading dose.

Widespread public interest and a proliferation of scientific publications regarding vitamin D stem from established autocrine and paracrine effects in most tissues as well as extensive observational data associating 25-hydroxyvitamin D levels with extraskeletal health outcomes. However, intervention trials have not convincingly demonstrated a benefit of vitamin D supplementation on most disease outcomes, suggesting that low 25-hydroxyvitamin D levels may be a marker rather than a cause of ill health.

KEY POINT

- Routine screening for vitamin D deficiency is not recommended in healthy populations; however, testing for deficiency is appropriate in groups at high risk or patients presenting with low bone mass, fractures, hypocalcemia, or hyperparathyroidism. **HVC**

Paget Disease of Bone

Although Paget disease of bone may present with localized symptoms, it is most commonly diagnosed in asymptomatic older patients presenting with elevated alkaline phosphatase levels or incidental radiographic findings. Commonly affected bones include the skull, spine, sacrum, pelvis, femur, and tibia. The skeletal site and extent of involvement including rate of bone turnover determine clinical features. Involvement of weight-bearing bones of the lower extremity may result in bone pain, deformity, or fracture. Involvement of a bone approximating a joint can contribute to degenerative joint disease (**Figure 19**). Expansion of Pagetic bone of the upper spine or skull base may cause spinal cord or cranial nerve compression.

Diagnosis is based on radiographic findings of thickening of cortical bone, coarsened trabecular markings, and distortion and expansion of involved bone. Biopsy is rarely needed. Serum alkaline phosphatase, a marker of increased bone turnover, is generally elevated but may not be elevated in some patients with longstanding disease that has become metabolically inactive. Alkaline phosphatase may be elevated in other

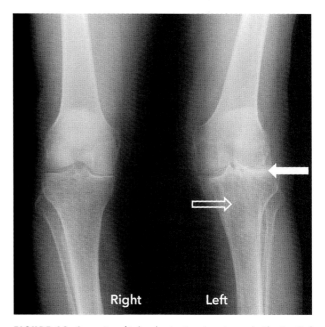

FIGURE 19. Coarsening of trabecular structures (*empty arrow*) without cortical deformity is diagnostic of Paget disease of bone in the proximal left tibia. Also shown is advanced degenerative arthritis in the adjacent left knee (*solid arrow*).

conditions, including vitamin D deficiency, other metabolic bone disease (such as osteomalacia), or recent fracture. Therefore, all patients with suspected Paget disease of bone require assessment of serum calcium, 25-hydroxyvitamin D, and a whole-body radionuclide bone scan. If the bone scan reveals other skeletal sites suspicious for Paget disease of bone, radiography of those sites is required for further evaluation.

Management of Paget disease is based on symptoms, location of involvement, and disease activity. Indications for treatment include: bone pain; risk for fracture and progressive deformity that could compromise bone, joint, or neurologic function; and elevated alkaline phosphatase concentrations. Bisphosphonates, particularly a one-time dose of 5 mg of intravenous zoledronic acid, often achieve the treatment goal of reducing pain and normalizing of alkaline phosphatase for up to 5 years. Oral bisphosphonates may also be used, but duration of treatment is variable.

Annual alkaline phosphatase levels should be monitored. Retreatment is indicated if previously normalized levels of alkaline phosphatase exceed normal levels. Imaging is required if there is a dramatic rise in alkaline phosphatase levels or acceleration in symptoms, which raises a concern for the rare sarcomatous transformation of Pagetic bone.

KEY POINTS

- Although Paget disease of bone may present with localized symptoms, it is most commonly diagnosed in asymptomatic older patients presenting with elevated alkaline phosphatase levels or incidental radiographic findings.

- Indications for treatment of Paget disease include bone pain; risk for fracture and progressive deformity that could compromise bone, joint, or neurologic function; and alkaline phosphatase concentrations.

- A one-time dose of intravenous zoledronic acid will often achieve the treatment goal of reducing pain and normalizing of alkaline phosphatase in patients with Paget disease of bone.

Bibliography

Disorders of Glucose Metabolism

American Diabetes Association. Standards of medical care in diabetes—2018. 2018; 41(Suppl 1): S1-S159.

Bergenstal RM, Klonoff DC, Garg SK, Bode BW, Meredith M, Slover RH, et al; ASPIRE In-Home Study Group. Threshold-based insulin-pump interruption for reduction of hypoglycemia. N Engl J Med. 2013;369:224-32. [PMID: 23789889] doi:10.1056/NEJMoa1303576

Cryer PE, Axelrod L, Grossman AB, et al. Evaluation and management of adult hypoglycemic disorders: an Endocrine Society Clinical Practice Guideline. J Clin Endocrinol Metabl. 2009; 94:709-28. [PMID: 19088155]

Duckworth W, Abraira C, Moritz T, Reda D, Emanuele N, Reaven PD, et al; VADT Investigators. Glucose control and vascular complications in veterans with type 2 diabetes. N Engl J Med. 2009;360:129-39. [PMID: 19092145] doi:10.1056/NEJMoa0808431

Garber AJ, Abrahamson MJ, Barzilay JI, et al. Consensus statement by the American Association of Clinical Endocrinologists and American College of Endocrinology on the comprehensive type 2 diabetes management algorithm-2018 executive summary. Endoc Pract. 2018; 24:91-120. [PMID: 29368965]

Hayward RA, Reaven PD, Wiitala WL, Bahn GD, Reda DJ, Ge L, et al; VADT investigators. Follow-up of glycemic control and cardiovascular outcomes in type 2 diabetes. N Engl J Med. 2015;372:2197-206. [PMID: 26039600] doi:10.1056/NEJMoa1414266

Holman RR, Paul SK, Bethel MA, Matthews DR, Neil HA. 10-year follow-up of intensive glucose control in type 2 diabetes. N Engl J Med. 2008;359:1577-89. [PMID: 18784090] doi:10.1056/NEJMoa0806470

Ismail-Beigi F, Craven T, Banerji MA, Basile J, Calles J, Cohen RM, et al; ACCORD trial group. Effect of intensive treatment of hyperglycaemia on microvascular outcomes in type 2 diabetes: an analysis of the ACCORD randomised trial. Lancet. 2010;376:419-30. [PMID: 20594588] doi:10.1016/S0140-6736(10)60576-4

Knowler WC, Barrett-Connor E, Fowler SE, Hamman RF, Lachin JM, Walker EA, et al; Diabetes Prevention Program Research Group. Reduction in the incidence of type 2 diabetes with lifestyle intervention or metformin. N Engl J Med. 2002;346:393-403. [PMID: 11832527]

Maldonado M, Hampe CS, Gaur LK, et al. Ketosis-prone diabetes: dissection of a heterogeneous syndrome using an immunogenetic and β-cell functional classification, prospective analysis, and clinical outcomes. J Clin Endocrinol Metab 2003;88:5090-98. [PMID: 14602731]

Marso SP, Daniels GH, Brown-Frandsen K, et al. Liraglutide and cardiovascular outcomes in type 2 diabetes. N Engl J Med. 2016; 375:311-322. [PMID:27295427]

Nathan DM, Cleary PA, Backlund JY, Genuth SM, Lachin JM, Orchard TJ, et al; Diabetes Control and Complications Trial/Epidemiology of Diabetes Interventions and Complications (DCCT/EDIC) Study Research Group. Intensive diabetes treatment and cardiovascular disease in patients with type 1 diabetes. N Engl J Med. 2005;353:2643-53. [PMID: 16371630]

Nathan DM, Zinman B, Cleary PA, Backlund JY, Genuth S, Miller R, et al; Diabetes Control and Complications Trial/Epidemiology of Diabetes Interventions and Complications (DCCT/EDIC) Research Group. Modern-day clinical course of type 1 diabetes mellitus after 30 years' duration: the diabetes control and complications trial/epidemiology of diabetes interventions and complications and Pittsburgh epidemiology of diabetes complications experience (1983-2005). Arch Intern Med. 2009;169:1307-16. [PMID: 19636033] doi:10.1001/archinternmed.2009.193

Neal B, Perkovic V, Mahaffey KW, de Zeeuw D, Fulcher G, Erondu N, et al; Canagliflozin and cardiovascular and renal events in type 2 diabetes. N Engl J Med. 2017;377:644-57. [PMID: 28605608]

Patel A, MacMahon S, Chalmers J, Neal B, Billot L, Woodward M, et al; ADVANCE Collaborative Group. Intensive blood glucose control and vascular outcomes in patients with type 2 diabetes. N Engl J Med. 2008;358:2560-72. [PMID: 18539916] doi:10.1056/NEJMoa0802987

Peters AL, Ahmann AJ, Battelino T, Evert A, Hirsch IB, Murad MH, et al. Diabetes technology-continuous subcutaneous insulin infusion therapy and continuous glucose monitoring in adults: an Endocrine Society Clinical Practice Guideline. J Clin Endocrinol Metab. 2016;101:3922-3937. [PMID: 27588440]

Qaseem A, Wilt TJ, Kansagara D, Horwitch C, Barry MJ, Forciea MA; Clinical Guidelines Committee of the American College of Physicians. Hemoglobin A1c targets for glycemic control with pharmacologic therapy for nonpregnant adults with type 2 diabetes mellitus: a guidance statement update from the American College of Physicians. Ann Intern Med. 2018 Mar 6. doi: 10.7326/M17-0939. [Epub ahead of print] PubMed PMID: 29507945.

Siu AL; U.S. Preventive Services Task Force. Screening for abnormal blood glucose and type 2 diabetes mellitus: U.S. Preventive Services Task Force recommendation statement. Ann Intern Med. 2015;163:861-868. [PMID: 26501513]

U.S. Department of Veterans Affairs/U.S. Department of Defense. VA/DoD Clinical Practice Guidelines for the management of diabetes mellitus in primary care. 2017. www.healthquality.va.gov/guidelines/cd/diabetes. Accessed May 16, 2018.

Whelton PK, Carey RM, Aronow WS, Casey DE Jr, Collins KJ, Dennison Himmelfarb C, et al; 2017 ACC/AHA/AAPA/ABC/ACPM/AGS/APhA/ASH/ASPC/NMA/PCNA guidelines for the prevention, detection, evaluation, and management of high blood pressure in adults: a report of the American College of Cardiology/American Heart Association Task Force on Clinical Practice Guidelines. J Am Coll Cardiol. 2017; doi: 10.1016/j.jacc.2017.11.006.

Zinman B, Wanner C, Lachin JM, et al. Empagliflozin, cardiovascular outcomes, and mortality in type 2 diabetes. N Engl J Med. 2015; 373: 2117-2128. [PMID: 26378978]

Disorders of the Pituitary Gland

Corsello SM, Barnabei A, Marchetti P, De Vecchis L, Salvatori R, Torino F. Endocrine side effects induced by immune checkpoint inhibitors. J Clin Endocrinol Metab. 2013;98:1361-75. [PMID: 23471977] doi:10.1210/jc.2012-4075

Fleseriu M, Hashim IA, Karavitaki N, Melmed S, Murad MH, Salvatori R, et al. Hormonal replacement in hypopituitarism in adults: an Endocrine Society Clinical Practice Guideline. J Clin Endocrinol Metab. 2016;101:3888-3921. [PMID: 27736313]

Freda PU, Beckers AM, Katznelson L, Molitch ME, Montori VM, Post KD, et al; Endocrine Society. Pituitary incidentaloma: an Endocrine Society Clinical Practice Guideline. J Clin Endocrinol Metab. 2011;96:894-904. [PMID: 21474686] doi:10.1210/jc.2010-1048

Guielman M, Basavilbaso, NG, Vitale M et al. Primary empty sella (PES). Pituitary. 2013;16:270-274. [PMID: 22875743]

Katznelson L, Laws ER Jr, Melmed S, Molitch ME, Murad MH, Utz A, et al; Endocrine Society. Acromegaly: an Endocrine Society Clinical Practice Guideline. J Clin Endocrinol Metab. 2014;99:3933-51. [PMID: 25356808] doi:10.1210/jc.2014-2700

Melmed S, Casanueva FF, Hoffman AR, Kleinberg DL, Montori VM, Schlechte JA, et al; Endocrine Society. Diagnosis and treatment of hyperprolactinemia: an Endocrine Society Clinical Practice Guideline. J Clin Endocrinol Metab. 2011;96:273-88. [PMID: 21296991] doi:10.1210/jc.2010-1692

Molitch ME, Clemmons DR, Malozowski S, Merriam GR, Vance ML; Endocrine Society. Evaluation and treatment of adult growth hormone deficiency: an Endocrine Society Clinical Practice Guideline. J Clin Endocrinol Metab. 2011;96:1587-609. [PMID: 21602453] doi:10.1210/jc.2011-0179

Nieman LK, Biller BM, Findling JW, Murad MH, Newell-Price J, Savage MO, et al; Endocrine Society. Treatment of Cushing's syndrome: an Endocrine Society Clinical Practice Guideline. J Clin Endocrinol Metab. 2015;100:2807-31. [PMID: 26222757] doi:10.1210/jc.2015-1818

Nieman LK, Biller BM, Findling JW, Newell-Price J, Savage MO, Stewart PM, et al. The diagnosis of Cushing's syndrome: an Endocrine Society Clinical Practice Guideline. J Clin Endocrinol Metab. 2008;93:1526-40. [PMID: 18334580] doi:10.1210/jc.2008-0125

Disorders of the Adrenal Glands

Bornstein SR, Allolio B, Arlt W, Barthel A, Don-Wauchope A, Hammer GD, et al. Diagnosis and treatment of primary adrenal insufficiency: an Endocrine Society Clinical Practice Guideline. J Clin Endocrinol Metab. 2016;101:364-89. [PMID: 26760044] doi:10.1210/jc.2015-1710

Fassnacht M, Arlt W, Bancos I, Dralle H, Newell-Price J, Sahdev A, et al. Management of adrenal incidentalomas: European Society of Endocrinology Clinical Practice Guideline in collaboration with the European Network for the Study of Adrenal Tumors. Eur J Endocrinol. 2016;175:G1-G34. [PMID: 27390021] doi:10.1530/EJE-16-0467

Funder JW, Carey RM, Mantero F, Murad MH, Reincke M, Shibata H, et al. The management of primary aldosteronism: case detection, diagnosis, and treatment: an Endocrine Society Clinical Practice Guideline. J Clin Endocrinol Metab. 2016;101:1889-916. [PMID: 26934393] doi:10.1210/jc.2015-4061

Lacroix A, Feelders RA, Stratakis CA, Nieman LK. Cushing's syndrome. Lancet. 2015 Aug 29;386(9996):913-27. doi: 10.1016/S0140-6736(14)61375-1. Epub 2015 May 21. Review. PubMed PMID: 26004339.

Lenders JW, Duh QY, Eisenhofer G, Gimenez-Roqueplo AP, Grebe SK, Murad MH, et al; Endocrine Society. Pheochromocytoma and paraganglioma: an Endocrine Society Clinical Practice Guideline. J Clin Endocrinol Metab. 2014;99:1915-42. [PMID: 24893135] doi:10.1210/jc.2014-1498

Libé R. Adrenocortical carcinoma (ACC): diagnosis, prognosis, and treatment. Front Cell Dev Biol. 2015;3:45. [PMID: 26191527] doi:10.3389/fcell.2015.00045

Nieman LK, Biller BM, Findling JW, Newell-Price J, Savage MO, Stewart PM, et al. The diagnosis of Cushing's syndrome: an Endocrine Society Clinical Practice Guideline. J Clin Endocrinol Metab. 2008;93:1526-40. [PMID: 18334580] doi:10.1210/jc.2008-0125

Rossi GP, Cesari M, Cuspidi C, Maiolino G, Cicala MV, Bisogni V, et al. Long-term control of arterial hypertension and regression of left ventricular hypertrophy with treatment of primary aldosteronism. Hypertension. 2013;62:62-9. [PMID: 23648698] doi:10.1161/HYPERTENSIONAHA.113.01316

Disorders of the Thyroid Gland

Alexander EK, Pearce EN, Brent GA, Brown RS, Chen H, Dosiou C, et al. 2017 Guidelines of the American Thyroid Association for the diagnosis and management of thyroid disease during pregnancy and the postpartum. Thyroid. 2017;27:315-389. [PMID: 28056690] doi:10.1089/thy.2016.0457

Burch HB, Cooper DS. Management of Graves disease: a review. JAMA. 2015;314:2544-54. [PMID: 26670972] doi:10.1001/jama.2015.16535

Cohen-Lehman J, Dahl P, Danzi S, Klein I. Effects of amiodarone therapy on thyroid function. Nat Rev Endocrinol. 2010;6:34-41. [PMID: 19935743] doi:10.1038/nrendo.2009.225

Cooper DS, Biondi B. Subclinical thyroid disease. Lancet. 2012;379:1142-54. [PMID: 22273398] doi:10.1016/S0140-6736(11)60276-6

De Leo S, Lee SY, Braverman LE. Hyperthyroidism. Lancet. 2016;388:906-18. [PMID: 27038492] doi:10.1016/S0140-6736(16)00278-6

Demers LM, Spencer CA. Laboratory medicine practice guidelines: laboratory support for the diagnosis and monitoring of thyroid disease. Clin Endocrinol (Oxf). 2003;58:138-40. [PMID: 12580927].

Fliers E, Bianco AC, Langouche L, Boelen A. Thyroid function in critically ill patients. Lancet Diabetes Endocrinol. 2015;3:816-25. [PMID: 26071885] doi:10.1016/S2213-8587(15)00225-9

Haugen BR, Alexander EK, Bible KC, Doherty GM, Mandel SJ, Nikiforov YE, et al. 2015 American Thyroid Association management guidelines for adult patients with thyroid nodules and differentiated thyroid cancer: the American Thyroid Association Guidelines Task Force on Thyroid Nodules and Differentiated Thyroid Cancer. Thyroid. 2016;26:1-133. [PMID: 26462967] doi:10.1089/thy.2015.0020

Hennessey JV. The emergence of levothyroxine as a treatment for hypothyroidism. Endocrine. 2017;55:6-18. [PMID: 27981511] doi:10.1007/s12020-016-1199-2

Kundra P, Burman KD. The effect of medications on thyroid function tests. Med Clin North Am. 2012;96:283-95. [PMID: 22443976] doi:10.1016/j.mcna.2012.02.001

Ross DS, Burch HB, Cooper DS, Greenlee MC, Laurberg P, Maia AL, et al. 2016 American Thyroid Association guidelines for diagnosis and management of hyperthyroidism and other causes of thyrotoxicosis. Thyroid. 2016;26:1343-1421. [PMID: 27521067]

Reproductive Disorders

Bhasin S, Brito JP, Cunningham GR, Hayes FJ, Hodis HN, Matsumoto AM, Snyder PJ, Swerdloff RS, Wu FC, Yialamas MA. Testosterone therapy in men with hypogonadism: an Endocrine Society Clinical Practice Guideline. J Clin Endocrinol Metab. 2018 May 1;103(5):1715-1744. [PMID: 29562364] doi: 10.1210/jc.2018-00229.

Bhasin S, Cunningham GR, Hayes FJ, Matsumoto AM, Snyder PJ, Swerdloff RS, et al; Task Force, Endocrine Society. Testosterone therapy in men with androgen deficiency syndromes: an Endocrine Society Clinical Practice Guideline. J Clin Endocrinol Metab. 2010;95:2536-59. [PMID: 20525905] doi:10.1210/jc.2009-2354

Bondy CA; Turner Syndrome Study Group. Care of girls and women with Turner syndrome: a guideline of the Turner Syndrome Study Group. J Clin Endocrinol Metab. 2007;92:10-25. [PMID: 17047017]

Brennan MJ. The effect of opioid therapy on endocrine function. Am J Med. 2013;126:S12-8. [PMID: 23414717] doi:10.1016/j.amjmed.2012.12.001

Fourman LT, Fazeli PK. Neuroendocrine causes of amenorrhea—an update. J Clin Endocrinol Metab. 2015;100:812-24. [PMID: 25581597] doi:10.1210/jc.2014-3344

Gordon CM. Clinical practice. Functional hypothalamic amenorrhea. N Engl J Med. 2010;363:365-71. [PMID: 20660404] doi:10.1056/NEJMcp0912024

Legro RS, Arslanian SA, Ehrmann DA, Hoeger KM, Murad MH, Pasquali R, et al; Endocrine Society. Diagnosis and treatment of polycystic ovary syndrome: an Endocrine Society Clinical Practice Guideline. J Clin Endocrinol Metab. 2013;98:4565-92. [PMID: 24151290] doi:10.1210/jc.2013-2350

Lindsay TJ, Vitrikas KR. Evaluation and treatment of infertility. Am Fam Physician. 2015;91:308-14. [PMID: 25822387]

Pope HG Jr, Wood RI, Rogol A, Nyberg F, Bowers L, Bhasin S. Adverse health consequences of performance-enhancing drugs: an Endocrine Society scientific statement. Endocr Rev. 2014;35:341-75. [PMID: 24423981] doi:10.1210/er.2013-1058

Transgender Hormone Therapy Management

American Psychological Association. Guidelines for psychological practice with transgender and gender nonconforming people. Am Psychol. 2015 Dec;70(9):832-64. doi: 10.1037/a0039906. PubMed PMID: 26653312. www.apa.org/practice/guidelines/transgender.pdf. Accessed May 15, 2018.

Center for Excellence for Transgender Health website. www.transhealth.ucsf.edu/trans?page=guidelines-home. Accessed May 15, 2018.

Coleman E, Bockting W, Botzer M, et al. Standards of care for the health of transsexual, transgender, and gender-nonconforming people, version 7. Int J Transgend. 2012;13:165.

Getahun D, Nash R, Flanders WD, Baird TC, Becerra-Culqui TA, Cromwell L, et al. Cross-sex hormones and acute cardiovascular events in transgender persons: a cohort study. Ann Intern Med. 2018 Jul 10. doi: 10.7326/M17-2785. [Epub ahead of print] PubMed PMID: 29987313.

Hembree WC, Cohen-Kettenis P, Delemarre-van de Waal HA, Gooren LJ, Meyer WJ 3rd, Spack NP, et al; Endocrine Society. Endocrine treatment of transsexual persons: an Endocrine Society Clinical Practice Guideline. J Clin Endocrinol Metab. 2009;94:3132-54. [PMID: 19509099] doi:10.1210/jc.2009-0345

Wylie K, Knudson G, Khan SI, Bonierbale M, Watanyusakul S, Baral S. Serving transgender people: clinical care considerations and service delivery models in transgender health. Lancet. 2016;388:401-11. [PMID: 27323926] doi:10.1016/S0140-6736(16)00682-6

Calcium and Bone Disorders

Adler RA, El-Hajj Fuleihan G, Bauer DC, Camacho PM, Clarke BL, Clines GA, et al. Managing osteoporosis in patients on long-term bisphosphonate treatment: report of a task force of the American Society for Bone and Mineral Research. J Bone Miner Res. 2016;31:1910. [PMID: 27759931] doi:10.1002/jbmr.2918

Bilezikian JP, Brandi ML, Eastell R, Silverberg SJ, Udelsman R, Marcocci C, et al. Guidelines for the management of asymptomatic primary hyperparathyroidism: summary statement from the Fourth International Workshop. J Clin Endocrinol Metab. 2014;99:3561-9. [PMID: 25162665] doi:10.1210/jc.2014-1413

Black DM, Rosen CJ. Postmenopausal osteoporosis [Letter]. N Engl J Med. 2016;374:2096-7. [PMID: 27223157] doi:10.1056/NEJMc1602599

Brandi ML, Bilezikian JP, Shoback D, Bouillon R, Clarke BL, Thakker RV, et al. Management of hypoparathyroidism: summary statement and guidelines. J Clin Endocrinol Metab. 2016;101:2273-83. [PMID: 26943719] doi:10.1210/jc.2015-3907

Buckley L, Guyatt G, Fink HA, Cannon M, Grossman J, Hansen KE, et al. 2017 American College of Rheumatology Guideline for the Prevention and Treatment of Glucocorticoid-Induced Osteoporosis. Arthritis & Rheumatology. 2017;69(8):1521-37.[PMID: 28585373] doi:10.1002/art.40137

Camacho PM, Petak SM, Binkley N, Clarke BL, Harris ST, Hurley DL, et al. American Association of Clinical Endocrinologist and American College of Endocrinology Clinical Practice Guidelines for the Diagnosis and Treatment of Postmenopausal Osteoporosis - 2016. Endocrine Practice. 2016;22(9):1111-8. [PMID 27643923] doi: 10.4158/EP161435.ESGL

Cosman F, de Beur SJ, LeBoff MS, Lewiecki EM, Tanner B, Randall S, et al; National Osteoporosis Foundation. Clinician's guide to prevention and treatment of osteoporosis. Osteoporos Int. 2014;25:2359-81. [PMID: 25182228] doi:10.1007/s00198-014-2794-2

Manson JE, Brannon PM, Rosen CJ, Taylor CL. Vitamin D deficiency - is there really a pandemic? N Engl J Med. 2016;375:1817-1820. [PMID: 27959647]

Singer FR, Bone HG 3rd, Hosking DJ, Lyles KW, Murad MH, Reid IR, et al; Endocrine Society. Paget's disease of bone: an Endocrine Society Clinical Practice Guideline. J Clin Endocrinol Metab. 2014;99:4408-22. [PMID: 25406796] doi:10.1210/jc.2014-2910

Endocrinology and Metabolism Self-Assessment Test

This self-assessment test contains one-best-answer multiple-choice questions. Please read these directions carefully before answering the questions. Answers, critiques, and bibliographies immediately follow these multiple-choice questions. The American College of Physicians (ACP) is accredited by the Accreditation Council for Continuing Medical Education (ACCME) to provide continuing medical education for physicians.

The American College of Physicians designates MKSAP 18 Endocrinology and Metabolism for a maximum of 19 *AMA PRA Category 1 Credits*™. Physicians should claim only the credit commensurate with the extent of their participation in the activity.

Successful completion of the CME activity, which includes participation in the evaluation component, enables the participant to earn up to 19 medical knowledge MOC points in the American Board of Internal Medicine's Maintenance of Certification (MOC) program. It is the CME activity provider's responsibility to submit participant completion information to ACCME for the purpose of granting MOC credit.

Earn Instantaneous CME Credits or MOC Points Online

Print subscribers can enter their answers online to earn instantaneous CME credits or MOC points. You can submit your answers using online answer sheets that are provided at mksap.acponline.org, where a record of your MKSAP 18 credits will be available. To earn CME credits or to apply for MOC points, you need to answer all of the questions in a test and earn a score of at least 50% correct (number of correct answers divided by the total number of questions). Please note that if you are applying for MOC points, you must also enter your birth date and ABIM candidate number.

Take either of the following approaches:

- Use the printed answer sheet at the back of this book to record your answers. Go to mksap.acponline.org, access the appropriate online answer sheet, transcribe your answers, and submit your test for instantaneous CME credits or MOC points. There is no additional fee for this service.

- Go to mksap.acponline.org, access the appropriate online answer sheet, directly enter your answers, and submit your test for instantaneous CME credits or MOC points. There is no additional fee for this service.

Earn CME Credits or MOC Points by Mail or Fax

Pay a $20 processing fee per answer sheet and submit the printed answer sheet at the back of this book by mail or fax, as instructed on the answer sheet. Make sure you calculate your score and enter your birth date and ABIM candidate number, and fax the answer sheet to 215-351-2799 or mail the answer sheet to Member and Customer Service, American College of Physicians, 190 N. Independence Mall West, Philadelphia, PA 19106-1572, using the courtesy envelope provided in your MKSAP 18 slipcase. You will need your 10-digit order number and 8-digit ACP ID number, which are printed on your packing slip. Please allow 4 to 6 weeks for your score report to be emailed back to you. Be sure to include your email address for a response.

If you do not have a 10-digit order number and 8-digit ACP ID number, or if you need help creating a username and password to access the MKSAP 18 online answer sheets, go to mksap.acponline.org or email custserv@acponline.org.

CME credits and MOC points are available from the publication date of December 31, 2018, until December 31, 2021. You may submit your answer sheet or enter your answers online at any time during this period.

Item 1

A 32-year-old woman is seen for follow-up evaluation of thyroid nodules. At her visit 2 weeks ago, a 3-cm right thyroid nodule and 2-cm right lateral neck mass were palpated on examination. The patient is asymptomatic. At age 12 she was treated with combination chemotherapy plus involved-field radiation for Hodgkin lymphoma. There is no family history of thyroid disease.

Laboratory studies show a serum thyroid-stimulating hormone level of 3.0 µU/mL (3.0 mU/L). Results of other laboratory studies are normal.

Thyroid ultrasound demonstrates a 3.1 × 2.8 × 1.6-cm hypoechoic solid right thyroid nodule with irregular margins. Right cervical lymphadenopathy was confirmed on ultrasonography.

Which of the following is the most likely diagnosis?

(A) Benign follicular thyroid nodule

(B) Follicular thyroid cancer

(C) Medullary thyroid cancer

(D) Papillary thyroid cancer

Item 2

A 45-year-old woman is evaluated for management of type 2 diabetes mellitus diagnosed 3 months ago. She was asymptomatic at diagnosis with an initial hemoglobin A_{1c} value of 9.7%. Her initial interventions included lifestyle modifications with weight loss and metformin. She is motivated to continue to lose weight. Medical history is significant for hypertension, hyperlipidemia, and frequent vulvovaginal candidiasis. She has no family history of thyroid or pancreatic malignancy. Medications are metformin, lisinopril, and atorvastatin.

On physical examination, vital signs are normal. BMI is 30. The remainder of the examination is unremarkable.

Results of laboratory studies show a hemoglobin A_{1c} level of 9.1%. Chemistry panel and creatinine levels are normal.

Which of the following is the most appropriate management for this patient's diabetes?

(A) Initiate empagliflozin

(B) Initiate glipizide

(C) Initiate insulin glargine

(D) Initiate liraglutide

Item 3

A 33-year-old man is evaluated for fatigue, headache, loss of appetite, and nausea for 6 months' duration. He has lost 9.1 kg (20 lb). Medical history is unremarkable, and he takes no medications.

On physical examination, temperature is normal, blood pressure is 118/70 mm Hg sitting and 98/68 mm Hg standing, pulse rate is 88/min sitting and 106/min standing, and respiration rate is 18/min. BMI is 19. The remainder of the physical examination is normal.

Laboratory studies:

Potassium	5.6 mEq/L (5.6 mmol/L)
Sodium	136 mEq/L (136 mmol/L)
Adrenocorticotropic hormone (ACTH)	450 pg/mL (99 pmol/L)
Cortisol, 8 AM	2.6 µg/dL (71.8 nmol/L)

Which of the following is the most appropriate next test?

(A) Cosyntropin stimulation test

(B) 21-Hydroxylase antibody measurement

(C) Pituitary MRI

(D) Serum aldosterone measurement

Item 4

A 23-year-old woman is seen in follow-up for evaluation of amenorrhea of 4 months' duration. Her only other medical problem is schizophrenia treated with risperidone.

On physical examination, vital signs and physical examination are normal.

Laboratory studies:

Prolactin	220 ng/mL (220 µg/L)
Thyroid-stimulating hormone	2.2 µU/mL (2.2 mU/L)
Thyroxine (T_4), free	1.2 ng/dL (15.5 pmol/L)
Urine human chorionic gonadotropin	Negative

Which of the following is the most appropriate next step?

(A) Obtain a pituitary MRI

(B) Start cabergoline

(C) Start an oral contraceptive

(D) Stop risperidone

Item 5

A 22-year-old woman is evaluated for loss of appetite and fatigue and 4.5-kg (10-lb) weight loss over the past 6 months. Medical history is otherwise unremarkable, and she takes no medications.

On physical examination, blood pressure is 100/70 mm Hg and pulse rate is 94/min. Other vital signs are normal. BMI is 22. The patient looks tanned, even in areas not exposed to the sun, and has buccal and palmar hyperpigmentation.

Laboratory studies:

Potassium	5.3 mEq/L (5.3 mmol/L)
Sodium	134 mEq/L (134 mmol/L)
Adrenocorticotropic hormone (ACTH)	650 pg/mL (143 pmol/L)
Cortisol	2.8 µg/dL (77.3 nmol/L)

Which of the following is the most appropriate treatment?

(A) Dexamethasone twice daily

(B) Hydrocortisone twice daily

(C) Hydrocortisone twice daily and fludrocortisone once daily

(D) Prednisone twice daily

(E) Prednisone twice daily and fludrocortisone once daily

Item 6

A 72-year-old man is evaluated during a follow-up office visit. Medical history is significant for prostate cancer managed with active surveillance since the age of 69 years. His only symptom is new-onset upper back pain. He takes no medication.

On physical examination, vital signs are normal. The upper spine is tender to palpation.

Laboratory studies show a serum calcium level of 9.9 mg/dL (2.5 mmol/L), serum creatinine level of 1.2 mg/dL (106.1 µmol/L), and prostate-specific antigen less than 4 ng/mL (4 µg/L).

Whole body radionuclide bone scan shows focal increased uptake at T7. There are no other abnormalities. Spine radiograph shows coarsening of trabeculae and expansion of body of T7 without cortical disruption consistent with Paget disease of bone.

Which of the following is the most appropriate management?

(A) Alkaline phosphatase measurement
(B) Bone mineral density testing
(C) Thoracic spine CT scan
(D) Zoledronic acid therapy

Item 7

A 25-year-old woman is evaluated for anterior neck pain, fatigue, exercise intolerance, excessive sweating, and tremors that began 6 weeks ago. Other than an upper respiratory infection 2 months ago, she has been healthy. Medical history is otherwise unremarkable, and she takes no medications.

On physical examination, pulse rate is 105/min. Other vital signs are normal. The patient's thyroid gland is tender to palpation and is without discrete nodules. No thyroid bruit is auscultated. Bilateral lid lag is noted, but there is no proptosis, conjunctival injection, or chemosis. There is a fine tremor of her outstretched hands. Deep tendon reflexes are brisk.

Laboratory studies show a serum thyroid-stimulating hormone (TSH) level less than 0.01 µU/mL (0.01 mU/L), a serum free thyroxine (T_4) level of 2.8 ng/dL (36.1 pmol/L), and a serum total triiodothyronine (T_3) level of 190 ng/dL (2.9 nmol/L). Urine pregnancy test is negative.

Which of the following is the most likely diagnosis?

(A) Graves disease
(B) Molar pregnancy
(C) Subacute thyroiditis
(D) Toxic multinodular goiter

Item 8

A 24-year-old woman is evaluated for management of type 1 diabetes mellitus. She was first diagnosed at 13 years of age. Having recently completed nursing school, the patient is motivated to gain control of diabetes to prevent complications, particularly diabetic neuropathy. Her only medication is insulin lispro, delivered through continuous subcutaneous insulin infusion pump therapy.

On physical examination, blood pressure is 142/92 mm Hg; the remainder of the vital signs is normal. BMI is 26. A comprehensive foot examination is normal.

Laboratory studies show hemoglobin A_{1c} level of 8.7% and an LDL cholesterol level of 110 mg/dL (2.8 mmol/L).

Which of the following is the most appropriate measure to reduce the risk of diabetic neuropathy?

(A) Improve blood pressure control
(B) Improve glycemic control
(C) Improve lipid control
(D) Initiate pregabalin
(E) Weight loss

Item 9

A 77-year-old woman is evaluated in the emergency department for new-onset generalized weakness and myalgia 2 days after receiving zoledronic acid for a recent diagnosis of osteoporosis. Medical history is significant for rheumatoid arthritis. She is mainly sedentary and uses a walker for ambulation. She lives alone and prepares her own meals. Her medications are zoledronic acid, methotrexate, prednisone, folic acid, and tramadol.

On physical examination, vital signs are normal; however, she develops hand spasm during the blood pressure measurement. BMI is 18. The patient is frail appearing. There is ulnar deviation at the metacarpophalangeal joints of both hands, but no signs of active synovitis.

Laboratory studies show a calcium level of 7.5 mg/dL (1.9 mmol/L).

Which of the following is the most likely diagnosis?

(A) Hungry bone syndrome
(B) Hyperphosphatemia
(C) Hypoparathyroidism
(D) Hypovitaminosis D

Item 10

A 65-year-old woman is evaluated for a 6-month history of increased facial and body hair and loss of scalp hair. Her voice has become deeper. Medical history is otherwise unremarkable, and she takes no medications. She has been menopausal since age 52 years.

On physical examination, blood pressure is 140/95 mm Hg and pulse rate is 82/min. Other vital signs are normal. BMI is 28. There are coarse dark hairs on the upper lip, chin, chest, and abdomen. She also has a deep voice, frontal hair loss, and clitoromegaly.

Laboratory studies show a total testosterone level of 89 ng/dL (3.1 nmol/L) and a dehydroepiandrosterone sulfate (DHEAS) level of 890 µg/dL (24.0 µmol/L) (normal <50-450 µg/dL [1.35-12.2 µmol/L]).

Which of the following is the most appropriate diagnostic test to perform next?

(A) Abdominal CT
(B) Adrenal vein sampling
(C) Pelvic MRI
(D) Pelvic ultrasound

Item 11

A 70-year-old man was admitted to the hospital 3 days ago with an ST-elevation myocardial infarction complicated by pulmonary edema and atrial fibrillation. He underwent emergency cardiac catheterization and left anterior descending (LAD) artery stent placement. Today the patient is feeling much better with complete resolution of his initial presenting symptoms.

Medications are aspirin, atorvastatin, clopidogrel, lisinopril, metoprolol, and low-molecular-weight heparin.

On physical examination, pulse rate is 92/min. Other vital signs are normal.

Cardiac examination reveals new findings of an irregularly irregular rhythm and an S_4. His physical examination is otherwise normal.

Laboratory studies obtained at the time of cardiac catheterization:

Thyroid-stimulating hormone (TSH)	0.2 µU/mL (0.2 mU/L)
Thyroxine (T_4), total	6.5 µg/dL (83.8 nmol/L)
Thyroxine (T_4), free	1.0 ng/dL (12.9 pmol/L)
Triiodothyronine (T_3), total	60 ng/dL (0.9 nmol/L)

Which of the following is the most likely diagnosis?

(A) Central hypothyroidism
(B) Heparin-induced thyroid function test abnormality
(C) Nonthyroidal illness syndrome
(D) Subclinical hyperthyroidism

Item 12

A 27-year-old woman was diagnosed with a 2-cm left cortisol-producing adrenal adenoma. She is admitted to the hospital for an adrenalectomy. Medical history is otherwise unremarkable, and she takes no medications.

On physical examination, blood pressure is 152/88 mm Hg; the remainder of the vital signs is normal. Centripetal obesity, facial plethora, fat deposition in the supraclavicular areas, and wide violaceous striae are present.

Which of the following is the most appropriate management following adrenalectomy?

(A) Epinephrine
(B) Fludrocortisone
(C) Hydrocortisone
(D) Phenoxybenzamine

Item 13

A 47-year-old man is evaluated during a follow-up visit to manage fatigue and decreased libido. Medical history is significant for hypertension and dyslipidemia. Medications are hydrochlorothiazide and atorvastatin.

On physical examination, vital signs are normal. He has normal hair distribution, no gynecomastia, and normal testicular examination.

Laboratory studies obtained at 3 PM revealed a total testosterone level of 275 ng/dL (9.5 nmol/L) and a luteinizing hormone level of 5 mU/mL (5 U/L).

Which of the following is the most appropriate management?

(A) Initiate testosterone replacement therapy
(B) Measure serum iron and total iron binding capacity
(C) Measure testosterone at 8 AM
(D) Obtain pituitary MRI

Item 14

A 58-year-old woman is evaluated during a follow-up visit 6 months after thyroidectomy for differentiated papillary thyroid cancer. She developed symptomatic hypocalcemia following surgery but is currently asymptomatic. Medications are calcium citrate, calcitriol, and levothyroxine.

Vital signs and physical examination are normal.

Laboratory studies:

Calcium	9.5 mg/dL (2.4 mmol/L)
Creatinine	1.0 mg/dL (88.4 µmol/L)
Phosphorus	4.5 mg/dL (1.5 mmol/L)
Magnesium	2.3 mg/dL (0.95 mmol/L)
Parathyroid hormone	<10 pg/mL (10 ng/L)

Which additional measurement is appropriate now?

(A) Bone mineral density
(B) 1,25-Dihydroxyvitamin D
(C) 24-Hour urine calcium
(D) 25-Hydroxyvitamin D
(E) Ionized calcium

Item 15

A 52-year-old woman is evaluated for a 1-year history of a 6.8-kg (15-lb) weight gain, easy bruising, hypertension, and worsening diabetes control. Medical history is also significant for a history of depression and anxiety. Medications are metformin and lisinopril.

On physical examination, blood pressure is 155/97 mm Hg and pulse rate is 82/min. Other vital signs are normal. BMI is 33. The patient has central obesity, supraclavicular and dorsocervical fat pads, and facial hirsutism. There are a few bruises on her arms and no abdominal striae.

Laboratory studies show a 24-hour urine free cortisol level of 205 µg/24 h, (564.9 nmol/24 h), midnight salivary cortisol of 298 ng/mL (821.2 nmol/L)(normal <100 ng/mL [275.6 nmol/L]), and adrenocorticotropic hormone (ACTH) less than 5 pg/mL (1.1 pmol/L).

Which of the following is the most likely cause of this patient's hypercortisolism?

(A) Adrenal tumor
(B) Bronchial carcinoid
(C) Pituitary tumor
(D) Psychiatric illness

Item 16

A 27-year-old man is evaluated for decreased libido. He is a professional body builder and reports longstanding use of anabolic steroids to improve physical appearance and muscular performance. His medical history is otherwise unremarkable, and he currently takes no medications other than anabolic steroids.

On physical examination, vital signs are normal. He has a muscular build, acne, bilateral symmetric gynecomastia, and small testes.

Laboratory studies:

Hematocrit	52%
Follicle-stimulating hormone	2 mU/mL (2 U/L)
Luteinizing hormone	3 mU/mL (3 U/L)
Testosterone, total (8 AM)	170 ng/dL (5.9 nmol/L)

Liver enzyme testing is normal.

Which of the following is the most appropriate management?

(A) Anastrozole

(B) Cessation of anabolic steroid use

(C) Clomiphene citrate

(D) Human chorionic gonadotropin

(E) Testosterone replacement

Item 17

A 25-year-old woman comes to the office to establish care. She is 5 weeks pregnant. She has hypothyroidism due to Hashimoto thyroiditis that was diagnosed 4 years ago. She is asymptomatic. Her only medications are levothyroxine and folic acid.

On physical examination, vital signs are normal. The patient's thyroid gland is nontender and diffusely enlarged without nodules. Pregnancy test is positive.

Serum thyroid-stimulating hormone level measured 4 months ago was 2.2 µU/mL (2.2 mU/L).

Which of the following is the most appropriate management of this patient's hypothyroidism?

(A) Check serum thyroid-stimulating hormone in 2 months

(B) Decrease levothyroxine dose by 30%

(C) Increase levothyroxine dose by 30%

(D) Stop levothyroxine and start liothyronine

Item 18

A 34-year-old transgender woman is evaluated during a routine examination. She desires gender-affirming hormone therapy. Her gender incongruence diagnosis has been made and confirmed by qualified medical providers. She smokes one pack of cigarettes per day, with a 15-pack-year history. Medical history is otherwise unremarkable. She takes no medications.

On physical examination, vital signs are normal. She has male hair distribution. Normal male genitalia are present. There are no evident inguinal hernias.

In addition to advising smoking cessation, which of the following is the most appropriate next step in management?

(A) Initiation of an androgen blocker

(B) Initiation of estradiol therapy

(C) Refer for gender confirmation surgery consultation

(D) Refer for discussion on fertility preservation options

(E) Return for treatment 1 year after living in desired gender role

Item 19

A 54-year-old woman is evaluated for flushing of the face of 1 year's duration. These episodes occur two or three times per week and last about 30 minutes. She went through menopause at age 50 and is on estrogen and progesterone hormone therapy. She also experiences episodes of anxiety, diaphoresis, and tachycardia. Medical history is significant for increasingly frequent migraine headaches, difficult to control hypertension, and gastroesophageal reflux disease. Medications are amitriptyline, chlorthalidone, metoprolol, conjugated estrogens, progesterone, and omeprazole.

On physical examination, blood pressure is 156/92 mm Hg; the remainder of the vital signs is normal. BMI is 32. The remainder of the examination is unremarkable.

Which of the following medications should be discontinued prior to screening for secondary causes of hypertension?

(A) Amitriptyline

(B) Chlorthalidone

(C) Metoprolol

(D) Omeprazole

(E) Progesterone

Item 20

A 74-year-old woman is seen in follow-up for osteoporosis diagnosed 5 years ago. She has been taking alendronate (70 mg weekly) without adverse effect for 5 years. Medical history is otherwise unremarkable. Alendronate is her only medication.

On physical examination, vital signs are normal. She has no kyphosis or height loss, and the remainder of her examination is also normal.

Her recent bone mineral density by dual-energy x-ray absorptiometry (DEXA) scan showed a lumbar spine T-score of –2.2 and femoral neck T-score of –2.4.

Which of the following is the most appropriate management?

(A) C-terminal peptide of type 1 collagen (CTx) measurement

(B) Continue alendronate for 5 additional years

(C) Decrease alendronate dose

(D) Discontinue alendronate

Item 21

A 67-year-old woman is evaluated for management of her type 2 diabetes mellitus. Medical history is significant for type 2 diabetes diagnosed 15 years ago, hypertension, hyperlipidemia, and obesity. She also has diabetic complications including nephropathy, retinopathy, and neuropathy. She does not have hypoglycemia. Medications are enalapril, atorvastatin, insulin glargine, insulin aspart, and metformin.

On physical examination, vital signs are normal. BMI is 31. Ophthalmoscopic examination reveals nonproliferative diabetic retinopathy. A foot examination reveals an insensate foot with intact skin. Vibratory sense is absent in the toes and ankle. The remainder of the physical examination is unremarkable.

Laboratory studies show a hemoglobin A_{1c} level of 7.7% and serum creatinine level of 1.4 mg/dL (123.8 µmol/L). She has had a gradual decline in her estimated glomerular filtration rate (eGFR) from 50 to 39 mL/min/1.73 m² over the last 5 years.

Which of the following is the most appropriate management?

(A) Continue current regimen

(B) Discontinue metformin dose

(C) Increase insulin glargine dose

(D) Increase glipizide dose

Item 22

A 19-year-old woman is evaluated for irregular menstrual cycles since menarche at 12 years of age, increasing amount of coarse facial hair, and acne. Symptoms have worsened since she stopped playing high school sports and subsequently gained weight. She is most concerned about the hair growth and acne. Medical history is otherwise unremarkable, and she takes no medications.

On physical examination, vital signs are normal. BMI is 31. She has coarse terminal hair on the upper lip and chin, acne on the face and back, and non-discolored striae on the abdomen. There is no galactorrhea and no other evidence of virilization such as deepening of the voice, clitoromegaly, or male pattern balding.

Laboratory studies show a total testosterone level of 73 ng/dL (2.5 nmol/L), dehydroepiandrosterone sulfate level of 1.8 µg/mL (4.9 µmol/L), and hemoglobin A_{1c} of 5.4%. Other laboratory results are normal. Serum pregnancy test is negative.

In addition to exercise and weight loss, which of the following is the most appropriate next step in management?

(A) Combined oral contraceptive therapy

(B) Metformin

(C) Pelvic ultrasound

(D) Spironolactone

Item 23

A 43-year-old man is evaluated for a change in his usual migraine headache. The headaches are now more frequent and respond poorly to his previously effective migraine headache medications. His medical history is otherwise unremarkable. Medications include ibuprofen and sumatriptan.

On physical examination, vital signs are normal. Physical examination including funduscopic examination is normal.

MRI reveals a 1-cm pituitary adenoma with suprasellar extension with no compression or abutment of the optic chiasm or optic nerves.

Laboratory studies show a cortisol level of 17 µg/dL (469.2 nmol/L), thyroid-stimulating hormone level of 2.6 µU/mL (2.6 mU/L), and thyroxine (T_4) level of 1.2 ng/dL (15.5 pmol/L).

Which of the following is the most appropriate diagnostic test to perform next?

(A) Measurement of prolactin and insulin-like growth factor 1 (IGF-1)

(B) Measurement of urine free cortisol

(C) Visual field examination

(D) No further evaluation is needed

Item 24

A 42-year-old woman is evaluated prior to surgery following a diagnosis of pheochromocytoma. Her symptoms are palpitations, hypertension, and sweating for 8 months' duration. Medications are lisinopril and hydralazine.

On physical examination, blood pressure is 155/98 mm Hg. Other vital signs and the remainder of the examination are normal.

Which of the following is the most appropriate next step in management?

(A) Increase hydralazine

(B) Increase lisinopril

(C) Start chlorthalidone

(D) Start metoprolol

(E) Start phenoxybenzamine

Item 25

A 60-year-old man is evaluated during a routine office visit. He was diagnosed with type 2 diabetes mellitus 6 years ago. Medical history is significant for coronary artery disease, hypertension, hyperlipidemia, and biliary pancreatitis. Medications are lisinopril, metoprolol, metformin, aspirin, and atorvastatin.

On physical examination, other than a blood pressure of 152/91 mm Hg, the vital signs are normal. BMI is 27. The remainder of the examination is normal.

Laboratory studies show a hemoglobin A_{1c} level of 8.2%.

Which of the following is the most appropriate treatment for this patient?

(A) Empagliflozin

(B) Glipizide

(C) Liraglutide

(D) Sitagliptin

Item 26

A 24-year-old woman is evaluated for a 6-month history of amenorrhea. Previously, menstrual cycles were regular. She also notes vaginal dryness. She reports no acne, stretch marks, breast discharge, or changes in weight. Medical history is otherwise unremarkable, and she takes no medications.

On physical examination vital signs are normal. BMI is 26. Vulvovaginal atrophy is noted on pelvic examination. The remainder of the examination is unremarkable.

Laboratory studies show undetectable beta-human chorionic gonadotropin. Prolactin and thyroid-stimulating hormone levels are within normal limits.

Which of the following is the most appropriate next diagnostic test?

(A) Dehydroepiandrosterone sulfate (DHEAS) measurement

(B) Follicle-stimulating hormone measurement

(C) Pelvic MRI

(D) Testosterone measurement

(E) Transvaginal ultrasound

Item 27

A 66-year-old woman was admitted to the hospital 24 hours ago with community-acquired pneumonia. Since admission, she has been confused and her oral intake has been poor. Appropriate antibiotics, intravenous fluids, and oxygen have been initiated. She has no other known medical problems.

On physical examination, temperature is 39 °C (102.2 °F), blood pressure is 142/88 mm Hg, pulse rate is 98/min, and respiration rate is 20/min. Oxygen saturation is 98% on oxygen, 2 L/min by nasal cannula. Crackles are evident in the right posterior thorax.

Laboratory studies show glucose values of 185 to 215 mg/dL (10.3-11.9 mmol/L) and a hemoglobin A_{1c} level is 5.5%.

A chest radiograph demonstrates a right lower lobe infiltrate.

Which of the following is the most appropriate management of this patient's hyperglycemia?

(A) Empagliflozin and sliding-scale insulin

(B) Metformin and sliding-scale insulin

(C) Scheduled basal insulin and correction insulin

(D) Sliding-scale insulin only

Item 28

A 45-year-old man is evaluated for anorexia, dizziness, and weakness. He was discharged from the hospital 5 days ago after transsphenoidal pituitary surgery for a pituitary macroadenoma abutting the optic chiasm. His postoperative course was uneventful, and his postoperative hormone evaluation was normal; he did not require any hormone replacement. He denies any polyuria or increase in thirst. He takes no medications.

On physical examination, vital signs and physical examination are normal.

Which of the following is the most appropriate diagnostic test to perform next?

(A) Antidiuretic hormone testing

(B) MRI of the pituitary

(C) Serum sodium measurement

(D) Thyroid-stimulating hormone measurement

Item 29

A 34-year-old woman is evaluated for new onset headaches of 4 months' duration. Her menstrual periods have been irreg-

ular for the last year. She has been trying to conceive for the last 6 months. Her last menstrual period was 7 weeks ago. She is otherwise healthy and takes no medications.

On physical examination, vital signs are normal. Visual field examination is normal. Examination of the optic discs and cranial nerve examination are normal. The remainder of the physical examination is noncontributory.

MRI obtained to evaluate her headaches reveals a partially empty sella with no evidence of pituitary tumor or other masses.

Laboratory studies:

Cortisol (8:00 AM)	15 µg/dL (414 nmol/L)
Estradiol	20 pg/mL (73.4 pmol/L)
Follicle-stimulating hormone	5 mU/mL (5 U/L)
Human chorionic gonadotropin, serum	Negative
Luteinizing hormone	4 mU/mL (4 U/L)
Prolactin	62 ng/mL (62 µg/L)
Thyroid-stimulating hormone	2.4 µU/mL (2.4 mU/L)
Thyroxine (T_4), free	1.3 ng/dL (16.8 pmol/L)
Serum human chorionic gonadotropin	Negative

Which of the following is the most appropriate management?

(A) Dopamine agonist therapy

(B) Neurosurgery consultation

(C) Oral contraceptive pill

(D) No treatment necessary

Item 30

A 21-year-old woman is seen in the office following parathyroidectomy for hyperparathyroidism. The pathology of three resected enlarged parathyroid glands showed hyperplasia. Her medical history is significant for oligomenorrhea. Family history is notable for hypercalcemia and kidney stones in her father, who died at age 49 from pancreatic cancer, and a pituitary tumor in her sister at age 16.

Her vital signs are normal. Skin findings include dermatofibroma. Her physical examination is normal with the exception of the surgical scar on her neck.

Which of the following is the most likely diagnosis?

(A) Familial hypocalciuric hypercalcemia

(B) Multiple endocrine neoplasia type 1 (MEN1)

(C) Parathyroid carcinoma

(D) Secondary hyperparathyroidism

(E) Tertiary hyperparathyroidism

Item 31

A 57-year-old woman is evaluated for cough, exertional dyspnea, and fatigue for 12 months' duration. Medical history is otherwise unremarkable, and she takes no medications.

On physical examination, temperature is 38.1 °C (100.6 °F), blood pressure is 132/78 mm Hg, pulse rate is 84/min, respiratory rate is 18/min; oxygen saturation is 95% breathing ambient air. The cardiac examination is normal. There are no wheezes or crackles on pulmonary examination. The remainder of the examination is unremarkable.

Laboratory studies:

Calcium	11.1 mg/dL (2.8 mmol/L)
Creatinine	1.2 mg/dL (106.1 µmol/L)
Phosphorus	4.7 mg/dL (1.5 mmol/L)
Parathyroid hormone	<10 pg/mL (10 ng/L)

Chest radiograph is shown.

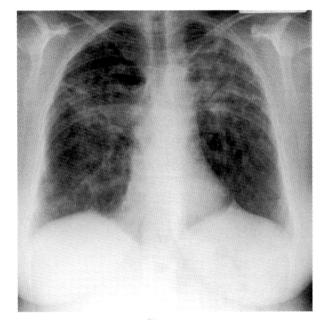

A tuberculin skin test is normal.

Which of the following is the most appropriate laboratory test to perform next?

(A) Alkaline phosphatase level
(B) Cortisol level
(C) 1,25-Dihydroxyvitamin D level
(D) Parathyroid hormone-related protein level

Item 32

A 28-year-old woman is evaluated for preconception counseling. She desires to achieve pregnancy in the next 6 months. Medical history is significant for type 1 diabetes mellitus diagnosed at 12 years of age. She has no known microvascular or macrovascular complications of diabetes. She is up to date on screening for microvascular complications with her last eye examination performed 11 months prior and a normal creatinine level, urine albumin-creatinine ratio, lipid panel, and foot examination 9 months prior. Thyroid-stimulating hormone level was 0.5 µU/mL (0.5 mU/L) 3 months ago. She is currently using a condom for contraception. Medical history also includes autoimmune thyroid disease. Medications are insulin lispro delivered through continuous subcutaneous insulin infusion and levothyroxine.

On physical examination, vital signs are normal. Nondilated retinal examination, thyroid examination, and monofilament testing are all normal.

Laboratory studies reveal that hemoglobin A_{1c} level is currently 6.7%, improved from 9% 3 months ago.

Which of the following is the most appropriate preconception management to perform next?

(A) Dilated eye examination
(B) Fasting lipid profile
(C) Nephrology referral
(D) Thyroid-stimulating hormone measurement
(E) Urine albumin-creatinine ratio

Item 33

A 38-year-old woman presents for first assessment of bone health 4 months into prednisone therapy. Medical history is significant for treatment of antiphospholipid syndrome with recurrent diffuse alveolar hemorrhage and secondary diabetes mellitus. She is not sexually active. She has had no fractures. Medications are prednisone, cyclophosphamide, neutral protamine Hagedorn (NPH) insulin, calcium citrate/vitamin D_3, sulfamethoxazole-trimethoprim, and omeprazole. She is expected to continue prednisone therapy, 7.5 mg or more, for at least the next 6 months.

On physical examination, vital signs are normal. BMI is 37. The remainder of the examination is normal.

Bone mineral density by dual-energy x-ray absorptiometry shows a lumbar spine Z-score of –2.1 and total hip Z-score of –3.1. Radiograph of the spine shows no vertebral compression.

Which of the following is the most appropriate treatment?

(A) Alendronate
(B) Teriparatide
(C) Zoledronic acid
(D) No additional therapy

Item 34

A 29-year-old woman is seen in follow-up for evaluation of abnormal thyroid laboratory results. She is currently 26 weeks pregnant. She was originally evaluated 1 week ago for concerns about lack of weight gain during pregnancy, palpitations, anxiety, and insomnia. There is no family history of thyroid or autoimmune disease. Medical history is unremarkable, and her only medication is a prenatal vitamin.

On physical examination, other than a pulse rate of 98/min, vital signs are normal. The patient is a thin, gravid woman with a mild tremor of the outstretched hands, lid lag, and small goiter. There is no exophthalmus.

Laboratory studies obtained last week show a thyroid-stimulating hormone level of 6.5 µU/mL (6.5 mU/mL) and a free thyroxine (T_4) level of 2.6 ng/dL (33.5 pmol/L).

Which of the following is the most likely diagnosis?

(A) Gestational thyrotoxicosis
(B) Graves disease
(C) Hypothyroidism
(D) Thyroid-stimulating hormone–secreting adenoma

Item 35

A 31-year-old woman is evaluated for amenorrhea. She stopped taking her oral contraceptive pill (OCP) 6 months ago with the goal of becoming pregnant. She has not had a menstrual cycle since stopping her OCP. Her cycles were regular prior to starting an OCP 6 years ago and while on the OCP. She notes a small amount of breast discharge with nipple stimulation; this has been a noted issue for approximately 3 months. Medical history is otherwise unremarkable. Her only medication is a folic acid supplement.

On physical examination, vital signs are normal. There is an elicitable milky discharge from the nipples bilaterally. Thyroid and skin examinations are normal. Visual field testing is normal.

Laboratory studies show a prolactin level of 75 ng/mL (75 µg/L). Serum pregnancy test is negative, and thyroid-stimulating hormone level, kidney function tests, and liver chemistry tests are normal.

MRI of the brain with and without contrast with fine cuts through pituitary reveals a 7-mm pituitary microadenoma.

Which of the following is the most appropriate management?

(A) Clomiphene citrate therapy
(B) Dopamine agonist therapy
(C) Pituitary surgery
(D) Resume oral contraceptive pill

Item 36

A 19-year-old man is evaluated during a follow-up evaluation of his type 1 diabetes mellitus. He was diagnosed 4 months ago with symptoms of hyperglycemia. His hemoglobin A_{1c} level at diagnosis was 11.1%, and antibodies to glutamic acid decarboxylase (GAD65) were positive. He was begun on prandial and basal insulin. He now reports progressive improvement in his glycemic control over the last 8 weeks without changes to his diet, activity level, or insulin doses. Data from his glucometer demonstrates an average fasting, preprandial, and bedtime blood glucose level of 80 mg/dL (4.4 mmol/L). He has several postprandial blood glucose values of approximately 60 mg/dL (3.3 mmol/L) associated with hypoglycemic symptoms. His current hemoglobin A_{1c} level is 5.0%. Medications are insulin glargine (8 U) and insulin aspart (2 U before meals).

His physical examination is notable for an increase in BMI from 18 at the time of his diabetes diagnosis, to now at 20. Vital signs and the remainder of the physical examination are normal.

Which of the following is the most appropriate management of this patient's diabetes?

(A) Continue insulin glargine dose, decrease insulin aspart dose
(B) Decrease insulin glargine dose, discontinue insulin aspart
(C) Discontinue insulin glargine, discontinue insulin aspart
(D) Discontinue insulin glargine, discontinue insulin aspart, add sliding-scale insulin regimen

Item 37

A 63-year-old woman was diagnosed with osteoporosis 6 years ago. Initial treatment with an oral bisphosphonate resulted in upper gastrointestinal symptoms, so subcutaneous denosumab twice yearly was prescribed. The patient has now completed 5 years of denosumab therapy. Medical history is otherwise unremarkable. Denosumab was last administered 6 months ago.

Vital signs and the remainder of the physical examination are normal.

Which of the following is the most appropriate management?

(A) Continue denosumab
(B) Dual-energy x-ray absorptiometry (DEXA) scan
(C) Osteoporosis drug holiday
(D) Switch to zoledronic acid

Item 38

A 55-year-old man with type 1 diabetes mellitus was admitted to the hospital for management of a non–ST-elevation myocardial infarction. He is clinically stable and eating well. He will begin fasting at midnight in preparation for a cardiac catheterization tomorrow. His current fasting blood glucose values range from 70 to 80 mg/dL (3.9-4.4 mmol/L), and his premeal blood glucose values range from 140 to 160 mg/dL (7.8-8.9 mmol/L) on his home doses of basal insulin glargine and prandial insulin aspart. His last hemoglobin A_{1c} value was 7.2%.

In addition to holding prandial insulin, which of the following is the most appropriate management for this patient's diabetes?

(A) Continue basal insulin dose
(B) Continue basal insulin dose and add correction insulin regimen
(C) Decrease basal insulin dose and add correction insulin regimen
(D) Hold basal insulin and add sliding-scale insulin regimen

Item 39

A 38-year-old woman is seen in follow-up to discuss the findings of an abdominal and pelvic CT scan done to evaluate renal colic, which has since resolved. The abdominal CT scan showed two small nonobstructing renal calculi in the right kidney and a 1.6-cm left adrenal mass with a density of 21 Hounsfield units (indeterminate for adrenal adenoma). Other than nephrolithiasis, the remainder of the medical history is unremarkable, and she takes no medications.

On physical examination, vital signs and the remainder of the examination are unremarkable.

Laboratory studies show normal serum electrolytes.

Which of the following is the most appropriate test to perform next?

(A) 24-Hour urine free cortisol measurement
(B) 24-Hour urine total metanephrine measurement
(C) Plasma aldosterone–plasma renin ratio (ARR) measurement
(D) Serum dehydroepiandrosterone sulfate (DHEAS) measurement

Item 40

A 57-year-old woman is evaluated during hospitalization following surgical fixation of a right femur neck pathologic fracture. Pathology of the femur shows a neoplasm containing numerous giant cells consistent with brown tumor.

On physical examination, vital signs are normal. There is a palpable mass on the lower left side of the right neck. There is an incision with surgical staples on the right hip. The remainder of the examination is unremarkable.

Laboratory studies:

Alkaline phosphatase	260 U/L
Calcium	13.2 mg/dL (3.3 mmol/L)
Creatinine	1.6 mg/dL (141.4 µmol/L)
Phosphorus	1.9 mg/dL (0.6 mmol/L)
Parathyroid hormone	1142 pg/mL (1142 ng/L)

Neck ultrasound shows a solid hypervascular mass $(6 \times 2.9 \times 3 \text{ cm})$ posterior to the left lobe of the thyroid, with compression and displacement of the trachea. A parathyroidectomy is planned.

Which of the following is the most appropriate test to perform next?

(A) 1,25-Dihydroxyvitamin D level
(B) 24-Hour urine calcium level
(C) 25-Hydroxyvitamin D level
(D) Ionized calcium level

Item 41

A 51-year-old woman underwent CT scan of the abdomen following a motor vehicle accident. This revealed a 2.5-cm right adrenal mass with a density of 6 Hounsfield units (compatible with adrenal adenoma). Medical history is significant for hypertension diagnosed 2 years ago. She is perimenopausal and has been experiencing sweating and hot flushes. Medications are hydrochlorothiazide and doxazosin.

On physical examination, blood pressure is 142/90 mm Hg, pulse rate is 90/min. Other vital signs are normal. BMI is 33. There are no supraclavicular fats pads or abdominal striae.

Laboratory studies show a cortisol level following a 1-mg overnight dexamethasone suppression test of 8 µg/dL (220.8 nmol/L), plasma aldosterone–plasma renin ratio (ARR) of 13, and plasma fractionated free metanephrines 32 pg/mL (0.17 nmol/L).

Which of the following is the most likely diagnosis?

(A) Non–hormone–secreting adrenal adenoma
(B) Pheochromocytoma
(C) Primary aldosteronism
(D) Subclinical Cushing syndrome

Item 42

A 48-year-old woman is evaluated for a 1-year history of 11.3-kg (25-lb) weight gain, fatigue, easy bruising, and difficulty remembering things. She works the night shift at a hotel reception desk. Medical history is significant for hypertension, type 2 diabetes mellitus, and menopausal hot flushes. Medications are lisinopril, estradiol, aspirin, and metformin.

On physical examination, blood pressure is 142/88 mm Hg. Other vital signs are normal. BMI is 34. The patient has central obesity and a dorsocervical fat pad is present. There are no abdominal striae, no proximal muscle weakness, and no supraclavicular fat pads.

Which of the following is the most appropriate next step in evaluation of this patient?

(A) 1-mg overnight dexamethasone suppression test
(B) 24-Hour urine free cortisol measurement
(C) Late night salivary cortisol measurement
(D) Morning serum total cortisol measurement

Item 43

A 52-year-old man is evaluated for gradual-onset breast tenderness and enlargement over the past 6 months. Medical history is significant for hypertension and symptomatic heart failure with reduced ejection fraction diagnosed 1 year ago. His medications are metoprolol, lisinopril, and spironolactone. He has noticed no change in his sexual function over the past year and reports the presence of morning erections.

On physical examination, vital signs are normal. BMI is 31. There is notable bilateral breast tenderness with rubbery concentric masses noted bilaterally at the areolae. There is no thyroid enlargement, hepatomegaly, or testicular abnormalities including atrophy or mass.

Which of the following is the most likely diagnosis?

(A) Breast cancer
(B) Germ cell tumor
(C) Hypogonadal-associated gynecomastia
(D) Pseudogynecomastia
(E) Spironolactone-induced gynecomastia

Item 44

A 24-year-old man is seen for follow-up management of hypothyroidism. He was diagnosed with hypothyroidism due to Hashimoto thyroiditis 8 years ago. Until 6 months ago, he had been euthyroid on the same dose of levothyroxine. More recently he has required escalating doses of levothyroxine to maintain euthyroidism. He reports that he is still taking levothyroxine as he always has–first thing in the morning on an empty stomach at least 1 hour before eating breakfast. At present, the patient admits to hypothyroid symptoms and intermittent crampy abdominal pain. He has an unintentional weight loss of 2.3 kg (5 lb) over the last 2 months and a new, very pruritic rash on his knees and elbows. His only medication is levothyroxine.

On physical examination, vital signs are normal. The patient's thyroid gland is normal to palpation without nodules. He has papules and excoriated blisters on his elbows, knees, and buttocks.

Laboratory studies show a serum thyroid-stimulating hormone level of 14 µU/mL (14 mU/L) and a free thyroxine (T_4) level of 0.9 ng/dL (11.6 pmol/L).

Which of the following is the most likely diagnosis?

(A) Celiac disease
(B) Medication noncompliance
(C) Primary adrenal insufficiency
(D) Thyroid hormone resistance

Item 45

A 37-year-old woman is unable to achieve pregnancy despite 7 months of unprotected intercourse. Her menstrual cycles are normal, occurring every 28 days with associated breast tenderness and bloating. There have been no prior pregnancies or attempts to achieve pregnancy by either the patient or her male partner. There is no history of previous sexually transmitted infections. She is otherwise healthy.

Medical history is significant for appendicitis at age 26 for which she had an uncomplicated appendectomy. Her only medication is a prenatal vitamin.

On physical examination, vital signs are normal. She has a well-healed abdominal scar. Thyroid, skin, and pelvic examinations are all unremarkable. There is no elicitable breast discharge, no signs of hyperandrogenism, and no visual field cuts.

Which of the following is the most appropriate management?

(A) Obtain midluteal phase serum progesterone level
(B) Obtain semen analysis
(C) Recommend an additional 5 months of unprotected intercourse
(D) Refer for laparoscopy

Item 46

A 55-year-old man is referred for evaluation of fatigue, weight gain, decreased libido, and difficulty maintaining an erection. Sexual functioning was normal until 6 months ago, and he has fathered two children. Medical history is significant for polysubstance abuse that is being managed with daily methadone. His medical history is otherwise unremarkable, and his only medication is methadone.

On physical examination, vital signs are normal. Neurological, genitalia, and the remainder of the physical examination are normal.

Laboratory studies:

Follicle-stimulating hormone	5 mU/mL (5 U/L)
Luteinizing hormone	4 mU/ml (4 U/L)
Prolactin	12 ng/mL (12 µg/L)
Testosterone	185 ng/dL (6.4 nmol/L)
Thyroid-stimulating hormone	2.4 µU/mL (2.4 mU/L)
Thyroxine (T$_4$), free	1.3 ng/dL (16.8 pmol/L)

Which of the following is the most likely cause of this patient's hypogonadism?

(A) Age-related decline in gonadal function
(B) Chronic opioid therapy
(C) Pituitary tumor
(D) Primary gonadal failure

Item 47

An 18-year-old woman is evaluated for absence of menarche. She has undergone some breast development (Tanner stage II). Medical history is unremarkable, and she takes no medications.

On physical examination, her height is 150 cm (59 in) and weight is 47 kg (103.6 lb). BMI is 21. Vital signs and the remainder of the physical examination, including pelvic examination, are normal.

Laboratory studies show a follicle-stimulating hormone level of 74 mU/mL (74 U/L). Serum beta-human chorionic gonadotropin level is undetectable. Thyroid-stimulating hormone and prolactin levels are normal.

On pelvic ultrasound, a uterus is present, but ovaries are difficult to visualize.

Which of the following is the most likely diagnosis?

(A) Functional hypothalamic amenorrhea
(B) Primary ovarian insufficiency
(C) Turner syndrome
(D) Vaginal agenesis

Item 48

A 47-year-old man is evaluated for intermittent episodes of anxiety, diaphoresis, and palpitations. These episodes occur approximately 4 hours after a meal. His first episode occurred while at work. A fingerstick blood glucose reading performed by the employee health nurse was 48 mg/dL (2.7 mmol/L). His symptoms resolved with juice. He has had three similar episodes over the last month. He has increased his consumption of snacks between meals in an attempt to avoid repeat episodes. He denies use of over-the counter supplements or illicit drug use. He does not consume alcohol. He is asymptomatic today. Medical history is significant for Roux-en-Y gastric bypass surgery 3 years ago. He takes no glucose-lowering medications.

On physical examination, vital signs are normal. BMI is 31. The remainder of his examination is normal.

His fingerstick blood glucose level is 85 mg/dL (4.7 mmol/L). Laboratory studies show a hemoglobin A$_{1c}$ level of 5%. All other laboratory results are normal.

Which of the following is the most appropriate diagnostic test to perform next?

(A) 72-Hour fast
(B) Mixed-meal testing
(C) Oral glucose tolerance test
(D) Pancreatic imaging

Item 49

A 65-year-old woman is admitted to the hospital for fatigue and weakness over the last 1 to 2 weeks. Medical history is significant for hypertension, type 2 diabetes mellitus, and rheumatoid arthritis. For the past 3 months, the patient's rheumatoid arthritis has been treated with methotrexate and prednisone. Because of inadequate control, etanercept was added 2 weeks ago. At that time, the patient decided to discontinue prednisone due to increased bruising of her skin.

CONT. Current medications are methotrexate, etanercept, amlodipine, folic acid, metformin, and aspirin.

On physical examination, blood pressure is 110/68 mm Hg sitting and 90/64 mm Hg standing, and pulse rate is 102/min sitting and 110/min standing. Symmetrical synovial bogginess is noted in the metacarpophalangeal joints and wrists bilaterally.

Laboratory studies show an 8 AM cortisol level of 2 µg/dL (55.2 nmol/L).

Which of the following is the most appropriate management?

(A) Initiation of hydrocortisone

(B) Initiation of hydrocortisone and fludrocortisone

(C) Performance of an adrenocorticotropic hormone (ACTH) stimulation test

(D) Performance of an ACTH stimulation test after administration of dexamethasone

Item 50

A 45-year-old woman comes to the office to review her thyroid function test results. Thyroid function testing was ordered in response to a recent diagnosis of hypercholesterolemia. The patient is otherwise well, and she takes no medications.

On physical examination, vital signs are normal. Her physical examination is normal with the exception of slowed relaxation phase of deep tendon reflexes.

Laboratory studies show a serum thyroid-stimulating hormone (TSH) level of 24 µU/mL (24 mU/L) and a free thyroxine (T_4) level of 0.65 ng/dL (8.4 pmol/L).

Which of the following is the most appropriate treatment?

(A) Desiccated thyroid extract

(B) Low-dose (25-µg) levothyroxine

(C) Weight-based replacement dose of levothyroxine

(D) No treatment

Item 51

A 24-year-old woman is evaluated for 6 months of amenorrhea, weight gain, and depressed mood. Medical history is otherwise unremarkable, and she takes no medications.

On physical examination, blood pressure is 134/86 mm Hg and pulse rate is 82/min. BMI is 31. Other vital signs are normal. The patient has facial plethora. Skin examination reveals multiple ecchymoses. There are wide pigmented striae on the abdomen as well as a dorsocervical fat pad.

Laboratory studies:

Cortisol, free, urine	
Initial measurement	120 µg/24 h (330.7 nmol/24 h)
Repeat measurement	240 µg/24 h (661.3 nmol/24 h)
Cortisol after 1 mg dexamethasone test	6.0 µg/dL (165.6 nmol/L)

Which of the following is the most appropriate diagnostic test to perform next?

(A) Adrenocorticotropic hormone (ACTH) level

(B) 8-mg Dexamethasone suppression test

(C) Inferior petrosal sinus sampling for ACTH

(D) Pituitary MRI

Item 52

A 56-year-old man is evaluated for palpitations and difficulty sleeping over the past month. His past medical history is significant for hypothyroidism following subtotal thyroidectomy 6 months ago for management of compressive symptoms from a multinodular goiter. Two months ago, he was diagnosed with hypogonadism and was prescribed intramuscular testosterone. He takes his levothyroxine on an empty stomach with a cup of coffee every morning. His medications are levothyroxine, testosterone enanthate, calcium carbonate, and omeprazole for gastroesophageal reflux disease.

On physical examination, his vital signs are normal. He has a well-healed anterior neck scar. There is a fine tremor of his outstretched hands. The remainder of the examination is normal.

Laboratory studies:

	2 Months Ago	Today
Serum thyroid-stimulating hormone	1.5 µU/mL (1.5 mU/L)	0.08 µU/mL (0.08 mU/L)
Thyroxine (T_4), free	1.1 ng/dL (14.2 pmol/L)	1.4 ng/dL (18.1 pmol/L)

Which of the following is the most likely explanation for the thyroid function test results?

(A) Calcium carbonate

(B) Levothyroxine with coffee

(C) Omeprazole

(D) Testosterone

Item 53

A 74-year-old woman is evaluated for back pain after a fall occurring 2 weeks ago. Medical history is significant for deep venous thrombosis 3 years ago following a 12-hour airplane flight. Medications are acetaminophen as needed for back pain and calcium carbonate with vitamin D.

On physical examination, vital signs are normal. She has minimal pain to percussion over T8. Her examination is otherwise normal.

Laboratory studies:

Alkaline phosphatase	82 U/L
Calcium, serum	9.9 mg/dL (2.5 mmol/L)
Creatinine, serum	1.1 mg/dL (97.2 µmol/L)
25-Hydroxyvitamin D	40 ng/mL (99.8 nmol/L)

Lateral spine radiograph shows 30% compression of T8, not present on prior radiographs. Bone mineral density by DEXA shows a lumbar spine T-score of –3.0 and femur neck T-score of –2.8.

Which of the following is the most appropriate treatment?

(A) Alendronate

(B) Calcitonin

(C) Denosumab

(D) Raloxifene

(E) Teriparatide

Item 54

A 78-year-old man with type 2 diabetes mellitus is evaluated during a routine follow-up examination. He reports hypoglycemia occurring approximately twice per week before dinner. It is worse if he plays golf in the afternoon. He has had three episodes in the last 3 months in which he required assistance from his wife. Medical history is significant for dyslipidemia, hypertension, and obesity. Medications are aspirin, atorvastatin, glyburide, lisinopril, and metformin.

On physical examination, vital signs are normal. BMI is 32. The remainder of the examination is normal.

Laboratory studies show a hemoglobin A_{1c} level of 6.5% and an estimated glomerular filtration rate (eGFR) of 50 mL/min/1.73 m^2.

Which of the following is the most appropriate management of hypoglycemia?

(A) Increase carbohydrate intake with the noon meal
(B) Prescribe glucagon
(C) Stop glyburide therapy
(D) Stop metformin therapy

Item 55

A 58-year-old man is evaluated for resistant hypertension. He was first diagnosed with hypertension 10 years ago, and his blood pressure has been increasingly difficult to control. Testing for secondary causes of hypertension will be undertaken. Medical history is otherwise unremarkable. Medications are lisinopril, spironolactone, hydrochlorothiazide, and metoprolol.

On physical examination, blood pressure is 149/93 mm Hg. Other vital signs are normal. BMI is 29. The remainder of the physical examination is unremarkable.

Which of the following should be discontinued prior to screening for secondary causes of hypertension?

(A) Hydrochlorothiazide
(B) Lisinopril
(C) Metoprolol
(D) Spironolactone

Item 56

A 75-year old man is evaluated for ongoing management of his type 2 diabetes mellitus. He was diagnosed with diabetes 11 years ago. In addition to diabetes, medical history is significant for hypertension, hyperlipidemia, and chronic kidney disease stage G3b. He had a myocardial infarction 6 months ago with subsequent placement of two drug-eluting stents. His hemoglobin A_{1c} level has decreased from 8.7% to 7.8% with adherence to lifestyle modifications and his basal and prandial insulin regimen. Medications are rosuvastatin, lisinopril, metoprolol, chlorthalidone, low-dose aspirin, and clopidogrel.

On physical examination, vital signs are normal. BMI is 29. Other than an S4, the cardiac examination and the remainder of the physical examination are normal.

According to the American Diabetes Association, which of the following is the most appropriate hemoglobin A_{1c} goal for this patient?

(A) Less than 7%
(B) 7% to less than 7.5%
(C) 7.5% to less than 8%
(D) 8% to less than 9%

Item 57

A 67-year-old man is evaluated for headache, fatigue, and weakness for the past several weeks. Medical history is significant for metastatic melanoma that is being treated with ipilimumab, which is his only medication.

On physical examination, vital signs are normal. There is a well-healed excisional scar on his posterior right shoulder. The remainder of the physical examination is normal.

MRI shows enlarged pituitary with homogeneous enhancement. There is no compression of the optic chiasm.

Laboratory studies:

Cortisol (8 AM)	3 µg/dL (82.8 nmol/L)
Prolactin	12 ng/mL (12 µg/L)
Thyroid-stimulating hormone	0.2 µU/mL (0.2 mU/L)
Thyroxine (T$_4$), free	0.6 ng/dL (7.7 pmol/L)

Which of the following is the most likely cause of this patient's findings?

(A) Ipilimumab-induced hypophysitis
(B) Lymphocytic hypophysitis
(C) Pituitary adenoma
(D) Primary hypothyroidism

Item 58

A 45-year-old man underwent abdominal CT imaging for evaluation of bloating and constipation. The CT scan shows a 5-cm right adrenal mass with a density of 42 Hounsfield units and absolute contrast washout of 38% at 10 minutes. Testing for pheochromocytoma and subclinical Cushing syndrome was negative. Medical history is otherwise unremarkable, and he takes no medications.

On physical examination, vital signs and the remainder of the physical examination are normal.

Which of the following is the most appropriate next step in management?

(A) Adrenal biopsy
(B) Adrenalectomy
(C) Mitotane therapy
(D) Repeat CT at 6 months

Item 59

A 55-year-old woman returns to the emergency department for persistent weakness, shakiness, and intermittent hand spasms. Three days ago, she was diagnosed with hypocalcemia, and vitamin D and calcium were initiated at that time.

Medical history is significant for metastatic ovarian cancer, currently treated with cisplatin and etoposide chemotherapy. Additional medications are calcium carbonate and vitamin D_3.

On physical examination, vital signs are normal. Tetany of the hand is noted during blood pressure assessment. Chvostek sign is positive.

Laboratory studies:

Albumin	3.5 g/dL (35 g/L)
Calcium	7.6 mg/dL (1.9 mmol/L)
Creatinine	1.0 mg/dL (88.4 µmol/L)
Parathyroid hormone	19 pg/mL (19 ng/L)
Potassium	4.2 mEq/L (4.2 mmol/L)

The laboratory results are similar to those obtained 3 days ago.

Electrocardiography shows a prolonged QTc interval.

Which of the following measurements is most appropriate to perform next?

(A) Bicarbonate

(B) Ionized calcium

(C) Magnesium

(D) Phosphorus

Item 60

A 60-year-old man is evaluated for management of type 2 diabetes mellitus. Three months ago he was diagnosed with type 2 diabetes mellitus and chronic kidney disease. At that time, he received diabetes education and began lifestyle modifications. Medical history is significant for chronic kidney disease, hypertension, and hyperlipidemia. His medications are lisinopril and atorvastatin.

On physical examination, his blood pressure is 146/88 mm Hg. BMI is 28.5. The remainder of his vital signs and physical examination are normal.

Laboratory studies show a hemoglobin A_{1c} level of 8.3%, serum creatinine level of 1.5 mg/dL (132.6 µmol/L), and estimated glomerular filtration rate of 48 mL/min/1.73 m².

Which of the following is the most appropriate treatment of this patient's diabetes?

(A) Empagliflozin

(B) Glipizide

(C) Metformin

(D) Saxagliptin

Item 61

A 55-year-old woman is seen during a follow-up evaluation for hyperthyroidism that was diagnosed 1 week ago. Thyroid examination revealed a palpable right thyroid nodule.

Thyroid-stimulating hormone (TSH) was less than 0.01 µU/mL (0.01 mU/L), free thyroxine (T_4) and total triiodothyronine (T_3) were 2.1 ng/dL (27.1 pmol/L) and 210 ng/dL (3.2 nmol/L), respectively. Atenolol was prescribed, and thyroid scintigraphy with determination of radioactive iodine uptake was ordered.

On physical examination, vital signs are normal. The neck and corresponding thyroid technetium-99 scan is shown.

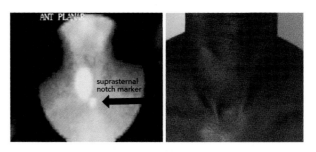

Uptake at 24 hours is 30% (normal 14% to 30%).

Which of the following is the most appropriate management?

(A) Fine-needle aspiration biopsy of the thyroid nodule

(B) Increase atenolol dosage

(C) Methimazole

(D) Radioactive iodine (^{131}I) therapy

Item 62

A 55-year-old man is evaluated during a follow-up visit after he was diagnosed with type 2 diabetes mellitus based on two hemoglobin A_{1c} measurements of 7.8%. His medical history is significant for dyslipidemia and hypertension. Medications are aspirin, atorvastatin, and lisinopril.

On physical examination, vital signs are normal. BMI is 33. The general physical examination, including nondilated eye examination, is normal.

The patient will initiate therapeutic lifestyle modifications, and metformin will be started.

In addition to spot urine albumin-creatinine ratio testing, which of the following screening tests should be done now?

(A) Comprehensive foot examination and dilated eye examination

(B) Fasting plasma glucose and 2-hour 75-g oral glucose tolerance test

(C) Serum B_{12} and folate concentrations

(D) 24-Hour urine protein and creatinine measurement

Item 63

A 45-year-man is seen in routine follow-up for his type 2 diabetes mellitus. He was diagnosed 5 years ago, and he does not have any diabetes-related complications. His current treatment includes insulin detemir, prandial insulin lispro, and metformin. His hemoglobin A_{1c} level has decreased to 7.4%. His fasting and preprandial blood glucose measurements range from 110 to 130 mg/dL (6.1-7.2 mmol/L). He has had no hypoglycemia. Medical history is significant for obesity. He wishes to reduce his hemoglobin A_{1c} level to below 7%, but he is reluctant to add another injectable medication to his regimen. Medications are insulin detemir, insulin lispro, and metformin.

On physical examination, vital signs are normal. BMI is 33. The remainder of the physical examination is unremarkable.

Which of the following is the most appropriate management of this patient's diabetes?

(A) Add liraglutide

(B) Continue current regimen

(C) Increase insulin detemir dose

(D) Measure postprandial blood glucose level

Item 64

A 65-year-old woman is evaluated for hypercalcemia that was incidentally discovered on routine blood testing for a new life insurance policy. She has no symptoms. Medical history is unremarkable. Her only medication is calcium carbonate taken as needed for occasional heartburn.

On physical examination, vital signs are normal. Height is unchanged from prior measurements. The remainder of her examination is normal.

Laboratory studies:

Estimate glomerular filtration rate	Greater than 60 mL/min/1.73 m²
Calcium	10.6 mg/dL (2.6 mmol/L)
Phosphorus	3.1 mg/dL (1.0 mmol/L)
Parathyroid hormone	72 pg/mL (72 ng/L)
25-Hydroxyvitamin D	35 ng/mL (87.4 nmol/L)
24-Hour urine calcium	240 mg/24 h (6 mmol/24 h)

Kidney-urinary-bladder radiograph is negative for kidney stones. Dual-energy x-ray absorptiometry (DEXA) bone mineral density scan shows femur neck T-score of –1.4, lumbar spine T-score of –1.4, and one-third radius T-score of –1.7.

Which of the following is the most appropriate management?

(A) Parathyroid sestamibi scan

(B) Reevaluate in 6 months

(C) Start alendronate

(D) Start cinacalcet

Item 65

A 45-year-old man is seen for follow-up evaluation for depression and to review the results of laboratory testing. He was seen 1 month ago for a 6-month history of depressed mood, difficulty sleeping, decreased appetite, 2.3-kg (5-lb) weight loss, and fatigue. Major depressive disorder was diagnosed, and escitalopram was prescribed. Today the patient reports a significant improvement in his mood, appetite, and the quality of his sleep since starting treatment.

On physical examination, vital signs and physical examination are normal. Screening laboratory studies from 1 month ago show a thyroid-stimulating hormone (TSH) level of 7 µU/mL (7 mU/L) and a free thyroxine (T$_4$) level of 1.0 ng/dL (12.9 pmol/L).

Which of the following is the most appropriate management?

(A) Measure thyroid peroxidase antibodies

(B) Measure thyrotropin receptor antibodies

(C) Measure serum triiodothyronine (T$_3$) level

(D) Prescribe levothyroxine

(E) Repeat serum TSH testing in 2 months

Item 66

A 52-year-old man is evaluated for difficult-to-control hypertension. Biochemical evaluation confirms a diagnosis of primary aldosteronism. Medications are amlodipine, losartan, and metoprolol.

On physical examination, blood pressure is 149/98 mm Hg and pulse rate is 75/min. The remainder of the vital signs and physical examination are unremarkable.

CT scan shows a 0.8-cm right adrenal mass with a density of 13 Hounsfield units.

Which of the following is the most appropriate management?

(A) Adrenal vein sampling

(B) Increase metoprolol

(C) Increase losartan

(D) Right adrenalectomy

Item 67

A 65-year-old woman comes to the office to establish care. Her medical history is notable for hypothyroidism due to Hashimoto thyroiditis treated with levothyroxine. She does not have any symptoms at this time. There is no history of head or neck radiation exposure.

On physical examination, vital signs are normal. The patient's thyroid gland is enlarged. The right lobe is larger than the left, and a mobile 2-cm nodule is palpable in the lower pole. There is no palpable cervical adenopathy.

Laboratory studies show a serum thyroid-stimulating hormone level of 2.0 µU/mL (2.0 mU/L).

Which of the following is the most appropriate diagnostic test to perform next?

(A) CT scan of the neck

(B) Fine-needle aspiration biopsy of the thyroid nodule

(C) Thyroid uptake and ^{131}I scan

(D) Ultrasound of the neck

Item 68

A 59-year-old woman is evaluated for fatigue and weight gain over the past 2 months. Her medical history is significant for a pituitary tumor, treated with surgery followed by radiation therapy, at age 54. She has recently self-initiated calcium and vitamin D and a multivitamin. Her only other medication is levothyroxine.

On physical examination, vital signs are normal. BMI is 31. The remainder of the physical examination is normal.

Which of the following is the most appropriate next step in management?

(A) Increase the levothyroxine dose

(B) Measure free thyroxine (T$_4$) level

(C) Measure thyroid-stimulating hormone level

(D) MRI of the brain

Item 69

A 53-year-old man returns for a follow-up visit for management of his type 2 diabetes mellitus. He was diagnosed with diabetes 10 years ago. In addition to diabetes, his medical history is significant for hypertension. Medications are enalapril and insulin glargine at bedtime and aspart insulin at meals.

On physical examination, blood pressure is 142/84 mm Hg. BMI is 27. The remainder of the vital signs and physical examination are unremarkable.

His fasting blood glucose level ranges from 150 to 180 mg/dL (8.3-10.0 mmol/L). His remaining premeal and bedtime blood glucose levels range from 110 to 130 mg/dL (6.1-7.2 mmol/L). He has intermittent episodes of hypoglycemia with recorded values ranging from 30 to 65 mg/dL (1.7-3.6 mmol/L). These occur once per week without a clear cause or pattern. For many episodes of hypoglycemia he experiences no symptoms, but he is able to detect hypoglycemia at blood glucose values less than 40 mg/dL (2.2 mmol/L). His most recent hemoglobin A$_{1c}$ level is 8.2%. He desires a hemoglobin A$_{1c}$ level less than 7%.

Which of the following is the most appropriate treatment of this patient's diabetes?

(A) Decrease all insulin doses

(B) Increase glargine insulin dose

(C) Initiate empagliflozin

(D) Initiate metformin

Item 70

A 42-year-old woman is evaluated in the office for osteoporosis because she was told her heel ultrasound screening test was abnormal at a health fair. She has no history of fractures. Family history is significant for osteoporosis in her mother, diagnosed at age 68 years; she has no history of fracture. Her only medication is a combination estradiol-levonorgestrel oral contraceptive pill.

On physical examination, vital signs are normal. BMI is 19. The remainder of her physical examination is normal.

Report of the quantitative heel ultrasound shows a Z-score of −0.5.

Which of the following is the most appropriate management?

(A) Lifestyle counseling for osteoporosis prevention

(B) Dual-energy x-ray absorptiometry (DEXA) scan

(C) Evaluation of secondary causes of bone loss

(D) Serial quantitative heel ultrasound testing

Item 71

A 27-year-old woman is seen in a follow-up visit for hyperthyroidism. Three months ago she was diagnosed with Graves disease, and methimazole was initiated. Today the patient reports an overall improvement in hyperthyroid symptoms, but over the past week she has developed a fever, sore throat, and painful swallowing. She reports no cough. Medications are methimazole and propranolol.

On physical examination, temperature is 38.7 °C (101.6 °F), blood pressure is 112/78 mm Hg, pulse rate is 98/min, and respiration rate is 18/min. The patient's posterior oropharynx is erythematous without exudates. Her examination is otherwise normal.

Which of the following is the most appropriate management?

(A) Begin empiric oral penicillin V

(B) Obtain a rapid antigen detection test for Group A streptococcus

(C) Obtain a throat culture

(D) Stop methimazole and obtain complete blood count with differential

Item 72

A 66-year-old man recently diagnosed with type 2 diabetes mellitus is evaluated in the emergency department for nausea, vomiting, and fatigue. He was diagnosed with type 2 diabetes 18 months ago. In the past month metformin was discontinued due to severe diarrhea, and glipizide and empagliflozin were initiated. In addition to type 2 diabetes, medical history is significant for coronary artery disease, hypertension, and dyslipidemia. Medications are aspirin, lisinopril, metoprolol, atorvastatin, glipizide, and empagliflozin.

On physical examination, temperature is normal, blood pressure is 90/60 mm Hg, pulse rate is 120/min, and respiration rate is 22/min. Dry mucous membranes are noted. There is diffuse abdominal tenderness to palpation without guarding. Other than tachycardia, the remainder of the examination is normal.

Laboratory studies:

Sodium	133 mEq/L (133 mmol/L)
Bicarbonate	10 mEq/L (10 mmol/L)
Glucose	150 mg/dL (8.3 mmol/L)
Anion gap	17 mEq/L (17 mmol/L)
β-hydroxybutyrate	Elevated

Which of the following is most likely responsible for the patient's findings?

(A) Atorvastatin

(B) Discontinuation of metformin

(C) Empagliflozin

(D) Glipizide

(E) Lisinopril

Item 73

A 32-year-old man is evaluated for decreased libido and fatigue. His symptoms have increased over the last 6 months.

His medical history is otherwise unremarkable, and he takes no medications.

On physical examination, vital signs are normal. BMI is 26. He has gynecomastia. Visual field acuity testing and testicular examination are normal. Smell is intact.

Laboratory studies:

Follicle-stimulating hormone	4 mU/mL (4 U/L)
Luteinizing hormone	5 mU/mL (5 U/L)
Prolactin	100 ng/mL (100 µg/L)
Testosterone	110 ng/dL (3.8 nmol/L)

Which of the following is the most appropriate diagnostic test to perform next?

(A) Karyotype analysis
(B) Pituitary MRI
(C) Screening for anabolic steroid abuse
(D) Serum ferritin measurement
(E) Sex hormone-binding globulin measurement

Item 74

A 74-year-old woman is evaluated in the emergency department for decreased responsiveness. She has become progressively confused and lethargic. She lives alone and stopped taking her medications at some time unknown. She was brought to the emergency department by a family member.

The patient had a near-total thyroidectomy for multinodular goiter 3 years ago.

On physical examination, temperature is 36.1 °C (97.0 °F), blood pressure is 80/45 mm Hg, pulse rate is 46/min, respiration rate is 10/min, and oxygen saturation is 92% breathing ambient air. BMI is 28. The patient is arousable with painful stimuli. She has a well-healed anterior neck scar. The patient's skin is cool and dry. She has periorbital edema and bipedal edema. Other than bradycardia, the cardiac examination is normal. The relaxation phase of her deep tendon reflexes is delayed.

Laboratory results show a sodium level of 129 mEq/L (129 mmol/L). Intravenous fluids are initiated.

Which of the following is the essential initial step in the management of this patient?

(A) Administer intravenous hydrocortisone
(B) Administer intravenous levothyroxine and liothyronine
(C) Administer norepinephrine
(D) Administer oral levothyroxine

Item 75

A 35-year-old woman is seen in follow-up evaluation for her type 2 diabetes mellitus. She was diagnosed 3 years ago. She checks her fasting and 2-hour postprandial blood glucose values several times per week. Her fasting blood glucose levels range from 100 to 110 mg/dL (5.5-6.1 mmol/L) and her 2-hour postprandial values are 120 to 165 mg/dL (6.7-9.1 mmol/L). Her review of symptoms is positive for chronic heavy menses. Medications are metformin and liraglutide.

On physical examination, blood pressure is 123/74 mm Hg and pulse rate is 76/min. BMI is 31.2. The examination is otherwise unremarkable.

Laboratory studies:

Hematocrit	33%
Iron studies	
Ferritin	11 ng/mL (11 µg/L)
Iron	40 µg/dL (7.2 µmol/L)
Iron-binding capacity, total	600 µg/dL (107.4 µmol/L)
Hemoglobin A_{1c}	7.3%

Which of the following is the most appropriate management of the elevated hemoglobin A_{1c} level?

(A) Basal insulin
(B) Empagliflozin
(C) Ferrous sulfate
(D) Hemoglobin electrophoresis

Item 76

A 69-year-old woman is seen in the office following a left thyroid lobectomy and isthmusectomy 1 week ago for management of compressive symptoms related to a large left thyroid nodule. The preoperative thyroid/neck ultrasound showed the nodule without suspicious features and no abnormal cervical lymph nodes. The pathology report describes a 4.5-cm left adenomatous nodule in a background of multinodular hyperplasia. There is a single focus of papillary thyroid carcinoma measuring 0.5 cm in the greatest dimension. No lymphovascular or extrathyroidal invasion is noted. Surgical margins are negative.

The patient is currently feeling well and reports complete resolution of her prior symptoms. Her medical history is otherwise unremarkable, and she takes no medications.

On physical examination, vital signs are normal. There is a well-healed anterior neck scar. Laboratory studies show a serum thyroid-stimulating hormone (TSH) level of 1.8 µU/mL (1.8 mU/L).

Which of the following is the most appropriate treatment?

(A) Levothyroxine to suppress serum TSH
(B) Radioactive iodine (^{131}I) therapy
(C) Resection of the remaining thyroid lobe
(D) No additional treatment

Item 77

A 37-year-old man is evaluated in the hospital for polyuria 1 day after transsphenoidal pituitary surgery for a craniopharyngioma. The patient reports increased thirst overnight. Urine output is currently 300 mL/hour for the last 12 hours. He takes no medications.

On physical examination, vital signs are normal. He has dry mucous membranes.

Laboratory studies show a sodium level of 146 mEq/L (146 mmol/L).

Which of the following is the most appropriate diagnostic test to perform next?

(A) Desmopressin challenge
(B) Urine and serum osmolality
(C) Urine electrolytes
(D) Water deprivation test

Item 78

A 22-year-old woman is evaluated for tachycardia, fever, agitation, and confusion 3 days following laparoscopic cholecystectomy for acute cholecystitis.

Medical history is significant for type 1 diabetes mellitus well controlled on basal-bolus insulin and Graves disease previously treated with methimazole. Methimazole was discontinued 6 months ago when she was considered to be in remission. Medications are insulin glargine and insulin aspart.

On physical examination, temperature is 39.0 °C (102.2 °F), blood pressure is 95/50 mm Hg, pulse rate is 132/min and irregular, and respiration rate is 24/min. The patient is confused and appears flushed and diaphoretic. Lid lag is noted. The thyroid gland is diffusely enlarged with an audible bruit. Her deep tendon reflexes are brisk. There is a fine tremor of her hands. Her examination is otherwise normal.

Which of the following is the most likely diagnosis?

(A) Adrenal crisis

(B) Malignant hyperthermia

(C) Myxedema coma

(D) Thyroid storm

Item 79

A 54-year-old man is evaluated at a follow-up visit after being diagnosed with type 2 diabetes mellitus 3 months ago. His initial hemoglobin A_{1c} level was 8.5%. He opted for lifestyle modifications initially. He has lost 4.5 kg (10 lb) in the interim after making significant changes to his diet and increasing his activity level. His average blood glucose level currently is 180 mg/dL (10 mmol/L). Medical history is otherwise unremarkable.

On physical examination, blood pressure is 130/74 mm Hg and pulse is 70/min. BMI is 27. The examination is otherwise unremarkable.

His repeat hemoglobin A_{1c} level today is 7.9%, but he would like it lower. Results of other laboratory studies are within normal ranges.

Which of the following is the most appropriate management?

(A) Continue current management

(B) Initiate empagliflozin

(C) Initiate liraglutide

(D) Initiate metformin

Item 80

A 22-year-old man was admitted to the intensive care unit 24 hours ago with nausea, vomiting, and lethargy of 2 days' duration. Medical history is unremarkable, and he takes no medications. His admission laboratory values were consistent with diabetic ketoacidosis, and he was initiated on intravenous fluids and intravenous insulin therapy. After 24 hours, he is currently receiving 0.45% normal saline at 250 mL/h with 20 mEq (20 mmol) of potassium chloride per liter and an insulin drip at 5 U/h. His nausea continues, but his vomiting has ceased. He is unable to eat.

On physical examination, vital signs are normal. He is alert and oriented, and the remainder of his physical examination is unremarkable.

Laboratory studies:

Electrolytes	
Sodium	141 mEq/L (141 mmol/L)
Potassium	4.0 mEq/L (4.0 mmol/L)
Chloride	104 mEq/L (104 mmol/L)
Bicarbonate	20 mEq/L (20 mmol/L)
Glucose	180 mg/dL (10 mmol/L)
pH	7.32

Which of the following is the most appropriate management?

(A) Continue current insulin drip rate

(B) Decrease insulin drip rate and add intravenous dextrose

(C) Discontinue intravenous potassium

(D) Transition insulin drip to subcutaneous insulin regimen

Item 81

A 68-year-old man is evaluated in the office for increasing shortness of breath, palpitations, difficulty sleeping, fatigue, generalized weakness, and 4.5-kg (10-lb) weight loss over the past month. His medical history is significant for heart failure and atrial fibrillation. For the past 2 years his medications have been metoprolol, lisinopril, amiodarone, and dabigatran.

On physical examination, the patient is afebrile, blood pressure is 140/80 mm Hg, pulse is 102/min, and respiration rate is 24/min. Deep tendon reflexes are brisk and symmetric. A fine tremor of his outstretched hands, bilateral lid lag, and an irregularly irregular heart rhythm are noted. Examination of the thyroid gland and remainder of the physical examination are normal.

Laboratory studies show a serum thyroid-stimulating hormone (TSH) level less than 0.01 μU/mL (0.01 mU/L), a free thyroxine (T_4) level of 3.1 ng/dL (40 pmol/L), and a serum total triiodothyronine (T_3) level of 190 ng/dL (2.9 nmol/L). TSH receptor antibodies are undetectable. Other laboratory studies are normal.

On thyroid ultrasound, the thyroid lobes and isthmus are normal in size. No thyroid nodules are seen. The background thyroid parenchyma demonstrates no demonstrable vascularity on color flow Doppler. Chest radiograph is normal.

In addition to increasing the metoprolol dose, which of the following is the most appropriate initial management?

(A) Discontinue amiodarone

(B) Begin methimazole

(C) Begin prednisone

(D) Thyroid scintigraphy with radioactive iodine uptake

Item 82

A 36-year-old woman is evaluated for new-onset hirsutism noted on the face, chest, and abdomen. Hirsute hair growth has rapidly progressed over the last 6 months. Additionally, she notes frontal hair loss. Menstrual cycles have become irregular over the same time course. Medical history is otherwise unremarkable, and she takes no medications.

On physical examination, her blood pressure is 142/88 mm Hg; the remainder of the vital signs is normal. BMI is 26. On skin examination, acne is noted. Dark terminal hair appears on the face, chest, and abdomen. The patient has diffuse hair thinning on top of the head. The remainder of the physical examination is noncontributory.

Laboratory studies:

Estradiol	68 pg/mL (249.6 pmol/L)
Follicle-stimulating hormone	12 mU/mL (12 U/L)
Human chorionic gonadotropin, serum	Negative
Prolactin	Normal
Testosterone, total	220 ng/dL (7.6 nmol/L)
Thyroid-stimulating hormone	Normal

Which of the following is the most appropriate management?

(A) Adrenal vein sampling for cortisol and androgens

(B) 24-Hour urine free cortisol

(C) Oral contraceptive therapy

(D) Pelvic ultrasound

Item 83

A 62-year-old woman is evaluated for management of her type 2 diabetes mellitus. She was diagnosed 2 years ago, and treatment was advanced to include lifestyle modifications, metformin, liraglutide, and empagliflozin, but it was not successful in reaching her hemoglobin A_{1c} goal. Her current regimen includes metformin and basal and prandial insulins. Her fasting and preprandial blood glucose values range from 150 to 200 mg/dL (8.3-11.1 mmol/L) with intermittent episodes of hypoglycemia. She has had a weight gain of 2.3 kg (5 lb) over the last 3 months. Medical history is also significant for hypertension, hyperlipidemia, and osteoarthritis. Medications are detemir insulin, lispro insulin, metformin, lisinopril, and atorvastatin.

On physical examination, blood pressure is 142/90 mm Hg and pulse rate is 63/min. BMI is 36. The remainder of the physical examination is unremarkable. Laboratory studies show a hemoglobin A_{1c} level of 8.8%.

Which of the following is the most appropriate management of this patient's diabetes?

(A) Add sitagliptin

(B) Add pioglitazone

(C) Increase insulin

(D) Metabolic surgery referral

Item 84

A 57-year-old woman is evaluated for progressive right upper leg pain for the past 2 years. The pain is worse with weight bearing. She is postmenopausal and otherwise in good health. She has no family history of fractures. She takes no medications.

On physical examination, vital signs are normal. BMI is 36. She has difficulty bearing weight and limps when walking. She has discomfort on palpation over the anterior tibia. The remainder of the physical examination is normal.

Laboratory studies:

Alkaline phosphatase	150 U/L
Calcium	8.2 mg/dL (2.0 mmol/L)
Creatinine	0.8 mg/dL (70.7 µmol/L)
Phosphorus	2.4 mg/dL (0.8 mmol/L)
Parathyroid hormone	176 pg/mL (176 ng/L)
25-Hydroxyvitamin D	<6 ng/mL (15.0 nmol/L)

Which of the following is the most likely diagnosis?

(A) Osteitis fibrosa cystica

(B) Osteogenesis imperfecta

(C) Osteomalacia

(D) Postmenopausal osteoporosis

Answers and Critiques

Item 1   Answer: D

Educational Objective: Diagnose radiation-induced papillary thyroid cancer.

The most likely diagnosis is papillary thyroid cancer. Radiation exposure of the thyroid during childhood is the strongest environmental risk factor for thyroid cancer. Patients under the age of 15, especially those younger than 5 years, have the highest risk of subsequently developing papillary thyroid cancer following a significant radiation exposure (>10 rads).

A benign follicular nodule is not the most likely diagnosis due to the history of radiation exposure in childhood, ultrasound findings (hypoechoic solid nodule with irregular margins), and cervical lymphadenopathy. Fine-needle aspiration biopsy (FNAB) of both the thyroid nodule and abnormal lymph nodes should be pursued to confirm the suspected diagnosis and inform surgical management. In addition to thyroidectomy, patients with thyroid cancer that has metastasized to cervical lymph nodes require dissection of the affected compartment (central neck dissection for central lymph node metastases, and central and lateral neck dissection for lateral metastases). Abnormal findings on sonography vary considerably in their specificity for predicting malignant lymph node involvement (range 43% to 100%). For this reason, FNAB of the thyroid nodule and any abnormal lymph nodes are usually performed simultaneously. The false-negative rate for lymph node FNAB is 6% to 8% overall, but increases to 20% for samples with inadequate cellularity. Inadequate cellularity is common for metastatic lymph nodes that have undergone cystic degeneration, which is common in papillary thyroid cancer. Measuring thyroglobulin in the aspirate can significantly improve diagnostic sensitivity of lymph node FNAB.

While radiation exposure is a risk factor for follicular thyroid cancer, this is a less likely diagnosis than papillary thyroid cancer. Follicular thyroid cancer is less common than papillary thyroid cancer, it tends to occur in older persons, and it rarely metastasizes to lymph nodes.

Medullary thyroid cancer is an unlikely diagnosis because it is the least common of the thyroid malignancies, representing about 1% to 2% of all thyroid cancers. Approximately 25% of medullary thyroid cancers are hereditary; all patients with medullary thyroid cancer should be screened with *RET* proto-oncogene sequencing. Medullary thyroid cancer may be associated with several syndromes, including multiple endocrine neoplasia type 2A (MEN2A) (which may include pheochromocytoma and hyperparathyroidism), MEN2B (marfanoid habitus and mucosal ganglioneuromas), or familial medullary thyroid cancer (medullary thyroid cancer alone).

KEY POINT

- Radiation exposure of the thyroid during childhood is the strongest environmental risk factor for thyroid cancer, most commonly papillary cancer.

Bibliography
Haugen BR, Alexander EK, Bible KC, Doherty GM, Mandel SJ, Nikiforov YE, et al. 2015 American Thyroid Association management guidelines for adult patients with thyroid nodules and differentiated thyroid cancer: The American Thyroid Association Guidelines Task Force on Thyroid Nodules and Differentiated Thyroid Cancer. Thyroid. 2016;26:1-133. [PMID: 26462967] doi:10.1089/thy.2015.0020

Item 2   Answer: D

Educational Objective: Treat type 2 diabetes mellitus in an obese patient.

According to the American Diabetes Association (ADA), this patient's goal hemoglobin A_{1c} level is less than 7% given that she is healthy and early in the disease course. The American College of Physicians (ACP) recommends a target hemoglobin A_{1c} level between 7% and 8% for most patients with type 2 diabetes. The ACP notes that more stringent targets may be appropriate for patients who have a long life expectancy (>15 years) and are interested in more intensive glycemic control despite the risk for harms, including but not limited to hypoglycemia, patient burden, and pharmacologic costs. Her hemoglobin A_{1c} level remains above goal despite 3 months of lifestyle modifications and metformin. The ADA recommends advancing to dual-therapy if the hemoglobin A_{1c} remains at 9% or above after 3 months of metformin therapy. Sequential therapeutic agents added to metformin should be selected based on the degree of hyperglycemia, comorbidities, weight, side effect profiles, cost, and patient preferences. Liraglutide, a glucagon-like peptide-1 (GLP-1) receptor agonist, is an appropriate adjunctive agent with metformin in this patient as it will improve glycemic control and contribute to desired weight loss. There are potential concerns for development of pancreatitis and medullary thyroid carcinoma with GLP-1 receptor agonists. The patient does not have a personal or family history of these abnormalities to preclude use of liraglutide.

Empagliflozin, a sodium-glucose transporter-2 (SGLT2) inhibitor, may be added to metformin when the hemoglobin A_{1c} remains above goal. SGLT2 inhibitor use improves glycemic control and induces weight loss, but it also increases the risk of genital mycotic infections. Empagliflozin should not be used in this patient because it may exacerbate her frequent vulvovaginal candidiasis infections.

Glipizide, a sulfonylurea, may also be added to metformin when the hemoglobin A_{1c} remains above goal. Glipizide will improve glycemic control, but it is associated with

Answers and Critiques

105

H
CONT.

weight gain that is not in concordance with the patient's desire for continued weight loss.

Basal insulin coverage can be provided with one to two daily injections of insulin detemir, glargine, or neutral protamine Hagedorn (NPH) insulin. Basal insulin may be added to metformin when the hemoglobin A_{1c} level remains above goal. Basal insulin will improve glycemic control, but it is associated with weight gain that is not in concordance with the patient's desire for continued weight loss.

KEY POINT

- Liraglutide is an add-on therapy to metformin to achieve improvement in hemoglobin A_{1c} level and weight loss.

Bibliography

American Diabetes Association. 8. Pharmacologic approaches to glycemic treatment: Standards of Medical Care in Diabetes-2018. Diabetes Care. 2018;41(Suppl 1):S73-S85. doi: 10.2337/dc18-S008. [PMID: 29222379]

Item 3 **Answer: B**

Educational Objective: Diagnose the cause of primary adrenal insufficiency.

The most appropriate next test is measurement of 21-hydroxylase antibodies. This patient has primary adrenal insufficiency as confirmed by the combination of low serum cortisol and elevated serum adrenocorticotropic hormone (ACTH). The most common cause of primary adrenal insufficiency in the United States is autoimmune adrenalitis, and positive 21-hydroxylase antibodies are found in approximately 90% of those cases.

Patients with autoimmune adrenalitis are at risk for the development of other autoimmune disorders including primary hypothyroidism, primary ovarian insufficiency, type 1 diabetes mellitus, celiac disease, and autoimmune gastritis. If 21-hydroxylase antibody measurement is negative, abdominal CT imaging should be performed. In autoimmune disease, the adrenal glands often appear atrophic, although normal-sized adrenal glands do not rule out this diagnosis. Other causes of primary adrenal insufficiency typically cause enlargement of the adrenal glands. These include infiltrative disorders such as lymphoma, sarcoidosis, histoplasmosis, or tuberculosis (the latter can be associated with normal-sized adrenal glands). Bilateral adrenal enlargement is also seen in primary adrenal insufficiency caused by bilateral adrenal hemorrhage. Metastatic disease to the adrenal glands rarely causes adrenal insufficiency.

Cosyntropin stimulation testing is used to diagnose the presence of adrenal insufficiency, but it will not help determine the underlying cause. In this patient, the diagnosis of primary adrenal insufficiency is confirmed by the presence of a serum cortisol level of less than 3 µg/dL (82.8 nmol/L) in combination with an elevated serum ACTH level. Hence, cosyntropin stimulation testing will not add further to the diagnosis or management.

MRI of the pituitary gland is not indicated in this patient with primary adrenal insufficiency, but it is the imaging modality of choice for investigation of secondary adrenal insufficiency. The latter is characterized by low serum cortisol in the setting of low or inappropriately normal serum ACTH levels.

Measurement of serum aldosterone would not help determine the underlying cause of this patient's primary adrenal insufficiency. Low or inappropriately normal serum aldosterone levels (associated with elevated plasma renin activity) are present in most patients with primary adrenal insufficiency due to destruction of the layers of the adrenal cortex by the underlying disease process. Aldosterone deficiency results in hyperkalemia, as noted in this patient, and hyponatremia may also be present.

KEY POINT

- The most common cause of primary adrenal insufficiency in the United States is autoimmune adrenalitis, and positive 21-hydroxylase antibodies are found in approximately 90% of those cases.

Bibliography

Bancos I, Hahner S, Tomlinson J, Arlt W. Diagnosis and management of adrenal insufficiency. Lancet Diabetes Endocrinol. 2015;3:216-26. [PMID: 25098712] doi:10.1016/S2213-8587(14)70142-1

Item 4 **Answer: A**

Educational Objective: Diagnose the cause of hyperprolactinemia.

The most appropriate next step in managing this patient is to obtain a pituitary MRI. The most common cause of hyperprolactinemia is physiologic; prolactin is released during pregnancy and postpartum to cause lactation. Another common cause of hyperprolactinemia is primary hypothyroidism. Hypothyroidism can cause diffuse hypertrophy of the pituitary gland that may resemble enlargement due to a pituitary adenoma on imaging. Nonfunctioning pituitary adenomas can also cause hyperprolactinemia by compressing the pituitary stalk and decreasing dopamine inhibition of prolactin secretion. Medications are a common cause of hyperprolactinemia. Antipsychotic agents cause hyperprolactinemia due to their antidopaminergic effect that interrupts the inhibition of prolactin by dopamine. Agents such as risperidone may raise the prolactin level above 200 ng/mL (200 µg/L). Evaluation for pituitary hypersecretion when a patient is taking a medication known to raise the prolactin level is difficult. When the prolactin level is only mildly elevated (<50 ng/mL [50 µg/L]), it may be reasonable to assume that hyperprolactinemia is a medication side effect. When significantly elevated (>100 ng/mL [100 µg/L]), either the medication needs to be withheld to further assess or a pituitary MRI obtained to evaluate for prolactinoma. Caution is warranted when discontinuation of an antipsychotic agent is being considered, and consultation with a psychiatrist is recommended prior to discontinuation. If the medication cannot be discontinued, a pituitary MRI is required to exclude the diagnosis of pituitary tumor.

Prolactinomas are treated with dopamine agonists. The two FDA-approved dopamine agonists are bromocriptine and cabergoline. Dopamine agonists typically decrease the size and hormone production of prolactinomas rapidly. Decreasing serum prolactin usually correlates with decreasing size of the tumor. Dopamine agonist therapy is not warranted without first diagnosing a prolactinoma with an MRI. Furthermore, addition of dopamine agonist therapy could worsen this patient's psychiatric disease.

Starting an oral contraceptive pill is inappropriate at this time since this patient needs a pituitary MRI to rule out a pituitary tumor prior to making a treatment decision. Once a pituitary tumor is ruled out, she can be started on an oral contraceptive pill to treat her estrogen deficiency caused by the hyperprolactinemia.

While stopping risperidone, or any psychiatric medication, may lead to decreased prolactin, this requires consultation and coordination of care with the patient's psychiatrist.

KEY POINT

- Antipsychotic agents cause hyperprolactinemia due to their antidopaminergic effect, which interrupts the inhibition of prolactin by dopamine; risperidone may raise the prolactin level above 200 ng/mL (200 µg/L).

Bibliography

Peuskens J, Pani L, Detraux J, De Hert M. The effects of novel and newly approved antipsychotics on serum prolactin levels: a comprehensive review. CNS Drugs. 2014;28:421-53. doi: 10.1007/s40263-014-0157-3. [PMID: 24677189]

Item 5   Answer: C

Educational Objective: Treat primary adrenal insufficiency.

This most appropriate treatment for this patient is hydrocortisone twice daily and fludrocortisone once daily. She has primary adrenal insufficiency, which affects all layers of the adrenal cortex, and therefore she requires both glucocorticoid and mineralocorticoid (aldosterone) therapy. Primary adrenal insufficiency is confirmed in this patient by the combination of low serum cortisol level and elevated serum adrenocorticotropic hormone (ACTH) level. Manifestations of aldosterone deficiency are hyponatremia and hyperkalemia. Some patients with primary adrenal insufficiency have normal serum electrolytes and therefore require measurement of plasma renin activity (high) and serum aldosterone (low or inappropriately normal) to confirm mineralocorticoid deficiency. The preferred glucocorticoid for treatment of adrenal insufficiency is hydrocortisone which, because of its shorter duration of action, can be prescribed two or three times daily to better mimic the circadian rhythm of endogenous cortisol secretion. The total daily recommended dose of hydrocortisone ranges from 15 to 25 mg. A higher dose of hydrocortisone (~15 mg) is given in the morning with the remaining dose (~5 mg) given in the afternoon (or in a thrice daily regimen, the second dose of hydrocortisone is given at noon with the

third, smaller dose taken later in the afternoon). For patients who have difficulty adhering to a twice-daily medication regimen, prednisone once daily in the morning may be substituted.

Dexamethasone has a long duration of action with the potential to cause comorbidities from excess glucocorticoid exposure and therefore should not be used long-term to treat adrenal insufficiency.

There are no adequate trial data to direct optimal dose and timing of glucocorticoid replacement. Measurement of serum cortisol and/or ACTH is not helpful. Glucocorticoid dosing is guided by patient symptoms. Administration of doses of glucocorticoid in excess of physiologic replacement can be associated with decreased bone mineral density and features of Cushing syndrome, with increased risk of metabolic syndrome, type 2 diabetes mellitus, hypertension, hyperlipidemia, obesity, and cardiovascular disease. Adequate mineralocorticoid replacement is indicated by normal blood pressure without orthostasis, absence of edema, and normal serum electrolytes.

Only glucocorticoid therapy is required in the treatment of secondary adrenal insufficiency. Fludrocortisone replacement is not required as aldosterone secretion is not under the control of ACTH. Hence, patients with secondary adrenal insufficiency do not develop hyperkalemia. Hyponatremia may be present in secondary adrenal insufficiency due to inappropriate antidiuretic hormone secretion and action, with resultant inability to excrete free water.

KEY POINT

- Patients with primary adrenal failure require both glucocorticoid and mineralocorticoid replacement therapy.

Bibliography

Bancos I, Hahner S, Tomlinson J, Arlt W. Diagnosis and management of adrenal insufficiency. Lancet Diabetes Endocrinol. 2015;3:216-26. [PMID: 25098712] doi:10.1016/S2213-8587(14)70142-1

Item 6   Answer: A

Educational Objective: Evaluate Paget disease of bone.

The laboratory results and findings on radiographs are most consistent with Paget disease of bone. Measurement of serum total alkaline phosphatase is the next step after radiographic diagnosis and delineation of which bones are affected. It reflects the metabolic activity of Paget disease of bone at diagnosis and is used in follow-up evaluation whether treatment is given or not. Occasionally, total alkaline phosphatase may be normal in newly diagnosed patients with radiographic and radionuclide bone scan evidence of Paget disease. This quiescent or "burnt-out" stage of the disease does not require treatment.

Many patients with Paget disease are older and may have risk factors for osteoporosis. These two conditions, however, are unrelated, have different treatment endpoints, and different bisphosphonate dosing. If bone mineral density were to be ordered, it would be for reasons independent of the evaluation and treatment of Paget disease.

CT imaging of bones provides greater resolution and is superior to conventional radiographs in detecting and characterizing some metabolic bone disorders. With the exception of clarifying the extent of basilar skull involvement and risk for cranial nerve impingement, clinically relevant Paget disease is readily detected and diagnosed by conventional radiographs and radionuclide bone scans.

Bisphosphonates, particularly intravenous zoledronic acid, are highly effective, often requiring a single dose to normalize alkaline phosphatase for several years in patients with Paget disease. Given the risk for spinal cord compression or compression fracture, involvement of T7 with Paget disease would be an indication for treatment unless the disease were metabolically inactive. Therefore, zoledronic acid would not be given prior to assessment of serum total alkaline phosphatase.

KEY POINT

- Serum alkaline phosphatase, a marker of increased bone turnover, should be measured after radiographic diagnosis of Paget disease of bone.

Bibliography

Singer FR, Bone HG 3rd, Hosking DJ, Lyles KW, Murad MH, Reid IR, et al; Endocrine Society. Paget's disease of bone: an Endocrine Society Clinical Practice Guideline. J Clin Endocrinol Metab. 2014;99:4408-22. [PMID: 25406796] doi:10.1210/jc.2014-2910

Item 7   Answer: C

Educational Objective: Diagnose subacute thyroiditis.

The most likely diagnosis is subacute thyroiditis. Subacute thyroiditis is an uncommon cause of thyrotoxicosis that presents following a viral upper respiratory tract infection and is distinguished by a tender or painful thyroid. This is a form of destructive thyroiditis resulting from the leakage of stored thyroid hormone from damaged thyroid follicles. The diagnosis can be confirmed by determining radioactive iodine uptake, which would be low (<10%). Management is aimed at controlling symptoms. This includes treatment with β-blockers and pain control with NSAIDs or, less commonly, glucocorticoids. In most cases, thyrotoxicosis typically lasts 2 to 6 weeks. It is followed by a hypothyroid phase after stored thyroid hormone is depleted, typically lasting 6 to 12 weeks. The patient may become clinically hypothyroid and require temporary levothyroxine therapy. Most patients with thyroiditis eventually recover to a euthyroid state.

Graves disease is the most common cause of thyrotoxicosis in the United States and most frequently affects young women. This patient does not have pathognomic features of Graves disease (thyroid bruit, eye disease, or dermopathy), making this an unlikely diagnosis.

Molar pregnancy is a rare cause of hyperthyroidism resulting from the binding of human chorionic gonadotropin (HCG) to the thyroid-stimulating hormone (TSH) receptor in the setting of very high HCG levels. The negative pregnancy test excludes this diagnosis.

Nodular thyroid disease (toxic adenoma and multinodular goiter) is the next most common cause of thyrotoxicosis after Graves disease and is more commonly seen in older adults. This patient lacks palpable thyroid nodules on examination, which is usually seen with hyperthyroidism from nodular thyroid disease. In addition, neither Graves disease nor nodular thyroid disease cause thyroid pain.

KEY POINT

- Subacute thyroiditis is an uncommon cause of thyrotoxicosis that presents following a viral upper respiratory tract infection and is distinguished by a tender or painful thyroid, suppressed thyroid-stimulating hormone, and elevated serum free thyroxine.

Bibliography

De Leo S, Lee SY, Braverman LE. Hyperthyroidism. Lancet. 2016;388:906-18. [PMID: 27038492] doi:10.1016/S0140-6736(16)00278-6

Item 8   Answer: B

Educational Objective: Reduce the risk of diabetic neuropathy in a patient with type 1 diabetes mellitus.

According to high-quality evidence, enhanced glucose control significantly prevents the development of clinical neuropathy and reduces nerve conduction and vibration threshold abnormalities in type 1 diabetes mellitus. Glycemic control can delay progression of neuropathy in type 2 diabetes. Other than glucose control, no other preventive strategies are available for diabetic neuropathy. Hemoglobin A_{1c} goals in patients with diabetes should be individually tailored taking into account the demonstrated benefits with regard to prevention and delay in microvascular complications with the risk of hypoglycemia. A reasonable goal of therapy might be a hemoglobin A_{1c} value less than or equal to 7% for most patients, with higher targets for older adult patients and those with comorbidities or a limited life expectancy and more stringent control for those patients with type 1 diabetes and during pregnancy.

The American Diabetes Association advocates for a target systolic blood pressure between 125 and 130 mm Hg in select patients (young, long life expectancy, increased risk of stroke), if this can be accomplished safely. While this patient will benefit from improved blood pressure control by reducing the risk of cardiovascular disease, it will have no impact on her risk for the development of diabetic neuropathy.

While lifestyle intervention to improve the lipid profile should be undertaken in all patients with diabetes, for patients without cardiovascular disease and under age 40 years, statin therapy should be considered only in those with multiple cardiovascular disease risk factors; the American College of Cardiology/American Heart Association risk calculator can determine the 10-year atherosclerotic cardiovascular disease risk to guide therapeutic management. Improved lipid control, while indicated and beneficial for the prevention of cardiovascular disease, does not assist in the prevention of diabetic neuropathy.

Although pregabalin is indicated to treat painful diabetic neuropathy, it does not prevent diabetic neuropathy.

Although weight loss should be discussed as part of a therapeutic lifestyle plan, there is no data to suggest weight loss prevents the development of diabetic neuropathy.

KEY POINT

- Enhanced glucose control significantly prevents the development of clinical neuropathy and reduces nerve conduction and vibration threshold abnormalities in type 1 diabetes mellitus.

Bibliography
Callaghan BC, Little AA, Feldman EL, Hughes RA. Enhanced glucose control for preventing and treating diabetic neuropathy. Cochrane Database Syst Rev. 2012:CD007543. [PMID: 22696371] doi:10.1002/14651858.CD007543.pub2

Item 9   Answer: D

Educational Objective: Identify vitamin D deficiency as a cause of hypocalcemia after antiresorptive therapy for osteoporosis.

The most likely diagnosis is vitamin D deficiency. Special populations will have lower levels of vitamin D owing to medical conditions or medication side effects. Obesity has been correlated with lower vitamin D levels possibly related to fat sequestration. Phenobarbital and phenytoin may increase the metabolism of vitamin D to inactive forms. Glucocorticoids can decrease vitamin D metabolism to active forms. Agents that decrease absorption such as orlistat can decrease vitamin D absorption. Malabsorption disorders, including celiac disease and bariatric surgery, can also result in vitamin D deficiency. This patient has multiple risk factors for vitamin D deficiency including age, possible malnutrition, glucocorticoid use, and being home bound. In the face of ongoing vitamin D deficiency, normocalcemia is maintained through increased bone resorption through increased osteoclastic activity. Antiresorptive drugs, especially the first dose of intravenous bisphosphonates and denosumab, rapidly suppress osteoclastic bone resorption and can precipitate hypocalcemia in these patients. Vitamin D sufficiency should be assessed prior to initiating antiresorptive drugs, especially those administered parenterally.

High baseline bone turnover and abrupt alteration in calcium flux between blood and bone are also features of hungry bone syndrome. However, this syndrome specifically occurs after parathyroidectomy for primary hyperparathyroidism. It is caused by rapid influx of calcium from the blood into the skeleton. In the absence of parathyroidectomy, hungry bone syndrome cannot explain this patient's findings.

Acute hyperphosphatemia from tumor lysis syndrome or phosphorus-containing bowel preparations may cause acute hypocalcemia. Chronic hyperphosphatemia associated with chronic kidney disease can also result in hypocalcemia. However, these conditions are not present and, in the case of chronic kidney disease, cannot account for the patient's rapid clinical deterioration.

In contrast to surgery, hypoparathyroidism due to autoimmunity, radiation, or infiltrative processes develops slowly and serum calcium declines gradually over months to years, which is not consistent with the precipitous drop seen in this patient over 2 days.

KEY POINT

- Potent antiresorptive drugs can cause severe hypocalcemia by impairing efflux of calcium from the skeleton in patients with vitamin D deficiency; it is important to assess vitamin D levels and correct deficiency before beginning treatment with an antiresorptive drug.

Bibliography
Kaur U, Chakrabarti SS, Gambhir IS. Zoledronic acid–induced hypocalcemia and hypophosphatemia in osteoporosis: a cause of concern. Curr Drug Saf. 2016;11:267-9. [PMID: 27113952]

Item 10   Answer: A

Educational Objective: Diagnose an androgen-producing adrenal tumor.

The most appropriate test to perform next is a CT scan of the abdomen. This postmenopausal woman has new-onset hyperandrogenism associated with significant elevation of serum dehydroepiandrosterone sulfate (DHEAS). The clinical picture of rapid-onset hirsutism and signs of virilization indicate an androgen-secreting tumor. Signs of virilization are deepening of the voice, clitoromegaly, hirsutism, and temporal hair loss. Under normal conditions, androgen production in women occurs in both the adrenal glands and ovaries, as well as by peripheral conversion. The major source of DHEAS is the adrenal gland, and an abdominal CT is recommended when serum DHEAS value is above 700 µg/dL (18.9 µmol/L).

DHEAS-secreting tumors of the adrenal gland are readily visible on CT imaging and adrenal vein sampling to localize the tumor is rarely required.

Pelvic MRI may be more sensitive at detecting small ovarian tumors and is often considered as second-line imaging when pelvic ultrasound is negative. If both pelvic ultrasound and MRI imaging are negative in the setting of suspicion for a testosterone-secreting ovarian tumor, ovarian vein sampling may be required to reveal the location of the tumor. Ovarian vein sampling is reserved for premenopausal women. Postmenopausal women can forego this invasive procedure and proceed directly to bilateral oophorectomy. Significant testosterone secretion can also be due to a non–tumorous condition called ovarian hyperthecosis. Hyperandrogenic symptoms are typically (but not always) of slower onset compared with that seen with androgen-secreting tumors.

A pelvic ultrasound is recommended as the first imaging study if testosterone is above 150 ng/dL (5.2 nmol/L). This patient's testosterone level was only mildly elevated, but the DHEAS was quite elevated making a testosterone-producing ovarian tumor less likely than an adrenal tumor.

KEY POINT

- Signs of androgen excess such as progressive hirsutism and virilization over a short period of time in female patients suggest the diagnosis of an androgen-producing adrenal or ovarian tumor.

Bibliography

Markopoulos MC, Kassi E, Alexandraki KI, Mastorakos G, Kaltsas G. Hyperandrogenism after menopause. Eur J Endocrinol. 2015;172:R79-91. [PMID: 25225480] doi:10.1530/EJE-14-0468

Item 11   Answer: C

Educational Objective: Diagnose nonthyroidal illness syndrome.

The most likely diagnosis is nonthyroidal illness syndrome (euthyroid sick syndrome), which is most often seen in critically ill hospitalized patients and is characterized by a reduced serum triiodothyronine (T_3) level, low or low-normal serum thyroxine (T_4) level, and normal or low (but detectable) serum thyroid-stimulating hormone (TSH) level. These findings result from changes in the peripheral uptake of thyroid hormones, reduced levels of thyroid hormone-binding proteins, and alterations in the expression and activity of deiodinases. Very low serum T_4 levels are associated with poor overall outcome. Treatment with levothyroxine or liothyronine is not indicated due to lack of evidence of benefit.

Central hypothyroidism is not the most likely diagnosis. The patient described here has no signs or symptoms suggestive of hypothyroidism. Characteristic biochemical findings in central hypothyroidism include low or inappropriately normal serum TSH in the setting of low total and free T_4 levels and reduced or low-normal serum T_3. In contrast to nonthyroidal illness, in which the T_3 to T_4 ratio is low, a high serum T_3 to T_4 ratio is seen in central hypothyroidism because conversion of T_4 to T_3 in peripheral tissues is maintained.

Heparin-induced thyroid function test abnormality is also incorrect. A single intravenous heparin injection may increase serum free T_4 up to 5 times the baseline value within minutes. This spurious laboratory finding is related to heparin-induced stimulation of lipoprotein lipase and generation of free fatty acids, which displace T_4 from binding proteins. Heparin has no effect on serum TSH, total T_4, or total T_3 values.

Subclinical hyperthyroidism is also not the most likely diagnosis. This patient has atrial fibrillation, but no other clinical findings suggestive of thyroid hormone excess. Although the low serum TSH level is consistent with this diagnosis, the total and free T_4 levels are near the lower limit of the normal range and total T_3 is reduced.

KEY POINT

- Nonthyroidal illness syndrome (euthyroid sick syndrome) is characterized by reduced serum T_3, low or low-normal serum T_4, and normal or low (but detectable) serum TSH levels.

Bibliography

Fliers E, Bianco AC, Langouche L, Boelen A. Thyroid function in critically ill patients. Lancet Diabetes Endocrinol. 2015;3:816-25. [PMID: 26071885] doi:10.1016/S2213-8587(15)00225-9

Item 12   Answer: C

Educational Objective: Manage Cushing syndrome with glucocorticoid therapy following adrenalectomy.

The most appropriate management of this patient following adrenalectomy for treatment of Cushing syndrome is hydrocortisone therapy. Patients who have undergone adrenalectomy for Cushing syndrome are at risk of secondary adrenal insufficiency due to hypercortisolism-induced suppression of the hypothalamic (corticotropin-releasing hormone [CRH]) and pituitary (adrenocorticotropic [ACTH] hormone) axis. Subsequent recovery of the hypothalamic-pituitary axis following removal of the source of excess cortisol secretion can take time, and hence endogenous cortisol production is impaired. In addition, cortisol-producing cells from the contralateral adrenal gland may have undergone atrophy due to lack of ACTH stimulation. Patients often require higher than physiologic doses of glucocorticoid therapy to prevent "glucocorticoid withdrawal syndrome," an ill-defined complex of symptoms of fatigue, loss of appetite, nausea, and/or myalgia. There is no agreed upon glucocorticoid regimen following adrenalectomy and treatment of Cushing syndrome. The process of tapering and eventual discontinuation of glucocorticoid therapy is guided by patient symptoms and can be a lengthy process, taking up to 1 year or longer for the remaining adrenal gland to produce adequate cortisol.

ACTH-dependent causes of Cushing syndrome also lead to suppression of endogenous CRH and ACTH production, and hence patients with these disorders also require glucocorticoid therapy following successful treatment of Cushing syndrome.

Epinephrine is also not under ACTH control, and therefore epinephrine replacement is not required after adrenalectomy. In addition, epinephrine replacement is not required following bilateral adrenalectomy, as lack of epinephrine is not known to be associated with clinical disease.

Likewise, fludrocortisone therapy is not required following adrenalectomy as mineralocorticoid secretion is not under ACTH control. Therefore, aldosterone secretion from the contralateral adrenal gland is not impacted by Cushing syndrome. Fludrocortisone therapy is required following bilateral adrenalectomy.

Phenoxybenzamine is used as a preoperative α-receptor blockade for 10 to 14 days before surgery for pheochromocytomas and paragangliomas to prevent hypertensive crises

CONT.

during surgery and is not indicated following adrenalectomy for Cushing syndrome.

KEY POINT

- Following adrenalectomy for Cushing syndrome, patients require daily glucocorticoid replacement therapy to allow recovery from prolonged suppression due to hypercortisolism; recovery of adrenal function may take up to 1 year or longer depending on the severity of Cushing syndrome.

Bibliography

Hochberg Z, Pacak K, Chrousos GP. Endocrine withdrawal syndromes. Endocr Rev. 2003;24:523-38. [PMID: 12920153]

Item 13   Answer: C

Educational Objective: Diagnose male hypogonadism.

The most appropriate management is to repeat testosterone measurement at 8 AM. The clinical diagnosis of hypogonadism is made on the basis of signs and symptoms consistent with androgen deficiency with the finding of low morning testosterone concentrations on at least two occasions. Timing of initial laboratory assessment is important due to the diurnal variation of testosterone. Additionally, assessment of hypogonadism should not be undertaken during acute illness. The next step in management of this patient would be to obtain a morning testosterone concentration; if low, testing should be confirmed with a repeat morning measurement. After the initial diagnosis, determination of primary or secondary hypogonadism is established by measurement of luteinizing hormone (LH) and follicle-stimulating hormone (FSH) levels. Elevated gonadotropin levels are seen in primary hypogonadism with LH and FSH levels low or inappropriately normal in secondary hypogonadism.

Based on Endocrine Society guidelines, men with hypogonadism should be treated with exogenous testosterone when they have consistent signs and symptoms of hypogonadism and low serum testosterone levels. Patients requiring testosterone replacement therapy should have testosterone levels monitored at 3 and 6 months after initiation and annually thereafter; the goal total testosterone level should be in the mid-normal range. Monitoring of the prostate specific antigen and hematocrit level should follow Endocrine Society guidelines. Before initiating testosterone therapy in this patient, the diagnosis of hypogonadism needs to be confirmed with two appropriately timed testosterone measurements.

The most sensitive and cost-effective initial diagnostic study in patients with suspected hemochromatosis is measurement of the fasting serum transferrin saturation (calculated as [serum iron/total iron binding capacity] ×100). Serum ferritin level measurement is indicated in patients with elevated transferrin saturation. Evaluation for hemochromatosis is only appropriate after the diagnosis of hypogonadism is established. The first diagnostic step for this patient is the collection of two properly collected serum testosterone levels to establish the diagnosis of hypogonadism.

If subsequent evaluation of the patient confirms the presence of hypogonadotrophic hypogonadism (low testosterone and low LH and FSH levels), MRI of the pituitary to detect a pituitary adenoma or other mass would be appropriate. A pituitary MRI would be premature at this point.

KEY POINT

- In men with specific signs and symptoms of hypogonadism, measuring an 8 AM total testosterone level is indicated; if the testosterone level is low, a second 8 AM confirmatory testosterone level is measured.

Bibliography

Basaria S. Male hypogonadism. Lancet. 2014;383:1250-63. [PMID: 24119423] doi:10.1016/S0140-6736(13)61126-5

Item 14   Answer: C

Educational Objective: Prevent complications of management of chronic hypoparathyroidism.

The most appropriate test to perform now is measurement of 24-hour urine calcium. In chronic hypoparathyroidism, goals of therapy are to eliminate symptoms while avoiding complications of therapy; monitoring of urine calcium excretion is mandatory because hypercalciuria often limits therapy. Without parathyroid hormone (PTH), urinary calcium excretion is higher than normal for any given serum calcium level. Complications of prolonged hypercalciuria include nephrolithiasis and impaired glomerular filtration rate. Serum calcium, magnesium, creatinine, and urine calcium levels should be assessed on a regular basis. The goal calcium levels should be low-normal without hypercalciuria. The magnesium level should ideally be greater than 2 mg/dL (0.83 mmol/L), and creatinine levels should remain in the normal range. If the urine calcium level is greater than 300 mg/24 h (hypercalciuria), calcium and/or vitamin D replacement needs to be decreased. Calcium is usually decreased first if the 25-hydroxyvitamin D level is within the normal sufficiency range (≥30 ng/mL [75 nmol/L]). Thiazide diuretics reduce urine calcium excretion and thus may permit sufficient calcium and vitamin D therapy to achieve goal calcium levels.

Hypoparathyroidism slows bone metabolism and is relatively protective against the development of postmenopausal osteoporosis. Further, osteoporosis medications would rarely be indicated in these patients. Therefore, bone mineral density testing is not indicated.

The dose of calcitriol administered is titrated by the serum calcium and/or phosphorus level rather than the serum 1,25-dihydroxyvitamin D level.

If serum PTH is not detectable 6 months after the onset of surgical hypoparathyroidism, it can be considered chronic. Without PTH, vitamin D activation, specifically the conversion of 25-hydroxyvitamin D to 1,25-dihydroxyvitamin D (calcitriol) in the kidney, is severely impaired. Although vitamin D nutritional status as assessed by 25-hydroxyvitamin D may be relevant for other health conditions, its measurement in not useful in the setting of chronic hypoparathyroidism unless residual PTH production remains.

Ionized calcium, rather than total calcium, is the relevant calcium fraction in the blood. However, in an otherwise healthy person in whom serum albumin concentrations are presumed to be normal, measurement of ionized calcium does not contribute to the management of hypoparathyroidism.

KEY POINT

- In chronic hypoparathyroidism, the goals of therapy are to eliminate symptoms while avoiding complications of therapy; monitoring urine calcium excretion is mandatory because hypercalciuria often limits therapy.

Bibliography

Brandi ML, Bilezikian JP, Shoback D, Bouillon R, Clarke BL, Thakker RV, Khan AA, Potts JT Jr. Management of hypoparathyroidism: summary statement and guidelines. J Clin Endocrinol Metab. 2016;101:2273-83. doi:10.1210/jc.2015-3907. [PMID: 26943719]

Item 15   Answer: A

Educational Objective: Diagnose adrenocorticotropic hormone (ACTH)-independent Cushing syndrome.

The most likely cause of this patient's hypercortisolism is adrenocorticotropic hormone (ACTH)-independent Cushing syndrome caused by an adrenal tumor. The diagnosis of Cushing syndrome is confirmed by the combination of clinical features (central obesity, dorsocervical and supraclavicular fat pads, new onset hypertension, and worsening diabetes control), in the setting of two positive diagnostic tests for Cushing syndrome: elevated 24-hour urine free cortisol level and elevated midnight salivary cortisol level. A 24-hour urine free cortisol that is three times the upper limit of the normal range (as in this patient) is considered to be confirmatory for Cushing syndrome if compatible clinical features are also present. Once Cushing syndrome is confirmed, the next step in the diagnosis is to categorize Cushing syndrome into ACTH-dependent and ACTH-independent types, which in turn governs subsequent localization tests. A low serum ACTH level, as in this patient, indicates ACTH-independent Cushing syndrome. Excluding glucocorticoid administration, the most common cause of ACTH-independent Cushing syndrome is a cortisol-secreting adrenal tumor. ACTH is suppressed in this situation due to elevated cortisol levels causing negative feedback at the level of the hypothalamus and pituitary gland, which inhibits ACTH production.

Cushing syndrome in the presence of a detectable or elevated serum ACTH indicates ACTH-dependent disease. Causes of ACTH-dependent Cushing syndrome include ACTH secretion from a pituitary tumor (most commonly) or from an ectopic source such as a bronchial carcinoid tumor.

Hypercortisolism in the absence of Cushing syndrome can occur with psychiatric illness. The mechanism of hypercortisolism associated with psychiatric illness is activation of the hypothalamic-pituitary axis; in this situation ACTH

production is not suppressed. In addition, patients do not manifest clinical features of Cushing syndrome. This patient's suppressed serum ACTH rules out psychiatric illness as the primary cause of her hypercortisolism.

KEY POINT

- Excluding glucocorticoid administration, the most common cause of adrenocorticotropic hormone (ACTH)-independent Cushing syndrome is an adrenal tumor.

Bibliography

Loriaux DL. Diagnosis and differential diagnosis of Cushing's syndrome. N Engl J Med. 2017;376:1451-1459. doi: 10.1056/NEJMra1505550. [PMID: 28402781]

Item 16   Answer: B

Educational Objective: Manage anabolic steroid-induced hypogonadism.

Cessation of anabolic steroid use is the appropriate management plan at this time. This patient presents with symptoms and signs suggestive of anabolic steroid-induced hypogonadism including decreased libido, acne, gynecomastia, small testes, and suppressed gonadotropins with resultant hypogonadism. Extratesticular effects may also be noted, including low HDL cholesterol level, hepatotoxicity, erythrocytosis, and increased risk of obstructive sleep apnea. Mood disorders are common in anabolic steroid users. He will remain hypogonadal for an undetermined amount of time after stopping exogenous androgens before recovery of his hypothalamic-pituitary-gonadal axis.

Anastrozole is an aromatase inhibitor. It blocks the conversion of androgens to estrogens leading to increased serum testosterone levels. Clomiphene is a selective estrogen receptor modulator that stimulates pituitary gonadotropins and consequently testosterone production. Human chorionic gonadotropin (HCG) binds to the luteinizing hormone (LH) receptor resulting in stimulation of testosterone secretion by Leydig cells. While all of these agents may be requested by patients to mitigate the effects of anabolic steroid-induced hypogonadism, there is no strong evidence supporting their effectiveness and safety for management of anabolic steroid-induced hypogonadism.

Testosterone therapy has been associated with increased hemoglobin and hematocrit levels, worsened obstructive sleep apnea, and decreased HDL cholesterol levels. Since this patient's hemoglobin level is already significantly elevated, testosterone replacement therapy might be potentially harmful. Also, testosterone replacement therapy would not resolve his acne, gynecomastia, or small testes. Furthermore, initiation of testosterone replacement therapy would delay resolution of the expected hypogonadism seen following the discontinuation of anabolic steroids.

KEY POINT

- Cessation of anabolic steroid use is the most appropriate management of steroid-induced hypogonadism.

Bibliography

Karavolos S, Reynolds M, Panagiotopoulou N, McEleny K, Scally M, Quinton R. Male central hypogonadism secondary to exogenous androgens: a review of the drugs and protocols highlighted by the online community of users for prevention and/or mitigation of adverse effects. Clin Endocrinol (Oxf). 2015;82:624-32. [PMID: 25333666] doi:10.1111/cen.12641

Item 17   Answer: C

Educational Objective: Treat hypothyroidism in pregnancy.

For women with hypothyroidism adequately treated with levothyroxine before pregnancy, dosing can be empirically increased by 30% when pregnancy is confirmed. Levothyroxine is the treatment of choice for the management of hypothyroidism during pregnancy. Patients can be counseled to start taking an additional two tablets of their prepregnancy levothyroxine dose per week, which is roughly equivalent to a 30% increase. In euthyroid women without thyroid disease, the total body thyroxine (T_4) pool increases by 40% to 50% during pregnancy. This is mediated by the stimulatory effects of thyroid-stimulating hormone (TSH) and placental human chorionic gonadotropin. Pregnant women with hypothyroidism are unable to augment thyroidal production of T_4 and triiodothyronine (T_3). The levothyroxine dose of hypothyroid women must therefore be adjusted to maintain a euthyroid state. Because T_4 requirements may begin to increase as early as 4 to 6 weeks of pregnancy, women with hypothyroidism should increase their levothyroxine dose or serum TSH should be measured as soon as pregnancy is confirmed. TSH should be measured every 4 weeks for the first half of pregnancy and around 30 weeks of gestation in all women with hypothyroidism. A TSH value in the lower half of the reference range should be targeted (equivalent to a TSH level below 2.5 µU/mL [2.5 mU/L]) both in preconception planning and during pregnancy.

Continuing the patient on her current dose of levothyroxine and checking serum TSH in 2 months or decreasing the patient's levothyroxine dose are both inappropriate management and could precipitate maternal or fetal hypothyroidism. The use of liothyronine or T_3-containing preparations including desiccated thyroid is contraindicated in pregnancy because the fetal central nervous system is relatively impermeable to T_3. Thyroid hormone is essential for normal fetal development and is especially critical for the fetal brain.

KEY POINT

- For women with hypothyroidism adequately treated with levothyroxine before pregnancy, dosing can be empirically increased by 30% when pregnancy is confirmed.

Bibliography

Alexander EK, Pearce EN, Brent GA, Brown RS, Chen H, Dosiou C, et al. 2017 Guidelines of the American Thyroid Association for the Diagnosis and Management of Thyroid Disease During Pregnancy and the Postpartum. Thyroid. 2017;27:315-389. [PMID: 28056690] doi:10.1089/thy.2016.0457

Item 18   Answer: D

Educational Objective: Understand risks associated with gender-affirming therapy.

Transgender medicine is the care of persons whose gender identity differs from the sex that was assigned at birth. Gender incongruence is persistent incongruence between gender identity and external sexual anatomy at birth absent of a confounding mental disorder. A transgender man is someone with a male gender identity and a female birth assigned sex; a transgender woman (as in this patient) is someone with a female gender identity and a male birth assigned sex.

The most appropriate next step in management is to refer the patient for discussion on fertility preservation options. Gender-affirming hormone therapy is the primary medical intervention sought by transgender people. Criteria for hormone therapy include persistent, well-documented gender dysphoria; capacity to make a fully informed decision; age of majority in a given country; and if present, control of significant medical or psychological conditions. Gender-affirmation hormone therapy limits fertility, thus reproductive options should be discussed with patients prior to initiation of hormone therapy.

While feminizing hormone therapy is typically estradiol with an androgen blocker, it would not be appropriate to initiate therapy without first considering its impact on fertility. Additionally, due to the risk of thromboembolic disease with estrogen therapy, smoking cessation must first be undertaken. Gender confirmation surgery is often the last step in the treatment process for gender dysphoria. It is recommended that individuals undergoing irreversible gender-affirming surgery, which affects fertility, engage in at least 1 year of satisfactory social role change as well as consistent and compliant hormone treatment, unless hormone therapy is not desired or medically contraindicated.

KEY POINT

- Because gender-affirming hormone therapy limits fertility, reproductive options should be discussed with patients prior to initiation.

Bibliography

Hembree WC, Cohen-Kettenis PT, Gooren L, et al. Endocrine treatment of gender-dysphoric/gender-incongruent persons: an Endocrine Society Clinical Practice Guideline. J Clin Endocrinol Metab 2017; 102:3869. [PMID: 28945902]

Item 19   Answer: A

Educational Objective: Recognize medications that can cause falsely elevated plasma free metanephrine levels.

Amitriptyline can cause falsely elevated normetanephrine levels and should be discontinued prior to screening for pheochromocytoma. Most pheochromocytomas secrete norepinephrine, resulting in episodic or sustained hypertension. Orthostatic hypotension can also be seen and likely reflects low plasma volume. In addition to the classic triad of diaphoresis, headache, and tachycardia, common symptoms include palpitations, tremor, pallor, and anxiety. Screening for pheochromocytoma is appropriate in this patient, following discontinuation of amitriptyline. Amitriptyline acts by inhibiting norepinephrine uptake into nerve terminals, with subsequent elevation of its metabolite, normetanephrine. False-positive elevation of plasma free normetanephrine levels can occur with other tricyclic medications such as nortriptyline or combination serotonin/norepinephrine uptake inhibitors such as venlafaxine or duloxetine. False-positive elevation of plasma normetanephrine and metanephrine levels can also occur with other medications including levodopa (a substrate for catecholamine synthesis); psychoactive medications such as buspirone, prochlorperazine, amphetamines; and over-the-counter decongestant medications that contain adrenergic receptor agonists. Plasma free metanephrines can also be elevated during acute or stressful medical situations including psychiatric illness. Therefore, unless there is significant suspicion for pheochromocytoma, testing should be delayed until the acute illness has passed. Medications that can interfere with catecholamine metabolism should be discontinued (with tapering if indicated) at least 2 weeks prior to testing for pheochromocytoma.

Omeprazole, chlorthalidone, metoprolol, and progesterone do not impact catecholamine metabolism and, therefore, can be continued during screening for pheochromocytoma.

KEY POINT

- Many medications cause falsely high levels of catecholamines or metanephrines including certain antidepressants that inhibit norepinephrine uptake; therefore discontinuation of these agents at least 2 weeks prior to testing for pheochromocytoma is recommended.

Bibliography

van Berkel A, Lenders JW, Timmers HJ. Diagnosis of endocrine disease: biochemical diagnosis of phaeochromocytoma and paraganglioma. Eur J Endocrinol. 2014;170:R109-19. [PMID: 24347425] doi:10.1530/EJE-13-0882

Item 20   Answer: D

Educational Objective: Manage a patient who has completed 5 years of oral bisphosphonate therapy.

The most appropriate management of this patient is to discontinue alendronate. The Fracture Intervention Trial Long-term Extension (FLEX) trial showed that continuing alendronate treatment for 10 years compared with stopping after 5 years resulted in a small decrease in the incidence of clinical vertebral fractures but not nonvertebral fractures. Subject characteristics most predictive of incident fracture after alendronate discontinuation were age older than 76 years, current femur neck T-score below −2.5, and prior osteoporotic fracture. Importantly, women with femur neck T-score below −3.5 or who fractured during the initial 5 years of alendronate therapy were not included in the FLEX trial. The authors concluded that patients at high risk of fracture may benefit

from continuing alendronate therapy for up to 10 years. There is inconsistency among expert groups regarding the need to monitor bone mineral density during osteoporosis therapy and at 5 years to inform decision making about discontinuation of therapy. Contrary to other groups, the American College of Physicians recommends against monitoring because data from several studies showed that women treated with antiresorptive treatment benefit from reduced fractures even if BMD did not increase.

The antiresorptive effect of alendronate can be assessed by bone turnover markers including serum C-terminal peptide of type 1 collagen (CTx). However, neither CTx levels on alendronate nor change with discontinuation predict which patients will fracture if alendronate is discontinued. Furthermore, serum CTx levels in patients taking alendronate vary widely and cannot be reliably interpreted without pretreatment values.

The FLEX trial included postmenopausal women who had taken 5 years of alendronate 5 mg daily (equivalent to 35 mg weekly) or 10 mg daily (equivalent to 70 mg weekly). There was no difference in outcomes based on alendronate dose. Therefore, the management decision to be made after 5 years of alendronate therapy is to continue or discontinue rather than to modify the dose.

KEY POINT

- For low-risk osteoporotic women, treatment with antiresorptive therapy for 5 years is sufficient.

Bibliography

Qaseem A, Forciea MA, McLean RM, Denberg TD; Clinical Guidelines Committee of the American College of Physicians. Treatment of low bone density or osteoporosis to prevent fractures in men and women: a Clinical Practice Guideline Update from the American College of Physicians. Ann Intern Med. 2017;166:818-839. doi: 10.7326/M15-1361. Epub 2017 May 9. [PMID: 28492856]

Item 21   Answer: A

Educational Objective: Manage type 2 diabetes mellitus in a patient with decreasing kidney function.

The most appropriate management of this patient's diabetes mellitus is to continue the current regimen. This is an older patient with multiple comorbidities. She is at her goal hemoglobin A_{1c} level of less than 8% per the American Diabetes Association guidelines with her current regimen. In contrast, the American College of Physicians recommends that clinicians should avoid targeting an hemoglobin A_{1c} level in patients with a life expectancy less than 10 years due to advanced age (80 years or older), residence in a nursing home, or chronic conditions (such as end-stage kidney disease) because the harms outweigh the benefits in this population.

The FDA previously considered serum creatinine levels of 1.4 mg/dL (123.8 µmol/L) or higher in women and 1.5 mg/dL (132.6 µmol/L) or higher in men a contraindication to metformin use due to concerns for development of lactic acidosis. After further review of safety data from multiple studies, the criteria for continued safe use of metformin have been revised by the FDA. The use of serum creatinine for determining safe use of metformin was replaced by estimated glomerular filtration rate (eGFR) to better estimate kidney function. Patients who have a decrease in eGFR to 30 to 45 mL/min/1.73 m² while treated with metformin may continue use after consideration of risks and benefits. If metformin is continued, frequent monitoring of kidney function (every 3 months) is recommended. Metformin should be discontinued if the eGFR falls below 30 mL/min/1.73 m².

Because she is at her goal hemoglobin A_{1c} level of less than 8%, intensifying her therapy with either insulin glargine or glipizide is unnecessary, In addition, increasing the insulin glargine or glipizide dose in the setting of worsening kidney function could increase the risk for hypoglycemia. Additional weight gain may also occur with an increased insulin glargine or glipizide dose.

KEY POINT

- Metformin may be continued in patients with an estimated glomerular filtration rate to 30 to 45 mL/min/1.73 m² after consideration of risks and benefits; if metformin is continued, frequent monitoring of kidney function (every 3 months) is recommended.

Bibliography
American Diabetes Association. 8. Pharmacologic approaches to glycemic treatment: Standards of Medical Care in Diabetes-2018. Diabetes Care. 2018;41(Suppl 1):S73-S85. doi: 10.2337/dc18-S008. [PMID: 29222379]

Item 22   Answer: A

Educational Objective: Treat polycystic ovary syndrome.

This patient has ovulatory dysfunction with clinical and biochemical evidence of hyperandrogenism. While this is suggestive of polycystic ovary syndrome, this is a diagnosis of exclusion. The prolonged clinical course and absence of the more concerning findings of virilization also support the diagnosis of polycystic ovary syndrome. Given that this patient is most concerned about hirsutism and acne, oral contraceptive therapy is the first-line therapeutic agent. Oral contraceptive therapy suppresses gonadotropin secretion and resultant ovarian androgen production. Additionally, the estrogen component increases sex hormone-binding globulin resulting in less androgen bioavailability. Oral contraceptives that contain 30 to 35 µg of ethinyl estradiol appear to be more effective in managing hirsutism than formulations containing less ethinyl estradiol. Furthermore, oral contraceptive therapy reduces new terminal hair growth, improves acne, and regulates menses to prevent endometrial hyperplasia.

Metformin minimally effects hirsutism and is not recommended for this indication. In patients with polycystic ovary syndrome, metformin could be considered for off-label treatment of prediabetes or treatment of type 2 diabetes, in addition to lifestyle modification.

Pelvic ultrasound and adrenal CT should be performed to exclude an ovarian or adrenal neoplasm if the serum total testosterone level is greater than 150 ng/dL (5.2 nmol/L), and adrenal CT is necessary to exclude an adrenal cortisol-secreting and/or androgen-secreting neoplasm if the plasma dehydroepiandrosterone sulfate (DHEAS) level is greater than 7.0 µg/mL (18.9 µmol/L). Pelvic ultrasound and adrenal CT are not indicated in this patient as her testosterone and DHEAS levels are not elevated to the degree that ovarian tumor is a consideration.

While spironolactone can reduce the growth of terminal hair, it is used as an add-on treatment to oral contraceptive therapy. This antiandrogen medication may disrupt organogenesis in a male fetus; thus, concomitant reliable contraception is mandated when initiating this treatment.

KEY POINT

- Oral contraceptive agents are first-line pharmacologic therapy for hirsutism, acne, and menstrual dysfunction unless fertility is desired in a patient with polycystic ovary syndrome.

Bibliography
McCartney CR, Marshall JC. Clinical practice: polycystic ovary syndrome. N Engl J Med. 2016;375:54-64. [PMID: 27406348] doi:10.1056/NEJMcp1514916

Item 23   Answer: A

Educational Objective: Evaluate a pituitary tumor for hypersecretion.

Measurement of prolactin and insulin-like growth factor 1 (IGF-1) is recommended for the evaluation of possible hypersecretion of an incidentally discovered pituitary tumor. When a pituitary tumor is incidentally noted, investigation must determine (1) whether it is causing a mass effect, (2) whether it is secreting excess hormones, and (3) whether it has a propensity to grow and cause problems in the future. After a thorough history and physical examination, biochemical testing can be undertaken in a targeted fashion based on the patient's clinical signs and symptoms. Although not generally useful in the differential diagnosis of a pituitary mass, all patients should be evaluated for hormone hyposecretion in order to identify and replace hormone deficiencies. Initial tests to evaluate for hormone deficiency should include measurement of 8 AM cortisol, thyroid-stimulating hormone (TSH), free (or total) thyroxine (T_4), follicle stimulating hormone (FSH), testosterone in men and menstrual history in women (normal menstrual cycles eliminates the need to measure hormone levels). Prolactin and IGF-1 are measured to rule out pituitary hormone hypersecretion. Screening for growth hormone excess in pituitary incidentalomas may allow early detection of a growth hormone secreting tumor therefore increasing the chance of a surgical cure. If the tumor is not causing mass effect and there is no evidence of hormone excess, a pituitary MRI should be repeated in 6 months for a macroadenoma (≥1 cm) and 12 months for a microadenoma (<1 cm) to assess for growth. If no growth occurs, MRIs should be repeated every 1 to 2 years for the next 3 years and then intermittently thereafter.

Measurement of urine free cortisol is not necessary in every patient with a pituitary tumor. This should be measured only when Cushing disease is suspected based on clinical history and physical examination findings. This patient has no physical features suspicious for Cushing disease nor does he have diseases associated with Cushing disease such as diabetes or hypertension.

Visual field examination is absolutely necessary in all patients with a macroadenoma that abuts or compresses the optic chiasm, but it is not necessary in patients with no evidence of involvement of the optic chiasm on MRI. This patient's tumor does not abut or compress the optic chiasm or optic nerves.

No further evaluation is inappropriate as pituitary hypersecretion should be evaluated in all pituitary tumors.

KEY POINT

- In patients with pituitary tumors, pituitary hypersecretion should be ruled out by biochemical testing.

Bibliography

Freda PU, Beckers AM, Katznelson L, Molitch ME, Montori VM, Post KD, et al; Endocrine Society. Pituitary incidentaloma: an Endocrine Society Clinical Practice Guideline. J Clin Endocrinol Metab. 2011;96:894-904. [PMID: 21474686] doi:10.1210/jc.2010-1048.

Item 24   Answer: E

Educational Objective: Manage a patient with pheochromocytoma prior to surgery.

The most appropriate preoperative management in this patient with a pheochromocytoma is an α-adrenergic blocking agent. An α-receptor blockade is required prior to adrenalectomy to prevent potential hypertensive crisis caused by catecholamine release during anesthesia induction and/or manipulation of the tumor. Phenoxybenzamine is started approximately 10 to 14 days prior to surgery, and the dose progressively increased to achieve a desired blood pressure of 130/80 mm Hg or lower when seated, and systolic pressure of 90 mm Hg or higher when standing. Because phenoxybenzamine causes vasodilation, an expected consequence of therapy is postural hypotension. To counteract this and allow appropriate dose escalation of phenoxybenzamine, patients are advised to drink plenty of fluids, eat high salt-containing foods, and to make liberal use of the salt shaker at meal times. If blood pressure is not adequately controlled with an α-receptor blockade (or prohibitive side effects occur with required higher doses), a calcium-channel blocker such as amlodipine can be added. A short-acting, selective α-blocker such as prazosin, doxazosin, or terazosin, can be considered alternatives to phenoxybenzamine, based on decreased cost and limited data suggesting similar patient outcomes.

Hydralazine or lisinopril do not provide the needed α-receptor blockade, and therefore increasing the dose of these medications would not be helpful before surgery.

Diuretics, such as chlorthalidone, should be avoided in patients with pheochromocytoma. These patients may have diminished intravascular volume secondary to intense vasoconstriction and further diuretic-induced volume depletion may lead to severe hypotension. Finally, diuretic treatment will not prevent hypertensive crisis during adrenalectomy.

Metoprolol or other β-blockers should never be started prior to adequate α-receptor blockade in patients with pheochromocytoma, as unopposed α-receptor stimulation can precipitate a hypertensive crisis. Once adequate α-receptor blockade has been achieved, however, a β-blocker is typically added to the medication regimen 2 to 3 days prior to surgery to counteract vasodilation-induced tachycardia.

In the case of very large tumors and/or significant metanephrine elevation, the catecholamine synthesis inhibitor metyrosine may also be added to the medication regimen. Metyrosine is not given routinely in the preoperative management of pheochromocytoma due to significant side effects associated with body-wide catecholamine deficiency.

KEY POINT

- An α-receptor blockade with phenoxybenzamine or another α-blocker is required prior to adrenalectomy for pheochromocytoma to prevent potential hypertensive crisis during anesthesia induction and/or manipulation of the tumor.

Bibliography

Lenders JW, Duh QY, Eisenhofer G, et al; Endocrine Society. Pheochromocytoma and paraganglioma: an Endocrine Society Clinical Practice Guideline. J Clin Endocrinol Metab. 2014 Jun;99(6):1915-42. doi: 10.1210/jc.2014-1498. PubMed PMID: 24893135.

Item 25   Answer: A

Educational Objective: Treat type 2 diabetes mellitus in a patient with cardiovascular disease.

The patient has uncontrolled diabetes in the setting of coronary artery disease, and empagliflozin is the most appropriate treatment. Empagliflozin increases excretion of glucose by the kidneys through inhibition of the sodium-glucose transporter-2 (SGLT2) receptors. Empagliflozin received approval from the FDA for patients with type 2 diabetes and established cardiovascular disease based upon the results of the Empagliflozin Cardiovascular Outcome Event Trial in Type 2 Diabetes Mellitus Patients (EMPA-REG OUTCOME). This study demonstrated a reduction in the primary composite outcome (cardiovascular-related death, nonfatal myocardial infarction, nonfatal stroke) and all-cause mortality when empagliflozin was added to standard care versus placebo. Empagliflozin has the additional potential benefit of inducing weight loss and blood pressure lowering in this overweight patient with uncontrolled hypertension.

Although the sulfonylurea, glipizide, could improve the patient's glycemic control, it has the potential side effect of weight gain; the combination of metformin plus an SGLT2 inhibitor is superior to metformin plus a sulfonylurea (mean between-group difference, 4.7 kg [CI, 4.4 to 5.0 kg]). The combination of metformin and an SGLT2 inhibitor reduces systolic blood pressure more than that of metformin and a sulfonylurea (between-group difference, 5.1 mm Hg [CI, 4.2 to 6.0 mm Hg]).

In patients with type 2 diabetes and cardiovascular risk factors, a significant reduction in the primary composite outcome (cardiovascular death, nonfatal myocardial infarction, or nonfatal stroke) and rates of cardiovascular death and all-cause mortality has also been associated with liraglutide. There have been postmarketing reports of fatal and nonfatal acute pancreatitis associated with liraglutide. While it is not known if liraglutide increases risk for development of pancreatitis in patients with a history of pancreatitis, many experts avoid its use in this patient population.

The dipeptidyl peptidase-4 (DPP-4) inhibitor, sitagliptin, could improve the patient's glycemic control; however, the combination of metformin and an SGLT2 inhibitor reduces systolic blood pressure more than metformin and a DPP-4 inhibitor (pooled between-group difference, 4.1 mm Hg [CI, 3.6 to 4.6 mm Hg]) and SGLT2 inhibitors reduced weight more than DPP-4 inhibitors (between group difference, 2.5 to 2.7 kg). There have been postmarketing reports of fatal and nonfatal acute pancreatitis associated with sitagliptin. While no causal relationship has been established, FDA labeling guidelines recommend that sitagliptin be used with caution in patients with a history of pancreatitis and some experts recommend against its use entirely in this population.

KEY POINT

- Empagliflozin has been shown to reduce cardiovascular-related events and all-cause mortality in patients with type 2 diabetes mellitus and cardiovascular disease.

Bibliography
Barry MJ, Humphrey LL, Qaseem A. Oral pharmacologic treatment of type 2 diabetes mellitus. Ann Intern Med. 2017;167:75-76. doi:10.7326/L17-0234. [PMID: 28672387]

Item 26   Answer: B
Educational Objective: **Evaluate secondary amenorrhea.**

This patient presents with secondary amenorrhea, defined as absence of menses for more than 3 months in women who previously had regular menstrual cycles. After ruling out pregnancy, the initial laboratory evaluation in secondary amenorrhea includes measurement of follicle-stimulating hormone (FSH), thyroid-stimulating hormone (TSH), and prolactin levels. Given negative pregnancy testing and normal TSH and prolactin levels in this patient, FSH testing is the remaining initial laboratory data point that has yet to be explored. If the FSH level is elevated, testing should be repeated in 1 month and accompanied by serum estradiol testing. If the FSH level is elevated on repeat testing and estradiol level is low, karyotype analysis is indicated to evaluate for Turner syndrome. Primary ovarian insufficiency is also associated with an elevated FSH and low estradiol levels. In women with normal or low FSH levels, the evaluation is typically directed by history and physical examination findings.

For example, a high BMI (≥30) and acne are frequently seen in women with polycystic ovary syndrome. In addition, a progestin withdrawal test can be performed to further assess the estrogen status of the patient. If a normal estrogen state is confirmed (bleeding within a week of stopping progesterone), hyperandrogenism should be considered.

Testosterone and dehydroepiandrosterone sulfate (DHEAS) are measured in patients with suspected hyperandrogenism as the cause of amenorrhea based on history, physical examination, and following initial laboratory evaluation (serum human chorionic gonadotropin, FSH, TSH, and prolactin).

Primary amenorrhea is the absence of menses by age 16 years accompanied by normal sexual hair pattern and normal breast development. Approximately 15% of patients presenting with primary amenorrhea may have an anatomic abnormality of the uterus, cervix, or vagina such as müllerian agenesis, transverse vaginal septum, or imperforate hymen. Digital vaginal examination, transvaginal ultrasound, or pelvic MRI may help to identify outflow tract anomalies. Because this patient has secondary amenorrhea, evaluation for anatomic abnormalities with transvaginal ultrasound or pelvic MRI is not indicated.

KEY POINT

- After ruling out pregnancy, the initial laboratory evaluation in secondary amenorrhea includes measurement of follicle-stimulating hormone, thyroid-stimulating hormone, and prolactin levels.

Bibliography
Klein DA, Poth MA. Amenorrhea: an approach to diagnosis and management. Am Fam Physician. 2013;87:781-8. [PMID: 23939500]

Item 27   Answer: C
Educational Objective: **Manage hyperglycemia in the hospital.**

The most appropriate management of this patient's hyperglycemia is to initiate scheduled basal insulin and correction insulin. Inpatient hyperglycemia, defined as consistently elevated plasma glucose values above 140 mg/dL (7.8 mmol/L), is associated with poor outcomes. Attempts to decrease morbidity and mortality with tight glycemic control (80-110 mg/dL [4.4-6.1 mmol/L]) have not consistently demonstrated improvements in adverse outcomes and, in some settings, have shown increased rates of severe hypoglycemic events and mortality. As a result, revised inpatient glycemic targets are less stringent than outpatient glucose targets to avoid both hypoglycemia and severe hyperglycemia that can lead to volume depletion and electrolyte abnormalities. Dietary modifications should be made once glucose levels exceed 140 mg/dL (7.8 mmol/L). At persistent glucose levels of 180 mg/dL (10.0 mmol/L) and higher, the American Diabetes Association recommends initiation of scheduled insulin with a blood glucose target of 140 to 180 mg/dL (7.8-10.0 mmol/L) for most critically ill and noncritically ill patients to decrease

CONT. the risk of adverse outcomes. Scheduled basal insulin or basal insulin plus correction insulin is appropriate for patients who are fasting or who have poor oral intake, such as this patient, with frequent bedside point-of-care monitoring every 4 to 6 hours for insulin adjustments. Scheduled basal and prandial insulin plus correction insulin are appropriate for patients who are eating.

The safety of oral antihyperglycemic agents, including empagliflozin, in the hospital setting has not been fully studied or established. In addition, sodium-glucose transporter-2 (SGLT2) inhibitors have been associated with diabetic ketoacidosis and should be avoided in situations that may produce ketone bodies, such as severe illness or prolonged fasting. Scheduled insulin therapy is the recommended treatment regimen for hyperglycemia in the hospital setting.

The safety of oral antihyperglycemic agents, including metformin, in the hospital setting has not been fully studied or established. Scheduled insulin therapy is the recommended treatment regimen for hyperglycemia in the hospital setting.

The sole use of correction insulin for the management of hyperglycemia is not recommended. It is a reactive approach to hyperglycemia that can lead to large fluctuations in glucose levels coupled with the near universal lag time between measurement of glucose and injection of insulin that occurs in most hospitals.

KEY POINT

- To manage in-patient hyperglycemia, scheduled basal insulin or basal insulin plus correction insulin is appropriate for patients who are fasting or who have poor oral intake.

Bibliography

American Diabetes Association. 14. Diabetes care in the hospital: Standards of Medical Care in Diabetes-2018. Diabetes Care. 2018;41(Suppl 1): S144-S151.doi: 10.2337/dc18-S014. [PMID: 29222385]

Item 28   Answer: C

Educational Objective: Diagnose syndrome of inappropriate antidiuretic hormone secretion (SIADH) following transsphenoidal pituitary surgery.

Serum sodium level should be measured in this patient. Sodium and water imbalance are common after pituitary surgery. Patients may exhibit findings of diabetes insipidus (DI) (polyuria, elevated or high normal serum sodium, and dilute urine) followed by syndrome of inappropriate antidiuretic hormone secretion (SIADH) followed again by DI. Central DI may be transient, lasting only a few weeks, or permanent. There is great variability in the presentation of these disorders; some patients manifest all phases, whereas others may manifest only DI or SIADH. During the postoperative hospital recovery, patients are assessed for hormone deficiency that may have occurred as the result of surgery and are then monitored by measuring fluid intake and output, serum sodium,

and urine osmolality. Following discharge, most experts measure serum sodium 1 week postoperatively to screen for SIADH. This patient denies any polyuria or polydipsia so it is unlikely that he has DI, but he is at risk for SIADH given the time frame of presentation. SIADH can occur 3 to 7 days after pituitary surgery. It is important to diagnose SIADH as treatment with fluid restriction will prevent further reduction in sodium levels.

Hyponatremia, defined as a serum sodium concentration less than 136 mEq/L (136 mmol/L), most often results from an increase in circulating antidiuretic hormone (ADH) in response to a true or sensed reduction in effective arterial blood volume with resulting fluid retention. Hyponatremia may also be caused by elevated ADH levels associated with SIADH. The first step in diagnosis of suspected SIADH is measurement of the serum sodium. The initial evaluation of patients with confirmed hyponatremia is measurement of plasma and urine osmolality and urine sodium as well as a careful assessment of the volume status. Measurement of antidiuretic hormone is not part of the diagnostic algorithm as ADH measurement is not quickly available, and results are difficult to interpret.

Pituitary MRI is unnecessary since the patient has no focal findings (cranial nerve deficit or fever) to suggest intracranial pathology or infection.

Measuring thyroid-stimulating hormone is incorrect as the result could be misleading in this patient following pituitary surgery. Measuring the free thyroxine (T_4) level would be more appropriate. In addition, given the long half-life of free T_4, testing is more appropriate 4 weeks after pituitary surgery to assess for secondary hypothyroidism. Symptoms occurring 5 days after pituitary surgery are not likely due to thyroid deficiency.

KEY POINT

- Syndrome of inappropriate antidiuretic hormone secretion (SIADH) is a common complication of pituitary surgery that may occur 3 to 7 days following surgery; treatment with fluid restriction will prevent further reduction in sodium levels.

Bibliography

Kiran Z, Sheikh A, Momin SN, Majeed I, Awan S, Rashid O, et al. Sodium and water imbalance after sellar, suprasellar, and parasellar surgery. Endocr Pract. 2017;23:309-317. [PMID: 27967227] doi:10.4158/EP161616.OR

Item 29   Answer: A

Educational Objective: Manage hypogonadotropic hypogonadism due to hyperprolactinemia.

The patient has hypogonadism due to hyperprolactinemia, and the most appropriate management is dopamine agonist therapy. Empty sella is diagnosed when the normal pituitary gland is not visualized or is excessively small on MRI. The pituitary sella is said to be "empty" because normal tissue is not seen. The finding may be primarily due to increased cerebrospinal fluid entering and enlarging the sella, or it may be secondary to a tumor, previous pituitary surgery, radiation, or infarction. When empty sella is found incidentally on imaging, an evaluation should be completed to determine if there is a known cause for secondary empty sella and if the patient has signs or symptoms of pituitary hormone deficiency. A patient without signs or symptoms should be screened for cortisol deficiency and hypothyroidism. The most common pituitary abnormality in empty sella is hyperprolactinemia. Hyperprolactinemia should be treated with dopamine agonist therapy in a woman with irregular menstrual periods who is trying to conceive. This normalizes the prolactin level and allows recovery of the gonadal axis.

Neurosurgical consultation is not necessary in the absence of signs/symptoms of increased intracranial pressure or visual deficit. Although this patient's original MRI was done for headache, she has no current signs of increased intracranial pressure or visual deficit on examination.

An oral contraceptive pill could be used for treatment if she were not trying to conceive. This is appropriate treatment for hypogonadism related to hyperprolactinemia in empty sella or in women with hyperprolactinemia secondary to a pituitary microadenoma to reduce her risk of developing osteoporosis.

Providing no treatment at this time is inappropriate given the patient's menstrual irregularity. In her case, she requires dopamine agonist therapy to treat her hypogonadism as she is trying to conceive; however, even if she were not trying to conceive, she would require treatment with either dopamine agonist therapy or an oral contraceptive pill to treat her hypogonadism and reduce her risk of developing osteoporosis.

KEY POINT

- Dopamine agonist therapy should be used to treat hyperprolactinemia in women with irregular periods who are trying to conceive.

Bibliography
Guitelman M, Garcia Basavilbaso N, Vitale M, Chervin A, Katz D, Miragaya K, et al. Primary empty sella (PES): a review of 175 cases. Pituitary. 2013;16:270-4. [PMID: 22875743] doi:10.1007/s11102-012-0416-6

Item 30   Answer: B

Educational Objective: Diagnose multiple endocrine neoplasia type 1 (MEN1).

Multigland hyperplasia causing primary hyperparathyroidism should lead to further investigation for an underlying disorder, especially in younger persons and those with a family history of primary hyperparathyroidism. Although there are several familial hyperparathyroidism syndromes, multiple endocrine neoplasia type 1 (MEN1) is the most common. In addition to genetic testing, MEN1 can be discriminated from other disorders by personal or family history of recurrent primary hyperparathyroidism and neoplasia in other endocrine tissues, most prominently neuroendocrine tumors arising from the pancreas and tumors of the pituitary gland.

In contrast, familial hypocalciuric hypercalcemia (FHH) presents as mild, stable hypercalcemia with normal parathyroid hormone (PTH) level and relatively low urine calcium excretion. PTH may be elevated in a small percentage of patients with coexistence of vitamin D deficiency. Kidney health is unaffected. A family history of persistent hypercalcemia despite parathyroidectomy is suggestive. Genetic testing may help to discriminate FHH from primary hyperparathyroidism prior to surgical exploration.

Parathyroid carcinoma is rare. Rapidly worsening or severe hypercalcemia accompanied by very high PTH levels, increased alkaline phosphatase, and locally invasive tumor arising from a single parathyroid gland are diagnostic.

Secondary hyperparathyroidism is a response to hypocalcemia often related to vitamin D deficiency or chronic kidney disease-related hyperphosphatemia. Left untreated, a chronic stimulus to PTH secretion may lead to parathyroid gland hyperplasia. Tertiary hyperparathyroidism is the result of long-standing secondary hyperparathyroidism in which the hyperplastic parathyroid glands exhibit autonomous function even after correction of underlying disease (for example, following kidney transplantation). Although the biochemical profile is similar to primary hyperparathyroidism, a history of preexisting and long-standing hypocalcemia or hyperphosphatemia is evident.

KEY POINT

- Primary hyperparathyroidism may be the first sign of multiple endocrine neoplasia syndrome 1 (MEN1) in persons with a family history of recurrent primary hyperparathyroidism and neuroendocrine tumors arising from the pancreas and tumors of the pituitary gland.

Bibliography
Thakker RV, Newey PJ, Walls GV, Bilezikian J, Dralle H, Ebeling PR, et al; Endocrine Society. Clinical Practice Guidelines for Multiple Endocrine Neoplasia Type 1 (MEN1). J Clin Endocrinol Metab. 2012;97:2990-3011. [PMID: 22723327] doi:10.1210/jc.2012-1230

Item 31   Answer: C

Educational Objective: Diagnose vitamin D–dependent hypercalcemia.

The most likely diagnosis is vitamin D–dependent hypercalcemia, and 1,25-dihydroxyvitamin D level should be measured. Vitamin D–dependent hypercalcemia is most commonly due to disorders associated with granulomatous inflammation. The patient's chest radiograph shows extensive infiltrates that are most prominent in the upper lung zones and are associated with hilar enlargement, highly suggestive of pulmonary sarcoidosis. Sarcoidosis is a multisystem granulomatous disease of unclear cause with a predilection for the lung; pulmonary involvement occurs in more than 90% of patients. Macrophages within granulomas convert 25-hydroxyvitamin D to 1,25-dihydroxyvitamin D without regulation by parathyroid hormone in contrast to renal conversion of vitamin D. An elevated 1,25-dihydroxyvitamin D level and suppressed parathyroid hormone is diagnostic of vitamin D-dependent hypercalcemia. As vitamin D enhances absorption of both calcium and phosphorus, concurrent elevation of serum calcium and phosphorus is also suggestive of vitamin D-dependent hypercalcemia.

There are two mechanisms of hypercalcemia of malignancy: local osteolytic and humoral. When lytic bone metastases are present, hypercalcemia is the result of increased mobilization of calcium from the bone. In these cases, the serum alkaline phosphatase level is typically elevated. Humoral hypercalcemia is less common and occurs when the tumor itself produces parathyroid-related protein (PTHrP) that binds to and activates the parathyroid receptor, raising serum calcium levels. Squamous cell carcinomas, breast cancers, and renal cell carcinomas are the tumors most commonly associated with hypercalcemia of malignancy. These diagnoses cannot explain the patient's prolonged clinical course, pulmonary infiltrates, and hilar lymphadenopathy.

When hypercalcemia is due to adrenal insufficiency, it is in the setting of adrenal crisis which is characterized by hypotension, fever, nausea, vomiting, abdominal pain, tachycardia, and even death. The patient's clinical course is not compatible with acute adrenal insufficiency.

KEY POINT

- An elevated 1,25-dihydroxyvitamin D level and suppressed parathyroid hormone is diagnostic of vitamin D-dependent hypercalcemia.

Bibliography

Donovan PJ, Sundac L, Pretorius CJ, d'Emden MC, McLeod DS. Calcitriol-mediated hypercalcemia: causes and course in 101 patients. J Clin Endocrinol Metab. 2013;98:4023-9. [PMID: 23979953] doi:10.1210/jc.2013-2016

Item 32   Answer: A

Educational Objective: Screen for diabetic retinopathy in a woman of childbearing age.

The most appropriate preconception management for this patient is a dilated eye examination. Women with type 1 or type 2 diabetes mellitus who are planning pregnancy should be counseled on the risk of development or progression of diabetic retinopathy. Additionally, rapid improvement in glycemic control in the setting of retinopathy is associated with temporary worsening of retinopathy. Given tight glycemic targets in pregnancy, this is often a time of intensified glycemic control for women placing them at greater risk for this complication. Dilated eye examinations should occur before pregnancy or in first trimester if not done prior to pregnancy. Patients should be monitored every trimester and then closely for 1 year postpartum as indicated by the degree of retinopathy.

This patient is up to date on lipid screening and additional screening as part of preconception management is not necessary.

Thyroid-stimulating hormone (TSH) levels should be monitored closely in pregnancy due to increased level of thyroid-binding globulin in pregnancy resulting in increased levothyroxine needs. This patient has had a TSH measurement with normal results 3 months ago. The dose of levothyroxine may need to be increased on average by 30% to 50% during pregnancy, and patients should have their TSH level checked as soon as a pregnancy test is positive.

A referral to a physician experienced in the care of kidney disease should be undertaken in patients with advanced kidney disease, which is not present in this patient as her most recent serum creatinine and urine albumin-creatinine ratio were normal.

KEY POINT

- Women with type 1 or type 2 diabetes mellitus who are planning pregnancy should be counseled on the risk of development or progression of diabetic retinopathy; rapid improvements in glycemic levels during pregnancy can temporarily worsen preexisting retinopathy.

Bibliography

American Diabetes Association. 10. Microvascular complications and foot care: Standards of Medical Care in Diabetes-2018. Diabetes Care. 2018;41(Suppl 1):S105-S118. doi: 10.2337/dc18-S010. [PMID: 29222381]

Item 33   Answer: A

Educational Objective: Treat glucocorticoid-induced osteoporosis.

The most appropriate treatment is alendronate. The American College of Rheumatology recommends that in all adults and children, an initial clinical fracture risk assessment for glucocorticoid-induced osteoporosis should be performed as soon as possible, but at least within 6 months of the initiation of long-term glucocorticoid treatment. Patients are categorized according to fracture risk. High fracture risk in patients younger than 40 years is defined as by a previous osteoporotic fracture. Moderate fracture risk is defined as hip or spine bone mineral density Z score less than –3 or rapid bone loss (>10% at the hip or spine over 1 year) and continuing glucocorticoid treatment at >7.5 mg/day for >6 months. Low risk is defined as no osteoporotic risk factors other than glucocorticoid use. Other criteria are used for defining low, moderate, and high fracture risk in patients age 40 years and older. Oral bisphosphonates are recommended as first-line therapy for patients with moderate to high fracture risk, such as this woman, regardless of age. This includes women of childbearing potential provided they are not planning a pregnancy during the period of bisphosphonate treatment.

Optimized calcium and vitamin D intake, lifestyle modifications, and reassessment of fracture risk including bone mineral density testing every 2 to 3 years is recommended over osteoporosis medications for patients younger than 40 at low risk of fracture. However, this patient is not low risk, and treatment with an oral bisphosphonate is indicated.

Teriparatide is indicated for the treatment of men and women with osteoporosis associated with sustained systemic glucocorticoid therapy at high risk for fracture. Although it increases bone mineral density at the spine and hip more than oral bisphosphonate therapy, it is less desirable due to expense and the requirement of daily injections.

Zoledronic acid is indicated for the treatment and prevention of glucocorticoid-induced osteoporosis in patients who cannot tolerate oral bisphosphonates. Due to uncertain impact on pregnancy outcomes, it is considered a third-line agent in younger women.

KEY POINT

- Oral bisphosphonates are recommended as first-line therapy in adult men and women on chronic glucocorticoid therapy with moderate to high fracture risk regardless of age.

Bibliography

Buckley L, Guyatt G, Fink HA, Cannon M, Grossman J, Hansen KE, Humphrey MB, Lane NE, Magrey M, Miller M, Morrison L, Rao M, Byun Robinson A, Saha S, Wolver S, Bannuru RR, Vaysbrot E, Osani M, Turgunbaev M, Miller AS, McAlindon T. 2017 American College of Rheumatology Guideline for the Prevention and Treatment of Glucocorticoid-Induced Osteoporosis. Arthritis Care Res (Hoboken). 2017;69:1095-1110. doi: 10.1002/acr.23279. Epub 2017 Jun 6. [PMID: 28585410]

Item 34   Answer: D

Educational Objective: Diagnose thyroid-stimulating hormone-secreting adenoma.

This patient most likely has a thyroid-stimulating hormone (TSH)-secreting adenoma. The initial evaluation based on clinical signs and/or symptoms of thyrotoxicosis should be measurement of serum TSH alone, followed by measurement of thyroxine (T_4) and triiodothyronine (T_3) levels if TSH is suppressed because the typical pattern of hyperthyroidism is TSH suppression with an elevated T_4 and/or T_3. However, this patient has signs and symptoms of hyperthyroidism with elevated TSH and free T_4 levels, which is concerning for a TSH-secreting adenoma. These tumors are extremely rare and are managed differently from other causes of thyrotoxicosis. Before this diagnosis is made, other causes of the laboratory abnormalities must be excluded (thyroid hormone resistance and familial dysalbuminemic hyperthyroxinemia). If there is no other explanation for elevated TSH and T_4 levels, a pituitary MRI should be performed. The patient's symptoms of hyperthyroidism and lack of family history of thyroid disease make a TSH-secreting adenoma more likely.

Serum TSH and human chorionic gonadotropin have a common α-subunit, allowing cross-reactivity at the TSH receptor. Gestational thyrotoxicosis typically occurs in the first trimester secondary to human chorionic gonadotropin (HCG) stimulation of the TSH receptor. Laboratory results would look similar to hyperthyroidism with suppressed TSH and elevated free T_4.

The clinical manifestations of hypothyroidism include fatigue, cold intolerance, constipation, heavy menses, weight gain, impaired concentration, dry skin, edema, depression, mood changes, muscle cramps, myalgia, and reduced fertility. Hypothyroidism is unlikely as her symptoms are not compatible and her TSH levels would be elevated with a normal or low free T_4 level.

The symptoms of thyrotoxicosis include heat intolerance, palpitations, dyspnea, tremulousness, menstrual irregularities, hyperdefecation, weight loss, increased appetite, proximal muscle weakness, fatigue, insomnia, and mood disturbances. The most common causes of hyperthyroidism are Graves disease and toxic adenoma(s). While the patient has thyrotoxicosis-related symptoms, hyperthyroidism due to Graves disease results in a suppressed TSH level with an elevated free T_4 level, which is not found in this case.

KEY POINT

- Signs and symptoms of a thyroid-stimulating hormone-secreting adenoma are those seen in hyperthyroidism, although laboratory evaluation reveals an elevated free thyroxine (T_4) level with an inappropriately normal or elevated thyroid-stimulating hormone level.

Bibliography

Amlashi FG, Tritos NA. Thyrotropin-secreting pituitary adenomas: epidemiology, diagnosis, and management. Endocrine. 2016;52:427-40. [PMID: 26792794] doi:10.1007/s12020-016-0863-3

Item 35   Answer: B

Educational Objective: Manage secondary amenorrhea due to a prolactinoma.

This patient has a prolactinoma resulting in amenorrhea and infertility due to the inhibitory effect of the elevated prolactin level on gonadotropin secretion. Prolactinomas are treated with dopamine agonists. The two FDA-approved dopamine agonists are bromocriptine and cabergoline. Cabergoline is much better tolerated and more effective at normalizing prolactin and tumor shrinkage, so it is typically the initial therapy chosen but is more expensive than bromocriptine. Dopamine agonists typically decrease the size and hormone production of prolactinomas rapidly. Response to therapy can be monitored by checking serum prolactin levels 1 month after initiating therapy and then every 3 to 4 months. Decreasing serum prolactin usually correlates with decreasing the size of the tumor. Normalization of prolactin concentrations with dopamine agonist therapy to allow spontaneous ovulation is the goal of management in women with microadenomas (<1 cm in size) considering pregnancy. Dopamine agonist therapy is effective at lowering prolactin levels, decreasing tumor size, and restoring gonadal function.

For women who do not ovulate with dopamine agonist therapy, clomiphene citrate therapy is sometimes added.

Unlike other pituitary tumors, medication rather than surgery is first-line therapy for prolactinomas. Even patients with severe mass effect such as vision loss are treated with medical therapy initially. Rarely, very large tumors or more invasive prolactinomas do not shrink with medical therapy and, also rarely, continue to grow. In these patients, surgery should be considered, followed by radiotherapy if growth recurs or continues. After being debulked, the prolactinoma may respond better to medical therapy.

Resuming an oral contraceptive pill will not correct the underlying disorder and would not assist this patient in becoming pregnant.

KEY POINT

- Symptomatic prolactinomas are treated with dopamine agonists.

Bibliography

Melmed S, Casanueva FF, Hoffman AR, Kleinberg DL, Montori VM, Schlechte JA, et al; Endocrine Society. Diagnosis and treatment of hyperprolactinemia: an Endocrine Society Clinical Practice Guideline. J Clin Endocrinol Metab. 2011;96:273-88. [PMID: 21296991] doi:10.1210/jc.2010-1692

Item 36   Answer: B

Educational Objective: Manage the "honeymoon phase" of type 1 diabetes mellitus.

The most appropriate management of this patient's diabetes is to decrease the insulin glargine dose and discontinue insulin aspart. The drastic reduction in endogenous insulin production secondary to pancreatic beta cell destruction in type 1 diabetes creates a glucose toxicity that induces a functional impairment of the remaining beta cells. As exogenous insulin therapy improves glycemic control, the remaining beta cells experience less metabolic stress, resulting in an improvement in the ability to produce insulin. This "honeymoon phase" may occur shortly after the diagnosis of diabetes and may last months to years. It is characterized by drastic improvements in glycemic control and reductions in insulin requirements, as seen in this patient. To prevent rapid return of glucose toxicity and to preserve the remaining beta cells as long as possible, insulin therapy should be continued during the "honeymoon phase" if possible without causing hypoglycemia. It is appropriate to decrease this patient's basal glargine insulin dose to improve his fasting hypoglycemia while also maintaining continuous insulin therapy. Given the symptomatic postprandial hypoglycemia he is experiencing on low doses of prandial insulin, it is appropriate to discontinue it at this time with close monitoring for postprandial hyperglycemia at the end of the "honeymoon phase."

Sole use of a sliding-scale insulin regimen is not recommended for glycemic control as it is reactionary in nature to elevated glucose values only. Using this strategy, it would be possible that the patient may not receive daily insulin during the "honeymoon phase," which would accelerate the risk of developing glucose toxicity again.

KEY POINT

- Continuing insulin, even at low doses, is recommended during the "honeymoon phase" of type 1 diabetes mellitus to reduce metabolic stress on functioning beta cells and preserve any residual function for as long as possible.

Bibliography

DeWitt DE, Hirsch IB. Outpatient insulin therapy in type 1 and type 2 diabetes mellitus: scientific review. JAMA. 2003;289:2254-64. [PMID: 12734137]

Item 37   Answer: A

Educational Objective: Manage postmenopausal osteoporosis in patients taking denosumab.

The most appropriate management for this patient is to continue denosumab. Denosumab, a monoclonal antibody against the receptor activator of nuclear factor κB ligand (RANKL), reduces bone resorption by inhibiting the development of osteoclasts. It circulates in the blood for up to 9 months after subcutaneous injection, but once cleared from the circulation, bone resorption transiently but dramatically increases, resulting in an abrupt decline in bone mineral density and, in some cases, vertebral fractures. Once initiated, there is no defined endpoint for cessation of denosumab therapy.

Although bone mineral density increases in response to denosumab therapy, it does not impact management with respect to dose and duration of treatment. Therefore, a DEXA scan is not necessary.

In the pharmacologic management of osteoporosis, drug holidays are considered during the course of bisphosphonate therapy. Due to their binding to bone tissue, bisphosphonates have durable effects on bone remodeling and fracture risk after discontinuation. After 5 years of treatment, patients at low risk for fracture can be considered for a bisphosphonate drug holiday. One study showed no cumulative difference in the risk for nonvertebral fractures in women continuing alendronate therapy for 5 versus 10 years. Post hoc analysis of this study showed that women with femoral neck T scores of –2.5 or worse and baseline prevalent vertebral fracture had reduced fracture risk by continuing alendronate therapy for 10 years versus stopping after 5 years compared with placebo.

Zoledronic acid is an intravenous bisphosphonate indicated for the treatment of osteoporosis especially in patients intolerant to oral bisphosphonates. Patients switched from zoledronic acid to denosumab experience further gains in bone mineral density suggesting additive benefit from this sequence of therapy. However, in patients receiving long-term denosumab, switching to zoledronic acid attenuated but did prevent loss of bone mineral density suggesting that denosumab therapy should be continued once initiated.

KEY POINT

- When administered subcutaneously twice yearly, denosumab suppresses bone resorption, increases bone density, and reduces the incidence of osteoporotic fractures in men and women; the effects of denosumab are not sustained when treatment is stopped.

Bibliography

Anastasilakis AD, Polyzos SA, Makras P, Aubry-Rozier B, Kaouri S, Lamy O. Clinical features of 24 patients with rebound-associated vertebral fractures after denosumab discontinuation: systematic review and additional cases. J Bone Miner Res. 2017;32:1291-1296. [PMID: 28240371] doi:10.1002/jbmr.3110

Item 38   Answer: C

Educational Objective: Manage type 1 diabetes mellitus in a hospitalized patient.

The most appropriate management of this patient's type 1 diabetes mellitus is to decrease basal insulin dose by 10% to 20% and add correction insulin regimen. This patient's fasting blood glucose values were already low on his home basal insulin doses, thus it is most appropriate to continue his basal insulin but at a reduced dose to avoid diabetic ketoacidosis and hypoglycemia. Correction insulin with basal insulin will treat hyperglycemia while he is fasting. Patients with type 1 diabetes must have continuous insulin therapy, particularly basal insulin, to avoid the development of DKA. Because of the requirement of continuous insulin, prolonged fasting in a patient with type 1 diabetes can be complicated by hypoglycemia. Proactive adjustments to insulin doses are required to avoid extreme fluctuations in glycemic control while in the fasting state.

This patient's fasting blood glucose value of 70 mg/dL (3.9 mmol/L) on the current basal insulin dose meets the American Diabetes Association's threshold value for downward titration of insulin doses to avoid hypoglycemia. The basal insulin dose should be decreased in addition to holding the prandial insulin in the fasting state. A sliding-scale insulin regimen should also be added to the basal insulin to help manage hyperglycemia that may occur while fasting.

Efficient glucose utilization is impaired when continuous insulin therapy, such as basal insulin, is held in type 1 diabetes. This may cause the development of diabetic ketoacidosis as a result of increased glycogenolysis and gluconeogenesis for fuel production. A sliding-scale insulin regimen alone is not physiologic and may cause large fluctuations in the blood glucose levels owing to the inherent reactive nature of its dosing, coupled with the near universal lag time between measurement of glucose and injection of insulin that occurs in most hospitals.

KEY POINT

- In fasting hospitalized patients with type 1 diabetes mellitus, the basal insulin dose should be decreased, the prandial insulin held to avoid hypoglycemia, and a correction insulin regimen should be added to help manage hyperglycemia.

Bibliography

Chiang JL, Kirkman MS, Laffel LM, Peters AL; Type 1 diabetes sourcebook authors. Type 1 diabetes through the life span: a position statement of the American Diabetes Association. Diabetes Care. 2014;37:2034-54. [PMID: 24935775] doi:10.2337/dc14-1140

Item 39   Answer: B

Educational Objective: Screen for adrenal hyperfunction in an incidentally noted adrenal mass.

The most appropriate next test to perform is a 24-hour urine total metanephrine measurement to screen for pheochromocytoma. Even though this patient does not have hypertension, she should be screened for pheochromocytoma, as these tumors may exist in the absence of typical symptoms or hypertension. Approximately 50% of pheochromocytomas are now first discovered as an incidental adrenal mass. An alternative screening test for pheochromocytoma is measuring the fractionated free plasma metanephrine level. This test has a false-positive rate of approximately 11%, and, therefore, may be considered more useful when suspicion for pheochromocytoma is high. This patient should also be screened for subclinical Cushing syndrome with a 1-mg overnight dexamethasone suppression test. The prevalence of incidentally noted adrenal masses increases with age and is estimated to be about 10% in the elderly. Most lesions are benign, nonfunctioning adenomas, and approximately 10% to 15% secrete excess hormones.

The 24-hour urine free cortisol test is not sensitive enough to diagnose subclinical autonomous cortisol secretion from an adrenal mass. The 24-hour urine free cortisol levels are usually within the normal range in subclinical Cushing syndrome.

The patient does not require screening for primary aldosteronism with a plasma aldosterone-plasma renin ratio (ARR) as she does not have hypertension. Only patients with an incidental adrenal mass and hypertension require screening for primary aldosteronism. Hypokalemia, traditionally thought to be a key feature of primary aldosteronism, is no longer a prerequisite for diagnosis because many patients with this disorder have normal potassium levels.

In women, rapid onset of hirsutism, menstrual irregularities, and virilization should raise suspicion for tumoral hyperandrogenism. Measurement of dehydroepiandrosterone sulfate (DHEAS) is not indicated in this patient, as she did not show signs of hyperandrogenism (hirsutism, deep voice, male pattern balding, clitoromegaly). Serum DHEAS may be measured if signs of significant hyperandrogenism are present in the setting of an adrenal mass that has radiologic features suspicious for malignancy (size >4 cm, heterogeneous enhancement with contrast administration, irregular margins, presence of calcifications or necrosis).

KEY POINT

- Biochemical testing for pheochromocytoma should be undertaken in all patients with an adrenal mass, even in the absence of typical symptoms or hypertension.

Bibliography

Fassnacht M, Arlt W, Bancos I, Dralle H, Newell-Price J, Sahdev A, et al. Management of adrenal incidentalomas: European Society of Endocrinology Clinical Practice Guideline in collaboration with the European Network for the Study of Adrenal Tumors. Eur J Endocrinol. 2016;175:G1-G34. [PMID: 27390021] doi:10.1530/EJE-16-0467

Item 40   Answer: C

Educational Objective: Manage a patient with severe primary hyperparathyroidism who is to undergo parathyroidectomy.

The most appropriate test to perform next for this patient is measurement of her 25-hydroxyvitamin D level. Vitamin D

H
CONT.

deficiency is common in patients with primary hyperparathyroidism (HPT) due to increased conversion of 25-hydroxyvitamin D to 1,25-dihydroxyvitamin D. Supplementation of vitamin D in patients with HPT has been shown to reduce parathyroid hormone levels, decrease bone turnover, and improve bone mineral density. Identifying and treating vitamin D deficiency perioperatively helps manage transient hypocalcemia, which routinely occurs after parathyroidectomy and especially in severe HPT where high bone turnover (as evidence by an elevated alkaline phosphatase) portends hungry bone syndrome.

Due to increased conversion, 1,25-dihydroxyvitamin D levels are frankly elevated in most instances of hyperparathyroidism and even in patients who are vitamin D deficient. It is not a useful test to identify and manage vitamin D deficiency in any circumstance and could be falsely reassuring in patients with HPT.

Given kidney excretion of calcium is the dominant mechanism by which hypercalcemia is corrected, urine calcium excretion can be assumed to be high in severe hypercalcemia with the exception of patients with severe acute kidney injury. Although guidelines suggest routine assessment of 24-hour urine calcium in the evaluation of HPT to exclude familial hypocalciuric hypercalcemia, the need for such screening primarily occurs when parathyroid hormone and calcium levels are mildly elevated. Additionally, a clinical diagnosis has already been established for this patient making 24-hour urine calcium measurement unnecessary.

Ionized calcium is the best test to assess the state of calcium homeostasis and is recommended by some experts when managing HPT. However, it is primarily of use when evaluating and managing hypocalcemia, especially when assumptions cannot be made regarding serum protein concentrations and blood pH.

KEY POINT

- In patients with primary hyperparathyroidism who are undergoing parathyroidectomy surgery, identifying and correcting vitamin D deficiency is important to avoid postoperative hypocalcemia, which occurs due to rapid flux of serum calcium into bone (hungry bone syndrome).

Bibliography

Kaderli RM, Riss P, Dunkler D, Pietschmann P, Selberherr A, Scheuba C, Niederle B. The impact of vitamin D status on hungry bone syndrome after surgery for primary hyperparathyroidism. Eur J Endocrinol. 2017 Sep 6. pii: EJE-17-0416. doi: 10.1530/EJE-17-0416. [Epub ahead of print] [PMID: 28877925]

Item 41   Answer: D

Educational Objective: Diagnose subclinical Cushing syndrome in a patient with an incidentally noted adrenal mass.

The most likely diagnosis in this patient with an incidentally discovered adrenal mass is subclinical Cushing syndrome. All patients with an incidental adrenal mass should be screened

for subclinical Cushing syndrome (SCS), a condition characterized by adrenocorticotropic hormone (ACTH)-independent cortisol secretion that may result in metabolic (hyperglycemia and hypertension) and bone (osteoporosis) effects of hypercortisolism, but not the more specific features of Cushing syndrome (centripetal obesity, facial plethora, abnormal fat deposition in the supraclavicular or dorsocervical areas, and wide violaceous striae). The preferred diagnostic test for SCS is a 1-mg overnight dexamethasone suppression test, with a morning cortisol level greater than 5 µg/dL (138 nmol/L) considered positive. Following a positive result for SCS, measurement of ACTH, dehydroepiandrosterone sulfate (DHEAS), urine free cortisol, and an 8-mg overnight dexamethasone suppression test are often required to confirm autonomous cortisol secretion. If SCS is confirmed, the risks and benefits of surgery need to be considered. Surgery for SCS has been associated with improvements in bone density and glucose, lipid, and blood pressure control.

This patient's serum cortisol level did not suppress to less than 5 µg/dL (138 nmol/L) following dexamethasone administration. Under normal conditions, exposure to dexamethasone results in suppression of ACTH secretion and hence suppression of adrenal cortisol secretion. In the setting of autonomous cortisol secretion from an adrenal mass, cortisol suppression following dexamethasone administration would not occur, as tumor production of cortisol is not under normal physiologic feedback control.

The patient's plasma free metanephrine levels were within the normal range. This test has excellent sensitivity, and a normal result rules out pheochromocytoma.

Primary aldosteronism is also unlikely based on a calculated plasma aldosterone-plasma renin ratio (ARR) of less than 20. Her blood pressure medications, hydrochlorothiazide and doxazosin, have minimal or mild effects on the ARR, and therefore the result can be reliably interpreted.

KEY POINT

- Initial testing for subclinical Cushing syndrome is a 1-mg overnight dexamethasone suppression test; a cortisol level greater than 5 µg/dL (138 nmol/L) is considered a positive test.

Bibliography

Fassnacht M, Wiebke A, Bancos, Dralle H, Newell-Price J, Sahdev A, Tabarin A, Terzolo M, Tsagarakis S, Dekkers OM. Management of adrenal incidentalomas: European Society of Endocrinology Clinical Practice Guideline in collaboration with the European Network for the Study of Adrenal Tumors. Eur J Endocrinol. 2016;175(2):G1–G34. PMID: 27390021.

Item 42   Answer: B

Educational Objective: Screen for Cushing syndrome in a patient with an alternate sleep schedule.

This patient should be screened for Cushing syndrome, and the best screening test in this patient is measurement of 24-hour urine free cortisol to quantify total daily cortisol secretion. Biochemical testing is used to establish the diagnosis of Cushing syndrome. It is critical that the biochemical diagnosis is firmly established prior to any imaging studies due to the relatively high prevalence of clinically insignificant pituitary and adrenal masses. Initial tests include the 1-mg overnight dexamethasone suppression test, 24-hour urine free cortisol, and late-night salivary cortisol. While the 1-mg overnight dexamethasone test and the late-night salivary cortisol test may be more convenient, they are likely to be less accurate in this patient because of her shift work and estrogen use. Measurement of 24-hour urine free cortisol is not impacted by estrogen therapy or sleeping patterns. A threefold or greater increase over normal values is diagnostic of Cushing syndrome if compatible clinical features are present (centripetal obesity, facial plethora, abnormal fat deposition in the supraclavicular or dorsocervical areas, and wide violaceous striae); if this increase is present, test results should be repeated to confirm the abnormal result.

The 1-mg overnight dexamethasone suppression test is also not reliable in this patient because it relies on serum cortisol measurement.

The late night salivary cortisol test is not a reliable screening test in this patient because she works a night shift and therefore her diurnal cortisol secretion will be reversed.

Measurement of morning serum cortisol is unreliable as a screening test for Cushing syndrome because normal secretion of cortisol is pulsatile and the normal range is broad. Hence, there is considerable overlap between serum cortisol levels seen in normal people, those with Cushing syndrome, and those with hypercortisolism due to psychological or medical stressors.

In addition, serum cortisol measurement is unreliable in this patient as she is on oral estrogen, which leads to an increase in cortisol binding proteins and subsequent elevation of serum total cortisol levels without impacting free cortisol levels.

KEY POINT

- The 24-hour urine free cortisol test for Cushing syndrome is not impacted by either estrogen therapy or sleeping patterns.

Bibliography

Loriaux DL. Diagnosis and differential diagnosis of Cushing's syndrome. N Engl J Med. 2017;376:1451-1459. doi: 10.1056/NEJMra1505550. [PMID:28402781]

Item 43   Answer: E

Educational Objective: Diagnose medication-induced male gynecomastia.

This patient most likely has spironolactone-induced gynecomastia. Gynecomastia occurs due to an imbalance between free estrogen and free androgen actions in breast tissue. Spironolactone is a known cause of gynecomastia. Spironolactone can increase the aromatization of testosterone to estradiol, decrease the testosterone production by the testes, and displace testosterone from sex hormone–binding globulin,

thereby increasing its metabolic clearance rate. Additionally, spironolactone also acts as an antiandrogen by binding to androgen receptors and displacing binding of testosterone and dihydrotestosterone to their receptors. Other recognized drug-related causes of gynecomastia include marijuana, alcohol, 5α-reductase inhibitors, H_2-receptor antagonists, digoxin, ketoconazole, calcium channel blockers, ACE inhibitors, antiretroviral agents, tricyclic antidepressants, and selective serotonin reuptake inhibitors.

Breast cancers are typically unilateral and nontender with a discrete fixed mass displaced from the nipple-areolar complex, whereas gynecomastia presents as a rubbery, concentric, subareolar mass. Gynecomastia is typically bilateral and often associated with breast tenderness.

Germ cell tumors account for 95% of testicular neoplasms with 6% of patients presenting with gynecomastia at time of diagnosis. The temporal association of gynecomastia with the initiation of a medication known to cause gynecomastia and a normal testicular examination makes germ cell tumor a much less likely diagnosis.

Hypogonadism, primary more so than secondary, is associated with gynecomastia due to an increase in estradiol relative to testosterone secretion. With primary hypogonadism, a rise in luteinizing hormone results in increased aromatization of testosterone to estradiol; this elevated luteinizing hormone is absent in secondary hypogonadism thus making gynecomastia a less prominent sign. This patient has unchanged sexual functioning, morning erections, and no evidence of testicular atrophy making hypogonadism an unlikely diagnosis.

Pseudogynecomastia is often seen in obese men. It occurs due to an increase in breast fat without any proliferation of glandular tissue. Gynecomastia and pseudogynecomastia are differentiated by examination. Pseudogynecomastia is characterized by the presence of subareolar adipose tissue, without glandular proliferation. True gynecomastia typically distorts the normally flat contour of the male nipple, causing it to protrude owing to the mass of glandular tissue beneath it. In pseudogynecomastia, the nipple is typically still flat but soft, and nondescript subcutaneous fat tissue is present in the breast area.

KEY POINT

- Gynecomastia can be an adverse effect of medications; spironolactone causes an imbalance between free estrogen and free androgen resulting in glandular breast tissue enlargement.

Bibliography

Dickson G. Gynecomastia. Am Fam Physician. 2012;85:716-22. [PMID: 22534349]

Item 44   Answer: A

Educational Objective: Diagnose celiac disease as a cause of thyroxine malabsorption.

The most likely diagnosis is celiac disease. The patient had been taking the same dose of levothyroxine for many years, but recently has required increasing doses to maintain euthyroidism. Despite his levothyroxine dose being increased, his serum thyroid-stimulating hormone (TSH) level remains elevated, his free thyroxine (T_4) is at the lower limit of the normal reference range, and he continues to have symptoms of thyroid hormone deficiency. Rising levothyroxine requirements in the absence of obvious medication noncompliance or inappropriate administration should alert the treating physician about possible malabsorption. Since levothyroxine is principally absorbed in the jejunum and ileum, any disease process affecting the small bowel can affect the fraction of an orally administered dose that is absorbed. The patient reports diarrhea, abdominal pain, and weight loss, and a rash that is characteristic of dermatitis herpetiformis, a finding that is unique to celiac disease. Patients with celiac disease frequently experience malabsorption of medications, vitamins, and other nutrients.

Medication noncompliance is a less likely explanation for this patient's escalating levothyroxine requirements given his prior history of being easily maintained on a stable dose of levothyroxine and self-reported adherence to his prescribed regimen. Medication noncompliance would not explain his associated symptoms of abdominal cramping, skin rash, and unintentional weight loss.

Autoimmune primary adrenal insufficiency occurs more commonly in patients with other autoimmune disorders, and this patient does report gastrointestinal symptoms and weight loss; however, he does not demonstrate hyperpigmentation or hypotension. Moreover, adrenal insufficiency would not provide an explanation for his rising levothyroxine dose requirements or skin rash.

Thyroid hormone resistance is also unlikely. The patient would not be expected to have had normal thyroid function test results previously, and his free T_4 would be elevated.

KEY POINT

- Malabsorptive disorders may decrease levothyroxine absorption resulting in higher than expected levothyroxine dose requirements.

Bibliography
Centanni M, Benvenga S, Sachmechi I. Diagnosis and management of treatment-refractory hypothyroidism: an expert consensus report. J Endocrinol Invest. 2017 Jul 10. doi: 10.1007/s40618-017-0706-y. [Epub ahead of print] [PMID: 28695483]

Item 45   Answer: B
Educational Objective: Manage infertility.

When evaluating infertility, both female and male factors should be considered concurrently. Thus, semen analysis is part of the initial diagnostic evaluation. Collection should occur after 2 to 3 days of sexual abstinence, but no longer to avoid decreased sperm motility. If semen analysis is abnormal, it should be repeated at least 2 weeks later, and if results are abnormal, referral to a reproductive endocrinologist is recommended.

Given that this patient has regular menses every 28 days with molimina symptoms (breast pain and bloating), her cycles appear to be ovulatory. Thus, laboratory assessment of ovulatory function is not needed at this time. In patients who do not have normal menstrual cycles with ovulation, laboratory assessment should be performed. A midluteal phase serum progesterone level, obtained approximately 1 week before the expected menses, is an effective way to assess ovulatory status. A progesterone level above 3 ng/mL (9.5 nmol/L) is evidence of recent ovulation. Measurement of serum thyroid stimulating hormone and prolactin levels is appropriate to exclude thyroid disease and hyperprolactinemia as causes of oligo-ovulation.

In women over the age of 35 years, an infertility evaluation is initiated after 6 months of unprotected intercourse; in women under the age of 35, an infertility evaluation is initiated after 1 year of regular unprotected intercourse. Recommending an additional 5 months of unprotected intercourse is unnecessary for this 37-year-old woman.

Laparoscopy for evaluation of pelvic adhesions or mild endometriosis may be warranted in patients with dysmenorrhea, history of sexually transmitted infections, or previous pelvic surgery. While assessment of tubal patency may be indicated in this patient given her prior history of appendicitis and abdominal surgery (putting her at risk for adhesions), laparoscopy is not indicated at this immediate time prior to moving forward with an initial noninvasive diagnostic evaluation.

KEY POINT

- When evaluating infertility, both female and male factors should be considered concurrently; semen analysis is part of the initial diagnostic evaluation.

Bibliography
Marshburn PB. Counseling and diagnostic evaluation for the infertile couple. Obstet Gynecol Clin North Am. 2015;42:1-14. [PMID: 25681836] doi:10.1016/j.ogc.2014.10.001

Item 46   Answer: B
Educational Objective: Recognize the effect of opioids on pituitary function.

This patient's opioid use is most likely responsible for his sexual dysfunction. Secondary hypogonadism is typically a result of insufficient gonadotropin-releasing hormone production by the hypothalamus or deficient luteinizing hormone (LH)/follicle-stimulating hormone (FSH) secretion by the anterior pituitary. This patient has symptoms of hypogonadism and a low testosterone level. Low or inappropriately normal FSH and LH levels in the presence of simultaneous low testosterone levels are diagnostic of secondary hypogonadism (hypogonadotropic hypogonadism). Untreated sleep apnea, exogenous testosterone administration, and obesity are common causes of secondary hypogonadism. Other acquired causes include hyperprolactinemia, chronic opioid use, glucocorticoid use, or infiltrative disease (lymphoma or hemochromatosis). Chronic opioid therapy is a well-established cause of hypogonadotropic hypogonadism. The mechanism of opioid-induced hypogonadism is thought to be central hypogonadism, with downregulation of gonadotropin-releasing hormone and subsequently LH and FSH. This, in turn, results in decreased testosterone production.

This patient's decline in gonadal function is not a result of his age. Although testosterone levels may decline with age, this patient's testosterone level of 185 ng/dL (6.4 nmol/L) is well below the normal range and below what would be expected for age-related decline in testosterone.

Although a pituitary tumor isn't completely ruled out without an MRI, the most likely cause of this patient's hypogonadism is the chronic opioid therapy. Testosterone levels greater than 150 ng/dL (5.2 nmol/L) are less likely to be related to a pituitary tumor. Patients with hypogonadotropic hypogonadism and testosterone levels less than 150 ng/dL (5.2 nmol/L) should have an MRI to evaluate for a pituitary tumor. The normal TSH and prolactin levels also argue against a pituitary or hypothalamic tumor.

In primary gonadal failure, there would be elevated FSH and LH levels with a low testosterone level. A low testosterone level with inappropriately normal or low FSH and LH levels is consistent with hypogonadotropic hypogonadism.

KEY POINT

• Chronic opioid use suppresses gonadotroph function, resulting in hypogonadotropic hypogonadism, which is increasingly recognized as a cause of secondary hypogonadism.

Bibliography
O'Rourke TK Jr, Wosnitzer MS. Opioid-induced androgen deficiency (opiad): diagnosis, management, and literature review. Curr Urol Rep. 2016;17:76. [PMID: 27586511] doi:10.1007/s11934-016-0634-y.

Item 47   Answer: C

Educational Objective: Diagnose Turner syndrome.

The most common cause of primary amenorrhea is gonadal dysgenesis caused by chromosomal abnormalities, most commonly those associated with Turner syndrome (TS). TS is caused by loss of part or all of an X chromosome (45,X0) occurring in 1 in 2500 live female births. In some studies, more than 20% of patients are diagnosed after 12 years of age; primary amenorrhea may be the presenting sign. The most consistent physical finding is short stature, as seen in this patient. Other findings may include neck webbing, hearing loss, aortic coarctation, and bicuspid aortic valve. Primary amenorrhea is seen in approximately 90% of women with TS. TS should be considered in women with primary or secondary amenorrhea, particularly those of short stature. Diagnosis is made by karyotype analysis.

Functional hypothalamic amenorrhea is caused by a functional disruption of the hypothalamic-pituitary-ovarian axis in which no anatomic or organic disease is identified. Disruption of the pulsatile release of hypothalamic gonad-

otropin-releasing hormone may occur due to stress, weight loss, or exercise; follicle-stimulating hormone (FSH) levels are not elevated in functional hypothalamic amenorrhea.

Primary ovarian insufficiency is considered when a woman younger than 40 years of age develops secondary amenorrhea with two serum FSH levels in the menopausal range (>35 mU/mL [35 U/L]). This condition impacts 1 in 100 women by the age of 40 years. If during the evaluation of secondary amenorrhea, an elevated FSH is found, it should be repeated in 1 month, along with a serum estradiol measurement. In young women, karyotype analysis is also indicated to rule out Turner syndrome.

Vaginal agenesis is the second most common cause of primary amenorrhea with an incidence of 1 in 5000. Vaginal agenesis is characterized by congenital absence of the vagina with variable uterine development. These women have a normal female karyotype and ovarian function, thus develop normal secondary sexual characteristics. Presentation is typically after age 15 years due to primary amenorrhea. Examination reveals normal external genitalia with a dimple or small pouch replacing the vagina. On laboratory testing, gonadotropins are unremarkable. This patient's normal pelvic examination eliminates this vaginal agenesis as a cause of primary amenorrhea.

KEY POINT

• The most common cause of primary amenorrhea is gonadal dysgenesis, most commonly associated with Turner syndrome (45,X0).

Bibliography
Pinsker JE. Clinical review: Turner syndrome: updating the paradigm of clinical care. J Clin Endocrinol Metab. 2012;97:E994-1003. [PMID: 22472565] doi:10.1210/jc.2012-1245

Item 48   Answer: B

Educational Objective: Evaluate postprandial hypoglycemia in a patient without diabetes.

The most appropriate diagnostic test to perform next is mixed-meal testing. Hypoglycemia in persons without diabetes is extremely rare and requires additional investigation. Causes of hypoglycemia in adults without diabetes include drug or alcohol use, critical illness, hormonal deficiency, non-islet cell tumor, endogenous hyperinsulinism, accidental or intentional hypoglycemia, and prior Roux-en-Y gastric bypass surgery. Postprandial hypoglycemia can develop 2 to 3 years after Roux-en-Y gastric bypass surgery. The patient either denies or does not have clinical evidence for the presence of many of these causes. The timing of the hypoglycemia can guide the appropriate next diagnostic test.

This patient is experiencing postprandial symptoms consistent with an increase in sympathetic activity within 5 hours of a meal. He meets two out of three criteria for a hypoglycemic disorder as defined by the Whipple triad: symptoms that can be attributed to hypoglycemia and resolution of symptoms with food consumption. He does not have documented hypoglycemia at the time of symptoms from a reliable laboratory method to meet the third criteria of the Whipple triad. Point-of-care fingerstick measurements lack precision to confirm hypoglycemia. An attempt should be made to recreate the scenario that is likely to cause the symptoms. Since his symptoms occur in the postprandial state, a mixed-meal test should be performed. The mixed-meal consists of food types that have induced the onset of symptoms in the past. The patient should have the following hypoglycemic laboratory tests measured at baseline and every 30 minutes for 5 hours after consuming the mixed-meal: plasma glucose, insulin, C-peptide, β-hydroxybutyrate (low in the presence of insulin), and proinsulin. He should also repeat these tests at the time of symptomatic hypoglycemia (<60 mg/dL [3.3 mmol/L]) before administering carbohydrates. If symptomatic hypoglycemia is documented during the mixed-meal testing, the patient should also be screened for insulin secretagogues (sulfonylureas and meglitinides) and insulin antibodies.

A 72-hour fast involves prolonged fasting while measuring the hypoglycemic laboratory test (plasma glucose, insulin, C-peptide, β-hydroxybutyrate, and proinsulin) every 6 hours, followed by every 1 to 2 hours once the glucose is less than 60 mg/dL (3.3 mmol/L) or the patient becomes symptomatic. Given that the patient is experiencing postprandial symptoms, the 72-hour fast would likely not induce hypoglycemia.

An oral glucose tolerance test (OGTT) consists of liquid caloric consumption that is usually not similar to the type of food that induces symptomatic postprandial hypoglycemia. The OGTT can produce unreliable results, particularly in those patients with altered gastric anatomy or gastric motility.

Pancreatic imaging should only occur after biochemical confirmation of endogenous hyperinsulinism.

KEY POINT

- A mixed-meal test consisting of the types of food that normally induce the hypoglycemia should be performed to determine the cause of postprandial hypoglycemia.

Bibliography

Cryer PE, Axelrod L, Grossman AB, Heller SR, Montori VM, Seaquist ER, et al; Endocrine Society. Evaluation and management of adult hypoglycemic disorders: an Endocrine Society Clinical Practice Guideline. J Clin Endocrinol Metab. 2009;94:709-28. [PMID: 19088155] doi:10.1210/jc.2008-1410

Item 49   **Answer:**   **A**

Educational Objective: Treat secondary adrenal insufficiency.

This patient has secondary adrenal insufficiency, and hydrocortisone is the most appropriate treatment. Oral, injectable (including joint injections), and occasionally even topical glucocorticoids are able to suppress adrenocorticotropic hormone (ACTH) secretion. Glucocorticoids prescribed at doses above physiologic replacement for longer than 3 weeks should be tapered when discontinued allowing recovery of the pituitary-adrenal axis; if therapy has lasted less than 3 weeks, no taper is required for pituitary-adrenal axis recovery. The diagnosis of adrenal insufficiency is based on demonstrating inappropriately low serum cortisol levels. Because most assays measure total cortisol, abnormalities in cortisol-binding protein or albumin can trigger spurious results. An early morning (8 AM) serum cortisol of less than 3 µg/dL (82.8 nmol/L) is consistent with cortisol deficiency, whereas values greater than 15 to 18 µg/dL (414.0-496.8 nmol/L) exclude the diagnosis when binding protein abnormalities and synthetic glucocorticoid exposure are excluded.

Fludrocortisone in addition to hydrocortisone is unwarranted as fludrocortisone is needed only in primary adrenal insufficiency. There is no mineralocorticoid deficiency in secondary adrenal insufficiency.

An ACTH stimulation test is not necessary in this patient since the cortisol level less than 3 µg/dL (82.8 nmol/L) is diagnostic of adrenal insufficiency. If an ACTH stimulation test were necessary, dexamethasone can be given prior to the ACTH stimulation test since dexamethasone is not measureable in the cortisol assay. That is unnecessary given this patient's cortisol level.

KEY POINT

- Oral, injectable (including joint injections), and even topical glucocorticoids are able to suppress adrenocorticotropic hormone (ACTH) secretion and result in secondary adrenal insufficiency.

Bibliography

Pazderska A, Pearce SH. Adrenal insufficiency - recognition and management. Clin Med (Lond). 2017;17:258-262. doi: 0.7861/clinmedicine.17-3-258. [PMID: 28572228]

Item 50   **Answer:**   **C**

Educational Objective: Treat hypothyroidism with weight-based dosing of levothyroxine.

This patient has hypothyroidism, and the most appropriate treatment is to prescribe a weight-based replacement dose of levothyroxine (1.6 µg/kg lean body weight). For patients with high body mass index values, an estimate of lean mass should be determined. Levothyroxine is the treatment of choice for thyroid hormone deficiency. Goals of therapy are to resolve signs and symptoms of hypothyroidism, normalize serum thyroid-stimulating hormone (TSH), and avoid overtreatment.

Although some patients express a preference for treatment with desiccated thyroid hormone (thyroid extract), there are potential safety concerns and lack of data on long-term outcomes. The physiologic ratio of thyroxine (T_4) to triiodothyronine (T_3) secreted by the human thyroid is approximately 15:1, whereas desiccated thyroid hormone, as originally derived from animal thyroid glands, contains supraphysiologic T_3 (T_4 to T_3 ratio 4:1). Patients taking desiccated thyroid hormone frequently experience low serum T_4

and supraphysiologic T$_3$ levels despite having a serum TSH within the reference range.

Although a full replacement dose of levothyroxine can be administered to most patients with overt hypothyroidism, older adults (age 65 years and older) and patients with cardiovascular disease should be prescribed a lower initial dose (25-50 µg/day) due to the effects of thyroid hormone on myocardial oxygen demand. The dose should be titrated based on TSH levels measured 6 to 8 weeks after any dose change. The patient described here is an otherwise healthy woman in her fifth decade of life. Prescribing a low initial dose of levothyroxine would unnecessarily delay correction of hypothyroidism.

Not prescribing treatment is also inappropriate. Although the patient does not currently report symptoms of thyroid hormone deficiency, she has overt hypothyroidism with physical findings consistent with this diagnosis (slowed reflexes) and evidence of metabolic complications (hypercholesterolemia). Hypothyroidism causes hypercholesterolemia through reduced cholesterol metabolism and contributes to the development cardiovascular disease. Treatment of patients with overt hypothyroidism and all nonpregnant adults with subclinical hypothyroidism and a serum TSH level above 10 µU/mL (10 mU/L) is indicated to ameliorate the risk of these complications.

KEY POINT

- Levothyroxine is the treatment of choice for thyroid hormone deficiency; for most younger adults without cardiac disease, a weight-based replacement dose of levothyroxine (1.6 µg/kg lean body weight) is recommended.

Bibliography

Hennessey JV. The emergence of levothyroxine as a treatment for hypothyroidism. Endocrine. 2017;55:6-18. [PMID: 27981511] doi:10.1007/s12020-016-1199-8

Item 51   Answer: A

Educational Objective: Diagnose the cause of Cushing syndrome.

The most appropriate diagnostic test for this patient is measurement of the adrenocorticotropic hormone (ACTH) level. Cushing disease is the term used to indicate excess cortisol production due to an ACTH-secreting pituitary adenoma. Cushing syndrome refers to hypercortisolism from any cause, exogenous or endogenous, ACTH-dependent or not. The most common cause of endogenous Cushing syndrome is Cushing disease. The initial step in evaluation for Cushing disease is to seek biochemical evidence of hypercortisolism. At least two first-line tests should be diagnostically abnormal before the diagnosis is confirmed. Initial tests include the overnight low-dose dexamethasone suppression test, 24-hour urine free cortisol, and late-night salivary cortisol. The 24-hour urine free cortisol and late night salivary cortisol tests should be performed at least twice to ensure reproducibility of results.

The abnormal dexamethasone suppression test and elevated urine free cortisol levels establish the diagnosis of Cushing syndrome in this patient. An ACTH measurement should be obtained once the diagnosis of Cushing syndrome is established to determine if it is ACTH dependent or ACTH independent.

Once ACTH-dependent Cushing syndrome is confirmed biochemically, a pituitary MRI should be obtained. If no pituitary tumor or a tumor less than 6 mm is visualized on MRI, an 8-mg dexamethasone suppression test is used to differentiate Cushing disease from an ectopic source of ACTH. Dexamethasone is administered at 11 PM, and cortisol is tested at 8 AM. A pituitary source of ACTH will respond to negative feedback from high doses of dexamethasone, suppressing plasma cortisol at 8 AM by more than 50%, whereas an ectopic source of ACTH will not have suppressible cortisol. However, this test has low sensitivity (88%) and specificity (57%) for Cushing disease, so inferior petrosal sinus sampling (IPSS) is often recommended before exploratory pituitary surgery. In IPSS, ACTH levels in the petrosal sinus are compared with those in the periphery after the administration of corticotropin-releasing hormone (CRH). A central to peripheral gradient greater than 2.0 before CRH or greater than 3.0 after CRH is diagnostic of Cushing disease.

An 8-mg dexamethasone suppression test, inferior petrosal sinus sampling, and pituitary MRI should follow, if necessary, ACTH testing. Their inclusion in the diagnostic algorithm at this point is premature and possibly unnecessary.

KEY POINT

- An adrenocorticotropic hormone (ACTH) measurement should be obtained once the diagnosis of Cushing syndrome is established to determine if it is ACTH dependent or ACTH independent.

Bibliography

Loriaux DL. Diagnosis and differential diagnosis of Cushing's syndrome. N Engl J Med. 2017;376:1451-1459. doi: 10.1056/NEJMra1505550. [PMID:28402781]

Item 52   Answer: D

Educational Objective: Diagnose testosterone-induced change in thyroxine-binding globulin.

The most likely explanation for the observed change in this patient's thyroid function test results is the initiation of testosterone. The administration of androgens and anabolic steroids leads to a reduction in thyroxine-binding globulin, which consequently increases the proportion of metabolically active free thyroxine that is available. Consequently, a reduction in levothyroxine dosing may be needed to prevent iatrogenic thyrotoxicosis. Conversely, higher levothyroxine doses are often required after the initiation of estrogen or selective estrogen receptor modulating therapies (tamoxifen and raloxifene) due to an increase in serum thyroxine-binding globulin concentrations.

Administering levothyroxine with coffee or calcium carbonate and treatment with omeprazole all decrease the absorption of thyroxine, resulting in reduced levels of free thyroxine (T_4) and elevated levels of thyroid-stimulating hormone. Calcium carbonate reduces the maximum absorption of levothyroxine by 25%. Because calcium and ferrous sulfate can bind levothyroxine, the ingestion of either medication, even as a component of a multivitamin, should be separated from levothyroxine by 4 hours. Administering levothyroxine with coffee, whether caffeinated or not, has been shown to reduce the absorption of levothyroxine. Ideally, levothyroxine should be taken 60 minutes before food or coffee is consumed. Oral levothyroxine is absorbed in the jejunum and ileum. The absorption of an orally administered dose is 70% to 80% under optimum fasting conditions, and an acidic gastric pH is important. Chronic therapy with omeprazole and other proton pump inhibitors impairs levothyroxine absorption by increasing gastric pH.

KEY POINT

- In patients receiving thyroxine replacement therapy, initiation of estrogen or raloxifene increases thyroxine-binding globulin levels whereas testosterone reduces thyroxine-binding globulin levels; in either situation a change in thyroxine dosage may be required.

Bibliography

Tahboub R, Arafah BM. Sex steroids and the thyroid. Best Pract Res Clin Endocrinol Metab. 2009 Dec;23(6):769-80. doi: 10.1016/j.beem.2009.06.005. [PMID: 19942152]

Item 53   Answer: A

Educational Objective: Treat postmenopausal osteoporosis.

The most appropriate treatment for this patient is alendronate. The American College of Physicians (ACP) recommends that clinicians offer pharmacologic treatment with alendronate, risedronate, zoledronic acid, or denosumab to reduce the risk for hip and vertebral fractures in women who have known osteoporosis. Individual patient factors and cost help decide which agent is initially used. Bisphosphonates are the most commonly prescribed first-line therapy as they have been shown to reduce the risk of fractures in large, randomized, placebo-controlled trials, and are generally well tolerated with low risk for serious adverse effects.

Although calcitonin increases spine bone mineral density in clinical trials, its anti-fracture efficacy is inconsistent at the spine. The availability of intravenous bisphosphonates and denosumab negates the argument for calcitonin in patients who cannot tolerate oral osteoporosis medications.

Denosumab is effective for prevention of vertebral fracture in postmenopausal women, yet it is expensive and, once started, should be continued indefinitely. Even if followed by intravenous bisphosphonate therapy, discontinuation results in loss of bone mineral density and has been associated with an increased risk of vertebral fracture. Denosumab may be

used safely in the setting of compromised kidney function (KDIGO stage G3b and G4). It may also be preferred in patients with poor adherence or tolerance of oral bisphosphonates.

Raloxifene is approved in postmenopausal women for the prevention and treatment of osteoporosis and the prevention of invasive breast cancer in those at high risk. However, raloxifene is contraindicated in those at increased risk of venous thromboembolism. ACP recommends against raloxifene for the treatment of osteoporosis in women.

Teriparatide and abaloparatide are anabolic therapies that reduce the risk of vertebral fracture in postmenopausal osteoporosis. Each increases bone mass and strength of the spine more than antiresorptive drugs and may be preferred if spine bone mineral density is severely low (T-score $\leq$ -3.5), in patients who fail bisphosphonate therapy, and in glucocorticoid-induced osteoporosis. Neither drug should be prescribed for patients who are at increased risk for osteosarcoma including those with a history of radiation therapy.

KEY POINT

- Alendronate, risedronate, zoledronic acid, and denosumab have been shown to reduce the risk for spine, hip, and nonvertebral fractures, and are generally well tolerated with low risk for serious adverse effects.

Bibliography

Qaseem A, Forciea MA, McLean RM, Denberg TD; Clinical Guidelines Committee of the American College of Physicians. Treatment of low bone density or osteoporosis to prevent fractures in men and women: A Clinical Practice Guideline Update From the American College of Physicians. Ann Intern Med. 2017;166:818-839. [PMID: 28492856] doi:10.7326/M15-1361

Item 54   Answer: C

Educational Objective: Manage medication-related hypoglycemia.

The most appropriate management of hypoglycemia for this patient is to stop glyburide therapy. Hypoglycemia can become a rate-limiting step in achieving glycemic goals for many persons. Clinicians should consider de-intensifying pharmacologic therapy in patients with type 2 diabetes who achieve hemoglobin A_{1c} levels less than 6.5%; furthermore, benefits of targeting a specific hemoglobin A_{1c} target level in patients with a life expectancy less than 10 years due to advanced age should be considered carefully because the harms outweigh the benefits in this population. Therapies must be adjusted to eliminate hypoglycemia, and glycemic goals should be individualized to accommodate targets that can be safely achieved. Several factors contribute to hypoglycemia including a mismatch of food consumption and insulin delivery, increased physical exertion, weight loss, worsening kidney impairment, abnormalities in gastrointestinal motility and absorption, and accidental/intentional overdose of insulin or other hypoglycemic agents such as sulfonylureas. Older adults are also at an increased risk for hypoglycemia. Sulfonylureas stimulate insulin secretion regardless of glycemic status. Thus, they pose risk for hypoglycemia, especially in drugs with long half-lives, such as glyburide, or in older persons. In light of this patient's age, kidney impairment, and frequency of hypoglycemia, glyburide should be stopped.

Immediate carbohydrate intake is the appropriate management of hypoglycemia in the alert individual; consumption of 15 grams of a fast-acting carbohydrate followed by a self-monitored blood glucose measurement 15 minutes later with repeat treatment if glucose is not improved. In this obese male, increased carbohydrate intake is not the appropriate way to manage this situation on a long-term basis as it can lead to further weight gain and increased insulin resistance.

If this patient was to remain on therapy that can induce hypoglycemia, glucagon should be prescribed. Glucagon should be provided to patients at risk for developing hypoglycemia and used intramuscularly by close contacts if the individual is not able to safely consume carbohydrates to correct hypoglycemia.

Metformin is the recommended first-line oral agent for type 2 diabetes due to known effectiveness and decreased hypoglycemia risk. Although this patient has a degree of kidney impairment, it is not such that metformin needs to be discontinued. After consideration of the risk and benefits, cautious continuation of metformin in kidney impairment may occur with an estimated glomerular filtration rate (eGFR) between 30 and 45 mL/min/1.73 m². Metformin should be discontinued if the eGFR falls below 30 mL/min/1.73 m².

KEY POINT

- Sulfonylureas stimulate insulin secretion, and they pose risk for hypoglycemia, especially drugs with long half-lives, such as glyburide, or in older persons.

Bibliography
Qaseem A, Wilt TJ, Kansagara D, Horwitch C, Barry MJ, Forciea MA, et al. Hemoglobin A_{1c} targets for glycemic control with pharmacologic therapy for nonpregnant adults with type 2 diabetes mellitus: a guidance statement update from tthe American College of Physicians. Ann Intern Med. [Epub ahead of print 6 March 2018]:. doi: 10.7326/M17-0939

Item 55   Answer: D

Educational Objective: Recognize medications that interfere with screening for primary aldosteronism.

Spironolactone can significantly interfere with interpretation of the plasma aldosterone-plasma renin ratio (ARR) and therefore should be discontinued approximately 6 weeks prior to screening for primary aldosteronism. Treatment-resistant hypertension is defined as blood pressure that remains above goal despite concurrent use of three antihypertensive agents of different classes, one of which is a diuretic. Possible situations in which screening for secondary causes of hypertension include: severe or resistant hypertension; young age of onset (in childhood or adolescence), especially in the absence of family history; abrupt worsening of blood pressure in a previously well-controlled patient; or clinical

features of an underlying disorder associated with hypertension (for example, cushingoid features). Hyperaldosteronism, usually from an aldosterone-producing adenoma or bilateral idiopathic hyperaldosteronism, may be present in up to 10% of patients with hypertension. Testing for primary aldosteronism should be considered in all patients with difficult to control hypertension. It should also be performed in patients with hypertension and an incidentally noted adrenal mass or spontaneous or diuretic-induced hypokalemia. Spironolactone and eplerenone cause elevation of renin levels and hence can result in a false-negative ARR. On stopping a mineralocorticoid antagonist, the patient may develop hypokalemia if the underlying diagnosis is primary aldosteronism. Potassium should be replaced accordingly prior to screening for primary aldosteronism, as hypokalemia results in lowering of aldosterone levels and hence impacts the ARR.

In general, most antihypertensive agents can be continued during screening for primary aldosteronism except for spironolactone, eplerenone, and high-dose amiloride therapy. Specifically, verapamil, doxazosin, and hydralazine have minimal impact on the ARR and, therefore, can be continued during screening for primary aldosteronism.

Other antihypertensive agents that have minor effects on the ARR can also be continued during screening for primary aldosteronism as long as the results of the ARR are interpreted with these effects in mind. The hallmark of primary aldosteronism is a suppressed renin level. Any medication that increases renin can result in a false-negative result. On the other hand, a suppressed renin in the presence of a medication that usually would raise renin (an ACE inhibitor) raises the suspicion for primary aldosteronism.

KEY POINT

- Spironolactone and eplerenone can significantly interfere with interpretation of the plasma aldosterone-plasma renin ratio (ARR) and therefore should be discontinued approximately 6 weeks prior to screening for primary aldosteronism.

Bibliography
Funder JW, Carey RM, Mantero F, Murad MH, Reincke M, Shibata H, et al. The management of primary aldosteronism: case detection, diagnosis, and treatment: an Endocrine Society Clinical Practice Guideline. J Clin Endocrinol Metab. 2016;101:1889-916. [PMID: 26934393] doi:10.1210/jc.2015-4061

Item 56   Answer: C

Educational Objective: Manage type 2 diabetes mellitus by individualizing glycemic targets.

This patient is an older adult with a complex/intermediate medical history. The American Diabetes Association (ADA) defines complex/intermediate medical history as the presence of at least three coexisting chronic illnesses serious enough to require medications or lifestyle management and may include arthritis, cancer, heart failure, depression, emphysema, falls, hypertension, incontinence, stage 3 or worse chronic kidney disease, myocardial infarction, and stroke. These patients are expected to have "intermediate life-expectancy," high treatment burden, hypoglycemia vulnerability, and fall risk. The ADA's recommended hemoglobin A_{1c} goal for a patient with similar characteristics and health status is 7.5% to 8%, if this can be achieved without significant hypoglycemia. Tighter glycemic control in this scenario would likely require an escalation in treatment burden with a subsequent increase in risks that may outweigh any potential long-term benefits. Additionally, the patient's reduced kidney function increases his hypoglycemia risk with more intense glycemic goals. The American College of Physicians (ACP) recommends that clinicians avoid targeting an hemoglobin A_{1c} level in patients with a life expectancy less than 10 years due to advanced age (80 years or older), residence in a nursing home, or chronic conditions (such as dementia, cancer, end-stage kidney disease, severe chronic obstructive pulmonary disease, or heart failure) because the harms outweigh the benefits in this population.

Intensive glycemic control early in the disease course in patients with type 2 diabetes may decrease the incidence of long-term cardiovascular events, as suggested from the 10-year follow-up from the UK Prospective Diabetes Study (UKPDS). Similar reductions in cardiovascular disease did not occur when tight glycemic control was applied to older adults with long-standing type 2 diabetes with prior cardiovascular events or cardiovascular risk factors in three landmark studies: Action to Control Cardiovascular Risk on Diabetes (ACCORD), Action in Diabetes and Vascular Disease: Preterax and Diamicron Modified Release Controlled Evaluation (ADVANCE), and Veterans Affairs Diabetes Trial (VADT). In addition, subjects in the intensive treatment arms had increased rates of hypoglycemia in all three studies and a higher rate of death in the ACCORD trial.

In an older healthy adult with little comorbidity, intact cognitive and functional status, the ADA recommends a hemoglobin A_{1c} goal of less than 7.5% given the expected longer life expectancy for that person. This patient does not meet these criteria. In contrast, the ACP recommends hemoglobin A_{1c} level between 7% and 8% in most patients with type 2 diabetes based on lack of mortality benefit for death or macrovascular events over 5 to 10 years and risk in substantial harms.

In patients with complex or poor health, a hemoglobin A_{1c} level less than 8.5% is recommended by the ADA, if it can be achieved without significant hypoglycemia. The ADA defines very complex or poor health requiring residence in a long-term care facility or end-stage chronic illnesses (stage 3-4 heart failure, oxygen-dependent lung disease, chronic kidney disease requiring dialysis, or uncontrolled metastatic cancer), moderate to severe cognitive impairment, or two or more activity of daily living dependencies.

Hemoglobin A_{1c} targets greater than 8.5% are generally not recommended due to an increased risk for hyperglycemia-related complications, such as dehydration from glycosuria, infections, and hyperglycemic hyperosmolar syndrome.

- A hemoglobin A_{1c} goal of 7.5% to 8% is recommended for older adults with complex medical history and significant comorbidities.

Bibliography

American Diabetes Association. 11. Older adults: Standards of Medical Care in Diabetes-2018. Diabetes Care. 2018;41(Suppl 1):S119-S125. doi:10.2337/dc18-S011. [PMID: 29222382]

Item 57   Answer: A

Educational Objective: Diagnose ipilimumab-induced hypophysitis.

In this patient, the most likely cause of pituitary enlargement and evidence of hypopituitarism is drug-induced hypophysitis. Ipilimumab is a checkpoint inhibitor that has been repeatedly associated with the development of hypophysitis in up to 17% of treated patients. Most patients present with the combination of headache, pituitary enlargement, and hypopituitarism occurring during the early phase of therapy, typically within 10 weeks. While the pituitary enlargement often resolves spontaneously, the panhypopituitarism appears to be permanent.

Lymphocytic hypophysitis is an autoimmune disease most commonly occurring in women during pregnancy and postpartum. It leads to pituitary enlargement, possible mass effect, and often deficiency of adrenocorticotropic hormone (ACTH). While the imaging and laboratory characteristics described could be consistent with lymphocytic hypophysitis, the patient's exposure to a drug known to cause hypophysitis and other aspects of the clinical history are not consistent with this diagnosis.

A pituitary adenoma is less likely given the homogeneous enhancement on MRI. Pituitary adenomas are usually evident on MRI after contrast administration. They appear as a relatively nonenhancing lesion within a homogeneously enhancing pituitary gland. This patient's MRI is not consistent with a pituitary adenoma.

Untreated primary hypothyroidism can cause pituitary enlargement due to thyrotroph hyperplasia and can mimic a pituitary adenoma. This patient's low thyroid-stimulating hormone and free thyroxine levels do not support a diagnosis of primary hypothyroidism.

- Checkpoint inhibitors such as nivolumab, ipilimumab, and pembrolizumab have been associated with the development of hypophysitis with most patients presenting with the combination of headache, pituitary enlargement, and hypopituitarism.

Bibliography

Byun DJ, Wolchok JD, Rosenberg LM, Girotra M. Cancer immunotherapy - immune checkpoint blockade and associated endocrinopathies. Nat Rev Endocrinol. 2017;13:195-207. [PMID: 28106152] doi:10.1038/nrendo.2016.205

Item 58   Answer: B

Educational Objective: Treat a large, indeterminate adrenal mass.

The most appropriate next step in management is adrenalectomy. The patient presented with an incidental adrenal mass with radiologic features that are indeterminate for adenoma and may indicate an adrenal malignancy (size >4 cm, density ≥10 Hounsfield units, and absolute contrast washout <50% at 10 minutes). Benign adrenal adenomas tend to be small (<4 cm), often have an intracytoplasmic fat content and appear less dense on noncontrast CT scan (<10 Hounsfield units), and exhibit rapid contrast washout during delayed contrast imaging (>50% at 10 minutes). These radiologic features are not diagnostic of malignancy, as one-third of benign adrenal masses are lipid poor (≥10 Hounsfield units) and many are larger than 4 cm. However, because adrenal carcinoma is an aggressive tumor and data indicate that prognosis may be more favorable when the disease is diagnosed and treated at an earlier stage, adrenalectomy is usually recommended.

Adrenal biopsy is not routinely indicated in the diagnostic evaluation of an incidentally discovered adrenal mass, even if the suspected diagnosis is primary adrenal malignancy, because adrenocortical carcinoma can be missed due to sampling error. Adrenal biopsy may be indicated when adrenal metastasis or an infiltrative disorder such as infection or lymphoma is suspected. Screening for pheochromocytoma should be performed prior to adrenal biopsy to avoid potential hypertensive crisis during the procedure.

Mitotane, an adrenolytic drug, may be used as adjuvant therapy following primary resection. Adrenalectomy is the first-line treatment of choice for patients with suspected adrenocortical carcinoma.

Repeat abdominal CT imaging at 6 months is suggested for adrenal masses that are small (<4 cm) and have benign radiologic features. The optimal time to repeat CT imaging in the radiologically benign-appearing, or even indeterminate-appearing, incidentally noted adrenal mass, is controversial. Repeat CT imaging is not indicated in this patient with high-risk features for adrenal carcinoma.

KEY POINT

- Adrenalectomy is recommended for incidental adrenal masses with radiologic features that suggest increased risk of an adrenal malignancy (size >4 cm, density ≥10 Hounsfield units, and absolute contrast washout <50% at 10 minutes).

Bibliography

Fassnacht M, Arlt W, Bancos I, Dralle H, Newell-Price J, Sahdev A, et al. Management of adrenal incidentalomas: European Society of Endocrinology Clinical Practice Guideline in collaboration with the European Network for the Study of Adrenal Tumors. Eur J Endocrinol. 2016;175:G1-G34. [PMID: 27390021] doi:10.1530/EJE-16-0467

Item 59   Answer: C

Educational Objective: Diagnose hypomagnesemia as the cause of hypocalcemia.

The most appropriate test to perform next is measurement of magnesium. Hypocalcemia is likely the result of hypoparathyroidism, which is most commonly caused by surgical injury. Autoimmune, infiltrative (hemochromatosis, Wilson disease, granulomas), and radiation-related injury can also cause acquired hypoparathyroidism. Other, less common causes of hypocalcemia include poor calcium intake, activating mutations in the calcium-sensing receptor (*CASR*) gene, parathyroid hormone (PTH) resistance, increased phosphate binding in vascular space (rhabdomyolysis or tumor lysis syndrome), increased citrate chelation with large volume blood transfusions, sepsis, vitamin D deficiency, and hypomagnesemia. Low levels of magnesium (due to medications, alcohol abuse, or malnutrition) activate G-proteins that stimulate calcium-sensing receptors and decrease PTH secretion. Functional hypoparathyroidism due to hypomagnesemia must be excluded before other diagnoses are pursued. Hypomagnesemia to the extent required to cause hypoparathyroidism is most commonly due to medications impairing renal handling of magnesium including platinum-based chemotherapeutic agents. Prompt resolution of hypocalcemia following correction of hypomagnesemia confirms the diagnosis.

Measurement of serum bicarbonate would allow assessment of acid-base derangements. Acute respiratory alkalosis causes transient symptomatic hypocalcemia due to a rapid increase in the fraction of intravascular calcium bound to albumin. However, changes in blood pH due to metabolic alkalosis are relatively small and gradual, allowing prevention of hypocalcemia by an increase in parathyroid hormone. This patient has a more compelling reason for persistent hypocalcemia, and measurement of serum bicarbonate is not necessary.

Approximately 40% to 45% of the calcium in serum is bound to protein, principally albumin, although the physiologically active form of calcium is in an ionized (or free) state. In most patients with relatively normal serum albumin levels, the total calcium usually accurately reflects the ionized calcium fraction. In this case, the patient's albumin level is normal and the patient's symptoms correspond to the measured calcium level, therefore measurement of ionized calcium is not needed.

Given phosphorus homeostasis and calcium homeostasis are closely linked, changes in serum phosphorus concentration should be routinely explored when evaluating hypocalcemia. Even so, hyperparathyroidism rather than hypoparathyroidism would be present if the primary cause of hypocalcemia was due to hyperphosphatemia.

KEY POINT

- Hypomagnesemia causes functional, reversible parathyroid hypofunction and must be excluded before a low or inappropriately normal parathyroid level is attributed to hypoparathyroidism.

Bibliography

Brandi ML, Bilezikian JP, Shoback D, Bouillon R, Clarke BL, Thakker RV, Khan AA, Potts JT Jr. Management of hypoparathyroidism: summary statement and guidelines. J Clin Endocrinol Metab. 2016;101:2273-83. doi:10.1210/jc.2015-3907. [PMID: 26943719]

Item 60   Answer: C

Educational Objective: Treat type 2 diabetes mellitus in a patient with chronic kidney disease.

The most appropriate treatment of this patient's diabetes mellitus is to initiate metformin. This patient's hemoglobin A_{1c} is above goal despite lifestyle modifications, and his treatment plan should be intensified. The first-line therapy recommended by the American Diabetes Association in conjunction with lifestyle modifications for treatment of type 2 diabetes is metformin. Previously, metformin use was contraindicated at serum creatinine levels of 1.4 mg/dL (123.8 µmol/L) or higher in women and 1.5 mg/dL (132.6 µmol/L) or higher in men. However, in a recent update the FDA concluded that metformin is considered to be safe in those with an estimated glomerular filtration rate (eGFR) greater than 45 mL/min/1.73 m² and is contraindicated in those with an eGFR less than 30 mL/min/1.73 m². The FDA recommends not initiating metformin for patients with eGFR greater than 30 mL/min/1.73 m² to less than 45 mL/min/1.73 m², or alternately, initiating metformin at a reduced dose (50%) with frequent monitoring of kidney function (every 3 months). The patient qualifies metformin therapy and frequent monitoring with his current kidney function.

Empagliflozin, a sodium-glucose transporter-2 (SGLT2) inhibitor, is a second-line agent after metformin initiation. In addition, SGLT2 inhibitors may cause hypotension due to intravascular volume depletion, especially in patients with kidney impairment, and acute kidney injury has been reported with its use. The FDA advises that risk factors for acute kidney injury (hypovolemia, chronic kidney disease, heart failure, and use of diuretics, ACE inhibitors, angiotensin receptor blockers, or NSAIDs) be considered before initiating this class of drugs.

The sulfonylurea, glipizide, is a second-line agent after metformin initiation. Glipizide could be considered as part of dual therapy if the glycemic goal is not reached with metformin. While sulfonylureas are the least expensive oral agent to add to metformin, they are associated with an increased risk for hypoglycemia as well as weight gain as compared with other potential combination therapies.

Saxagliptin, a dipeptidyl peptidase-4 (DPP-4) inhibitor, is a second-line agent after metformin initiation. Saxagliptin could be considered as part of dual therapy if the glycemic goal is not reached with metformin. However, the FDA has warned that the DPP-4 inhibitors saxagliptin and alogliptin may increase the risk for heart failure, especially in patients who already have heart or kidney disease.

KEY POINT

- Metformin is considered to be safe in those with an estimate glomerular filtration rate (eGFR) greater than 45 mL/minute/1.73 m² and is contraindicated in those with an eGFR less than 30 mL/min/1.73 m².

Bibliography

Barry MJ, Humphrey LL, Qaseem A. Oral pharmacologic treatment of type 2 diabetes mellitus. Ann Intern Med. 2017;167:75-76. doi:10.7326/L17-0234. [PMID: 28672387]

Item 61   Answer: D

Educational Objective: Treat toxic adenoma with radioactive iodine.

The most appropriate management is radioactive iodine (¹³¹I) therapy. The patient's examination findings and thyroid scintigraphy results are consistent with a diagnosis of toxic adenoma. Toxic adenoma and multinodular goiter are the second most common cause of hyperthyroidism overall and are most frequently seen in older adults. These autonomously functioning nodules synthesize and secrete thyroid hormones independent of thyroid-stimulating hormone (TSH) stimulation as a result of activating mutations of the TSH receptor or $G_{s\alpha}$. They are usually large and can be easily palpated on examination. First-line treatment options include radioactive iodine therapy or surgery. Radioactive iodine is the most commonly used first-line treatment. The radioisotope ¹³¹I emits both gamma and beta radiation. Gamma radiation can be detected by the camera to determine radioactive iodine uptake and create an image of the thyroid gland during thyroid scintigraphy, whereas beta radiation yields the therapeutic effect by triggering thyroid follicular cell death. If a patient has a particularly large goiter with compressive symptoms or if there is concern for malignancy, surgery is recommended as first-line therapy.

Autonomous nodules are associated with a very low risk of malignancy (<1%), and fine-needle aspiration biopsy is not indicated. If biopsy is performed, it frequently yields indeterminate cytology results, such as suspicion for follicular neoplasm, and generates inappropriate concern and unnecessary recommendations for follow-up examinations and biopsies.

Increasing the atenolol dosage and prescribing methimazole are also not the best management options. While β-blockers ameliorate adrenergic symptoms, they do not address the underlying cause. This patient has a normal heart rate and blood pressure on her current dose of atenolol, so increasing this further is not indicated.

Antithyroid drugs (methimazole) are not first line for managing hyperthyroidism because spontaneous remission does not occur and treatment would have to be continued indefinitely.

KEY POINT

- First-line therapy for toxic adenoma is radioactive iodine (¹³¹I) therapy or surgery.

Bibliography

Haugen BR, Alexander EK, Bible KC, Doherty GM, Mandel SJ, Nikiforov YE, Pacini F, Randolph GW, Sawka AM, Schlumberger M, Schuff KG, Sherman SI, Sosa JA, Steward DL, Tuttle RM, Wartofsky L. 2015 American Thyroid Association Management Guidelines for Adult Patients with Thyroid Nodules and Differentiated Thyroid Cancer: The American Thyroid Association Guidelines Task Force on Thyroid Nodules and Differentiated Thyroid Cancer. Thyroid. 2016;26:1-133. doi:10.1089/thy.2015.0020. [PMID: 26462967]

Item 62   Answer: A

Educational Objective: Screen for neuropathy and retinopathy in type 2 diabetes mellitus.

This patient requires a comprehensive foot examination and dilated eye examination. Patients with diabetes mellitus require monitoring for complications. A thorough foot examination should be done annually in patients with type 2 diabetes. Although this patient had an unremarkable visual foot inspection, he has not yet had a comprehensive foot examination, which is indicated at the time of diagnosis of type 2 diabetes and then annually thereafter. A comprehensive foot examination includes inspection of the skin, assessment of foot deformities, neurologic assessment (10-g monofilament testing with at least one other nerve assessment–pinprick, temperature, vibration, or ankle reflexes), and vascular assessment including pulses in the legs and feet. In patients with type 1 diabetes mellitus, a dilated comprehensive eye examination 5 years after diagnosis is appropriate; however, in patients with type 2 diabetes, a dilated comprehensive eye examination is indicated at time of diagnosis.

Prediabetes and diabetes can be diagnosed based on the elevated results from one of the following screening tests repeated on two separate occasions: fasting plasma glucose, 2-hour postprandial glucose during an oral glucose tolerance test, or hemoglobin A_{1c}. This patient has two abnormal hemoglobin A_{1c} measurements and additional testing with a fasting plasma glucose test and oral glucose tolerance test for the purposes of diagnosis is not warranted.

Although long-term use of metformin may be associated with vitamin B_{12} deficiency and periodic measurement of vitamin B_{12} levels should be considered in metformin treatment patients, B_{12} and folate measurements are not recommended at time of initiation of metformin therapy.

Annual screening for albuminuria in patients with type 2 diabetes should be undertaken starting at the time of diagnosis; this is done on a random spot urine sample as planned in this patient, not a 24-hour urine collection for protein and creatinine.

KEY POINT

- Screening for dyslipidemia, hypertension, a dilated eye examination, spot urine albumin-creatinine ratio, and a comprehensive foot examination should be performed at the time of diagnosis of type 2 diabetes.

Bibliography

American Diabetes Association. 10. Microvascular complications and foot care: Standards of Medical Care in Diabetes-2018. Diabetes Care. 2018;41(Suppl 1):S105-S118. doi: 10.2337/dc18-S010. [PMID: 29222381]

Item 63   Answer: D

Educational Objective: Diagnose hyperglycemia in a patient meeting preprandial glycemic targets.

Measuring postprandial blood glucose level is the most appropriate management of this patient's diabetes. This patient is healthy with few comorbidities. His preprandial blood glucose target is 80 to 130 mg/dL (4.4-7.2 mmol/L). Despite meeting his preprandial glycemic targets, his hemoglobin A_{1c} level remains above his goal of less than 7%. Postprandial hyperglycemia has a greater effect on hemoglobin A_{1c} when it is near 7%. Measuring postprandial blood glucose levels in this patient may identify undetected hyperglycemia that could be treated with an increase in his prandial insulin lispro dose.

Liraglutide is an injectable glucagon-like peptide-1 (GLP-1) receptor agonist with several mechanisms of action: slows gastric emptying, glucose-dependent increase in insulin secretion, and glucose-dependent suppression of glucagon secretion. Although liraglutide has the potential to aid with weight loss in this obese patient and improve his hemoglobin A_{1c} to goal, adding another injectable agent to the regimen of a patient who is reluctant to do this does not take into consideration patient preferences. In addition, liraglutide has not been approved by the FDA for combination use with prandial insulin.

Continuing his current regimen will not allow him to achieve his target hemoglobin A_{1c} goal. The American Diabetes Association recommends a hemoglobin A_{1c} goal of less than 6.5% to 7% for healthy persons with type 2 diabetes mellitus with few comorbidities to decrease the incidence of diabetes-related complications in the future. The American College of Physicians (ACP) recommends a target hemoglobin A_{1c} level between 7% and 8% for most patients with type 2 diabetes. ACP notes that more stringent targets may be appropriate for patients who have a long life expectancy (>15 years) and are interested in more intensive glycemic control despite the risk for harms.

The patient has reached the recommended preprandial glycemic goal of 80 to 130 mg/dL (4.4-7.2 mmol/L). Increasing his insulin detemir dose may increase his risk of developing hypoglycemia and would not adequately treat postprandial hyperglycemia that may be contributing to the elevated hemoglobin A_{1c}.

KEY POINT

- Measuring postprandial blood glucose levels may identify undetected hyperglycemia when preprandial blood glucose values are at target goal, but the hemoglobin A_{1c} is above goal.

Bibliography

American Diabetes Association. 6. Glycemic targets: Standards of Medical Care in Diabetes-2018. Diabetes Care. 2018;41(Suppl 1):S55-S64. doi:10.2337/dc18-S006. [PMID: 29222377]

Item 64   Answer: B

Educational Objective: Manage a patient with asymptomatic primary hyperparathyroidism.

The most appropriate management for this patient is to reassess the patient in 6 to 12 months. Guideline-recommended indications for parathyroidectomy include increase in serum calcium level ≥1 mg/dL (0.25 mmol/L) above upper limit of normal; creatinine clearance <60 mL/min, 24-hour urine calcium >400 mg/day (>10 mmol/day), or increased stone risk by biochemical stone risk analysis; presence of nephrolithiasis or nephrocalcinosis by radio-graph, ultrasound, or CT; T-score (on DEXA scan) of less than or equal to -2.5 at any site or evidence of vertebral fracture; and age younger than 50 years. Parathyroid-ectomy is also indicated in patients in whom medical surveillance is neither desired nor possible, and those with complications of hyperparathyroidism including significant bone, kidney, gastrointestinal, or neuromuscular symptoms. Patients without indications for parathyroid-ectomy require periodic reassessment that includes serum calcium and creatinine every 6 to 12 months and bone mineral density of the lumbar spine, hip, and distal radius every 2 years.

Although imaging tests such as parathyroid sestamibi scan may be performed as part of evaluation of primary hyperparathyroidism, it is most appropriate once surgery is indicated. The results of imaging do not influence the management of nonsurgical patients.

Primary hyperparathyroidism is associated with increased bone turnover and decreased bone strength. Although alendronate suppresses bone resorption and improves bone mineral density at the lumbar spine in patients with primary hyperparathyroidism, it has not been shown to reduce fracture risk or to reduce serum calcium levels. Patients at high risk of fracture (T-score ≤-2.5 and/or prevalent fragility fracture) at presentation or during monitoring should undergo parathyroid-ectomy.

Cinacalcet is indicated to treat symptomatic, severe hypercalcemia in adults with primary hyperparathyroidism for whom parathyroidectomy cannot be performed. Although it may be used chronically, cinacalcet is more commonly used until surgery is feasible.

KEY POINT

- Patients with primary hyperparathyroidism who do not undergo surgery require monitoring of serum calcium and creatinine every 6 to 12 months and bone mineral density of the lumbar spine, hip, and distal radius every 2 years.

Bibliography

Bilezikian JP, Brandi ML, Eastell R, Silverberg SJ, Udelsman R, Marcocci C, et al. Guidelines for the management of asymptomatic primary hyperparathyroidism: summary statement from the Fourth International Workshop. J Clin Endocrinol Metab. 2014;99:3561-9. [PMID: 25162665] doi:10.1210/jc.2014-1413

Item 65   Answer: E

Educational Objective: Manage subclinical hypothyroidism.

This patient has subclinical hypothyroidism, and the most appropriate management is to repeat serum thyroid-stimulating hormone (TSH) testing in 2 months. Free thyroxine (T_4) and thyroid peroxide antibodies could also be measured at that time. Subclinical hypothyroidism is an early form of primary hypothyroidism affecting up to 10% of the population and is characterized by a serum TSH level above the upper limit of the reference range and normal free T_4 level. Before making this diagnosis; however, transient elevation of serum TSH levels should be ruled out by repeating the measurement of TSH in 2 to 3 months.

Thyroid peroxidase (TPO) antibodies are frequently seen in the setting of Hashimoto thyroiditis, the most common cause of hypothyroidism in the United States. TPO antibody positivity would support a diagnosis of primary hypothyroidism, predict risk of progression to overt hypothyroidism, and may impact treatment decisions accordingly. However, the most appropriate next step in the management of this patient is to confirm the diagnosis of subclinical hypothyroidism by documenting persistent serum TSH elevation.

Thyrotropin receptor antibodies would be more consistent with Graves disease and testing for these antibodies would not be appropriate in this setting.

Measurement of serum triiodothyronine (T_3) in patients with known or suspected primary hypothyroidism is generally not indicated. Elevation of serum TSH is the earliest biochemical change observed in the setting of primary hypothyroidism. Reductions in serum T_3 are not usually seen until after free T_4 levels are low. Measuring serum T_3 has little to no impact on diagnosis or management decisions.

More severe subclinical hypothyroidism, serum TSH greater than 10 μU/mL (10 mU/L), may increase the risk of coronary artery disease and heart failure, whereas serum TSH levels below 7 to 10 μU/mL (7-10 mU/L) are not associated with increased morbidity or mortality. Treatment with levothyroxine would be considered if the patient's serum TSH is similar or higher on reassessment, but this is not the most appropriate next step in management.

KEY POINT

- Subclinical hypothyroidism is characterized by a serum thyroid-stimulating hormone (TSH) level above the upper limit of the reference range and normal free thyroxine (T_4) level; before making this diagnosis, however, transient elevation of serum TSH should be ruled out by repeating the measurement of TSH in 2 to 3 months.

Bibliography

Peeters RP. Subclinical hypothyroidism. N Engl J Med. 2017 Jun 29; 376(26):2556-2565. doi: 10.1056/NEJMcp1611144. [PMID: 28657873]

Item 66   Answer: A

Educational Objective: **Diagnose the cause of primary aldosteronism.**

The next step in this patient's management is adrenal vein sampling. Once the diagnosis of primary aldosteronism has been confirmed biochemically, radiographic localization with abdominal CT is indicated. CT is recommended over MRI in most cases due to similar efficacy and lower cost. Adrenal hyperplasia and adenomas secreting excess aldosterone, however, may not always be visualized. Adrenal vein sampling is, therefore, needed in most patients to determine the source of aldosterone secretion when imaging is unrevealing and to confirm lateralization when imaging demonstrates an adrenal adenoma, such as in this case. Adrenal vein sampling is especially important in older patients because of a higher frequency of nonfunctioning adrenal incidentalomas. Patients with an aldosterone-secreting adenoma are usually offered adrenalectomy, whereas those with primary aldosteronism due to bilateral adrenal hyperplasia are treated medically. Omission of adrenal vein sampling can lead to misdiagnosis in approximately 25% of cases, and subsequent unnecessary adrenalectomy, or medical therapy when adrenalectomy could be offered. Right adrenalectomy should not be performed in this patient without further confirmation of the source of primary aldosteronism.

Aldosterone likely exerts direct toxic effects on cardiac cells as evidenced by a higher prevalence of left ventricular hypertrophy and decreased left ventricular function when compared with matched control patients with similar levels of hypertension. These deleterious effects are likely mediated by mineralocorticoid receptors in the heart, coronary arteries, aorta, and other blood vessels. Increasing this patient's losartan or metoprolol dose may lead to better control of his hypertension, but neither of these medications blocks the aldosterone receptor. Therefore, the patient would still be subject to the deleterious effects of excess stimulation of aldosterone receptors, which may lead to cardiac disease.

KEY POINT

- Most patients with biochemically confirmed primary aldosteronism should undergo adrenal vein sampling to confirm the source of the hyperaldosteronism.

Bibliography

Rossi GP, Auchus RJ, Brown M, Lenders JW, Naruse M, Plouin PF, et al. An expert consensus statement on use of adrenal vein sampling for the subtyping of primary aldosteronism. Hypertension. 2014;63:151-60. [PMID: 24218436] doi:10.1161/HYPERTENSIONAHA.113.02097

Item 67   Answer: D

Educational Objective: **Evaluate a thyroid nodule with neck ultrasonography.**

The most appropriate diagnostic test to perform next is ultrasound of the neck. Ultrasound can confirm the presence of thyroid nodules palpated on examination and those detected on other imaging studies. Ultrasound must be performed prior to fine-needle aspiration biopsy (FNAB) to confirm the presence of a nodule, determine that biopsy is indicated, ensure that there are no additional nonpalpable nodules that warrant FNAB, and assess the cervical lymph nodes. In patients with solitary palpable nodules, 15% will have no corresponding nodule on ultrasound, and a similar proportion will have an additional nodule measuring 1 cm or larger.

Performing a CT scan of the neck is a more costly test, exposes the patient to unnecessary radiation, and is inferior to ultrasound at assessing the thyroid gland.

FNAB should not be performed prior to thyroid/neck ultrasound. Whether or not FNAB is indicated depends on the size and sonographic appearance of the nodule, clinical risk factors for malignancy, and presence of pathologic lymph nodes. Nodules that are predominantly cystic or posteriorly located within the thyroid gland are prone to sampling error.

Measurement of serum thyroid-stimulating hormone (TSH) is also part of the initial evaluation of a thyroid nodule. The purpose of measuring TSH is to evaluate for the presence of autonomously functioning or "hot" nodules, which account for 5% to 10% of palpable thyroid nodules. Autonomous nodules may cause hyperthyroidism and are associated with a very low risk of malignancy. Autonomous nodules can be confirmed by performing a thyroid uptake and scan. They concentrate radioactive iodine to a greater extent than normal thyroid tissue, which shows absent or diminished uptake. The TSH in this patient is normal, which does not support a diagnosis of an autonomously functioning thyroid nodule; therefore performing a thyroid uptake and ^{131}I scan is not indicated.

KEY POINT

- Ultrasound can confirm the presence of thyroid nodules palpated on examination and based on findings can help to determine if fine-needle aspiration is needed to assess for malignancy.

Bibliography

Haugen BR, Alexander EK, Bible KC, Doherty GM, Mandel SJ, Nikiforov YE, et al. 2015 American Thyroid Association Management Guidelines for Adult Patients with Thyroid Nodules and Differentiated Thyroid Cancer: The American Thyroid Association Guidelines Task Force on Thyroid Nodules and Differentiated Thyroid Cancer. Thyroid. 2016;26:1-133. [PMID: 26462967] doi:10.1089/thy.2015.0020

Item 68   Answer: B

Educational Objective: **Manage secondary hypothyroidism.**

The most appropriate next step in management is measurement of the free thyroxine (T$_4$) level. Thyroid-stimulating hormone (TSH) deficiency leads to secondary or central hypothyroidism. Secondary hypothyroidism symptoms are clinically identical to primary hypothyroidism symptoms. Secondary hypothyroidism is diagnosed by demonstrating a simultaneously inappropriately normal or low TSH and low T$_4$ (free or total). Patients are treated with levothyroxine replacement in the same manner as primary hypothyroidism; however, the serum TSH cannot be used to monitor and assess for adequacy of thyroid hormone replacement dosing. Instead, the levothyroxine dose is adjusted based on free T_4 levels with the goal of obtaining a value within the normal reference range. The patient's recent symptoms of fatigue and weight gain may be due to hypothyroidism resulting from impaired absorption of levothyroxine after recently starting a calcium supplement. A low T_4 level will confirm the diagnosis. In general the therapeutic goal is to keep the free T_4 in the upper half of the normal range. To improve gastrointestinal absorption, levothyroxine should be taken on an empty stomach, 1 hour before or 3 hours after ingestion of food. Medications that would interfere with absorption, such as calcium- or iron-containing supplements should be separated by 4 hours.

Increasing the levothyroxine would not be appropriate without first documenting the presence of hypothyroidism by measuring the T_4 level. In addition, the preferred initial therapy may simply be to discontinue the calcium, if not warranted, or to separate ingestion of calcium and levothyroxine by at least 2 to 3 hours.

The patient has no symptoms suggestive of a pituitary mass effect or other indication to recommend pituitary imaging.

KEY POINT

- Serum thyroid-stimulating hormone level cannot be used to monitor and assess for adequacy of thyroid hormone replacement dosing in secondary hypothyroidism; the levothyroxine dose is adjusted based on free thyroxine (T_4) levels with the goal of obtaining a value within the upper half of the normal reference range.

Bibliography

Beck-Peccoz P, Rodari G, Giavoli C, Lania A. Central hypothyroidism - a neglected thyroid disorder. Nat Rev Endocrinol. 2017;13:588-598. doi:10.1038/nrendo.2017.47. Epub 2017 May 26. [PMID: 28549061]

Item 69   Answer: A

Educational Objective: Treat hypoglycemic unawareness.

The most appropriate treatment of this patient's diabetes is to decrease all insulin doses. He is having hypoglycemia at least once per week with some of these events qualifying as clinically significant per the American Diabetes Association with glucose values less than 54 mg/dL (3.0 mmol/L). He is developing hypoglycemia unawareness as evidenced by his inability to detect decreases in his blood glucose until it is less than 40 mg/dL (2.2 mmol/L). This is secondary to an ineffective response of the autonomic system to hypoglycemia, in addition to an inadequate release of counterregulatory hormones to correct hypoglycemia. Blood glucose targets should be relaxed, and insulin dosing should be decreased in the setting of hypoglycemia unawareness. Avoidance of hypoglycemia for

several weeks may restore the ability to detect hypoglycemia in some patients. Since the hypoglycemia is intermittent and without a pattern for this patient, all insulin doses should be decreased to avoid hypoglycemia.

The patient has fasting hyperglycemia and a hemoglobin A_{1c} level above goal. Increasing the dose of his glargine insulin could lower his glucose values, but it may potentially exacerbate his hypoglycemia.

Empagliflozin could improve this patient's hyperglycemia while also improving his blood pressure control and inducing weight loss; however, it may also exacerbate the hypoglycemia when used in conjunction with insulin.

Metformin could improve hyperglycemia for this patient, particularly fasting hyperglycemia secondary to hepatic gluconeogenesis. Given the clinically significant hypoglycemia experienced by this patient, that should be addressed first by relaxing his glycemic goals.

KEY POINT

- Treatment for hypoglycemic unawareness is to reduce the insulin dose and avoid hypoglycemia in order to provide the body an opportunity to restore the ability to detect hypoglycemia.

Bibliography

American Diabetes Association. 6. Glycemic targets: Standards of Medical Care in Diabetes-2018. Diabetes Care. 2018;41(Suppl 1):S55-S64. doi:10.2337/dc18-S006. [PMID: 29222377]

Item 70   Answer: A

Educational Objective: Avoid inappropriate screening for osteoporosis.

The most appropriate management for this patient is lifestyle counseling for osteoporosis prevention. Lifestyle measures include adequate calcium and vitamin D, exercise, smoking cessation, counseling on fall prevention, and avoidance of heavy alcohol use.

Most guidelines recommend screening for osteoporosis with dual-energy x-ray absorptiometry (DEXA) scan in women 65 years of age and older. Screening of younger women may be indicated if one or more risk factors for osteoporosis are present. In premenopausal women without risk factors, assessment of bone mineral density (BMD) for fracture risk is not advised or validated. However, if testing is done in an otherwise healthy person, such as this patient, results that are below age- and gender-matched averages (Z-score <0) generally do not require further evaluation or serial monitoring. The discovery of below average BMD could lead to a discussion regarding osteoporosis prevention with lifestyle modification and assessment of BMD after menopause, but prior to age 65, when screening might otherwise occur.

Testing for secondary causes of bone loss is unnecessary when BMD is normal for age. Below average BMD in adults may in fact represent below average peak bone mass rather than loss of bone.

Although BMD measured by quantitative heel ultrasound is predictive of osteoporotic fracture in older women and men, BMD measurement by DEXA scan remains the gold standard for diagnosis of osteoporosis and fracture risk assessment. Therefore, abnormal ultrasound results in these populations should be confirmed by DEXA scan. Even so, a DEXA scan should not be performed in this patient given that screening is not indicated and the heel ultrasound result is within the normal range.

KEY POINT

- Screening for osteoporosis in premenopausal women is not indicated in the absence of risk factors.

Bibliography

Cosman F, de Beur SJ, LeBoff MS, Lewiecki EM, Tanner B, Randall S, et al; National Osteoporosis Foundation. Clinician's guide to prevention and treatment of osteoporosis. Osteoporos Int. 2014;25:2359-81. [PMID: 25182228] doi:10.1007/s00198-014-2794-2

Item 71   Answer: D

Educational Objective: Diagnose methimazole-induced agranulocytosis.

The most appropriate management is to stop methimazole and order a complete blood count with differential. The patient has been receiving methimazole for treatment of Graves hyperthyroidism over the past 3 months. She has both a sore throat and a fever, which can be seen in patients with methimazole-induced agranulocytosis. Agranulocytosis affects between one in 300 and one in 500 patients taking antithyroid drug therapy. Agranulocytosis from methimazole usually occurs within the first several months of initiating therapy but generally is not seen with doses below 20 mg per day. Suspected agranulocytosis should be managed with cessation of the offending drug and assessment of the patient's neutrophil count. An absolute neutrophil count below $500/\mu L$ $(0.5 \times 10^9/L)$ confirms the diagnosis. Management of agranulocytosis may include hospitalization, broad-spectrum antibiotics, and hematopoietic growth factor therapy. Patients should be counseled regarding agranulocytosis as a potential side effect at the initiation of therapy and instructed to contact the prescribing physician immediately with occurrence of any suggestive symptoms.

Diagnosis and treatment of patients with Group A streptococcus (GAS) pharyngitis has traditionally been aided by the four-point Centor criteria: (1) fever, (2) absence of cough, (3) tonsillar exudates, and (4) tender anterior cervical lymphadenopathy. The Centor criteria have a low positive predictive value for GAS infection; according to the Infectious Disease Society of America, these criteria may be used to determine which patients have a low likelihood of GAS pharyngitis and require no further testing. No additional testing or treatment is needed for patients who meet fewer than three criteria. Patients who meet three or more criteria should have a confirmatory test (either a rapid antigen detection test for GAS or throat culture). Penicillin or amoxicillin is first-line treatment for GAS pharyngitis. However, the clinical situation of most immediate concern is the possibility of methimazole-induced agranulocytosis, a potentially fatal condition. The most appropriate management is to stop the drug and measure the neutrophil count.

KEY POINT

- Antithyroid drug-related agranulocytosis affects between one in 300 and one in 500 patients taking therapy and may present with fever and sore throat; initial management includes stopping the drug and assessment of the neutrophil count.

Bibliography

Vicente N, Cardoso L, Barros L, Carrilho F. Antithyroid drug-induced agranulocytosis: state of the art on diagnosis and management. Drugs R D. 2017;17:91-96. doi: 10.1007/s40268-017-0172-1. [PMID: 28105610]

Item 72   Answer: C

Educational Objective: Diagnose diabetic ketoacidosis associated with a sodium-glucose cotransporter 2 (SGLT2) inhibitor.

Sodium-glucose cotransporter 2 (SGLT2) inhibitors (canagliflozin, dapagliflozin, and empagliflozin) improve glycemia by increasing excretion of glucose by the kidney. SGLT2 is expressed in the proximal tubule and mediates reabsorption of approximately 90% of the filtered glucose load. SGLT2 inhibitors promote excretion of glucose by the kidneys and thereby modestly lower elevated blood glucose levels in patients with type 2 diabetes. Euglycemic diabetic ketoacidosis has been reported in patients with type 2 diabetes taking SGLT2 inhibitors. Because of this, the FDA issued a Drug Safety Communication that warns of an increased risk of diabetic ketoacidosis with uncharacteristically mild to moderate glucose elevations (euglycemic diabetic ketoacidosis) associated with the use of all the approved SGLT2 inhibitors. SGLT2 inhibitors should be discontinued in patients who develop acidosis on these agents.

Statins may cause myopathy and liver aminotransferase elevations and are associated with an increased risk of diabetes and, possibly, cognitive dysfunction. The incidence of these adverse effects ranges from 1% to 10%, but permanent disability related to statin intolerance is rare. Statin therapy is not associated with ketoacidosis.

According to labeling guidelines, initiation of metformin therapy is not recommended if the estimated glomerular filtration rate (eGFR) is between 30 and 45 mL/min/1.73 m² and is contraindicated if the eGFR is less than 30 mL/min/1.73 m² due to the risk of lactic acidosis. Metformin should be used cautiously in patients with heart failure or hepatic impairment. The discontinuation of metformin is not associated with the development of lactic acidosis or ketoacidosis.

Glipizide is a sulfonylurea. Sulfonylurea agents work by stimulating insulin secretion. Sulfonylurea agents are associated with weight gain, and they can cause hypoglycemia.

Answers and Critiques

CONT.

They are not, however, associated with the development of ketoacidosis in patients with type 2 diabetes.

A common adverse effect of ACE inhibitors is a dry, nonproductive cough. Other common adverse effects include hyperkalemia and, occasionally, worsening kidney function. ACE inhibitors can cause life-threatening angioedema but not ketoacidosis.

KEY POINT

- An increased risk of diabetic ketoacidosis with mild to moderate glucose elevations has been associated with the use of all the approved sodium-glucose transporter-2 (SGLT2) inhibitors (canagliflozin, dapagliflozin, and empagliflozin).

Bibliography

FDA Drug Safety Communication. FDA warns that SGLT2 inhibitors for diabetes may result in a serious condition of too much acid in the blood. May 15, 2015 https://www.fda.gov/downloads/drugs/drugsafety/ucm446954.pdf. Accessed March 1, 2018.

Item 73   Answer: B

Educational Objective: Evaluate secondary hypogonadism.

The most appropriate test for this patient is a pituitary MRI. With a low testosterone level and low serum luteinizing hormone (LH) and follicle-stimulating hormone (FSH) concentrations, this patient has secondary hypogonadism. Hyperprolactinemia is the most likely cause of his hypogonadism; hyperprolactinemia leads to secondary hypogonadism through suppression of gonadotropin-releasing hormone synthesis and secretion. This patient is on no medications that might cause hyperprolactinemia. In the absence of a culprit drug, the most likely cause of his hyperprolactinemia is a lactotroph adenoma; therefore a pituitary MRI is indicated.

A karyotype analysis is not indicated in the evaluation of secondary hypogonadism; however, it should be considered in men and women who have primary hypogonadism.

Anabolic steroid use will result in low or normal gonadotropin levels, a low testosterone level, and clinical evidence of hyperandrogenism such as excessive muscle bulk, acne, gynecomastia, and decreased testicular volume. Anabolic steroid abuse, however, would not cause hyperprolactinemia as seen in this patient.

Most patients with hereditary hemochromatosis are diagnosed in the presymptomatic phase when iron test results are abnormal. In patients with symptoms, clinical presentation varies and often includes nonspecific findings such as chronic fatigue, weakness, nonspecific abdominal pain, arthralgia, and elevated liver enzymes. Endocrine organs are commonly affected, and diabetes mellitus, hypothyroidism, and gonadal failure may occur. Laboratory evaluation of hemochromatosis-related gonadal failure most commonly demonstrates a hypogonadotropic state (low LH and FSH levels). While this patient is hypogonadotrophic, he has an elevated prolactin level, and a pituitary MRI is the best next diagnostic test.

Obesity results in decreased concentrations of sex hormone-binding globulin (SHBG); if SHBG is low, free testosterone should be measured in patients with low total testosterone concentrations. This patient is not obese and has evidence of secondary hypogonadism (low testosterone level and low serum LH and FSH concentrations), making determination of SHBG concentration unnecessary.

KEY POINT

- Secondary hypogonadism is characterized by low testosterone level and low or inappropriately normal serum luteinizing hormone and follicle-stimulating hormone concentrations; MRI of the pituitary is typically performed to evaluate secondary hypogonadism in the absence of obvious reversible causes such as drugs.

Bibliography

Basaria S. Male hypogonadism. Lancet. 2014;383:1250-63. [PMID: 24119423] doi:10.1016/S0140-6736(13)61126-5.

Item 74   Answer: A

Educational Objective: Treat myxedema coma.

The most appropriate next step in the management of this patient is to administer intravenous hydrocortisone. This patient has myxedema coma, which has a very high mortality rate if there is a delay in treatment. Myxedema coma is more common in elderly women; it may occur in those with a history of hypothyroidism or no antecedent illness. Myocardial infarction, infection, stroke, trauma, and gastrointestinal bleeding are common precipitating events. Mental status changes and hypothermia are the most common clinical manifestations. Ventilatory drive is decreased, resulting in hypoxemia and hypercapnia. Additional signs include bradycardia, hypoglycemia, hyponatremia, and/or hypotension. This patient's condition was likely precipitated by recent nonadherence with her prescribed medications. The serum cortisol level should be checked as soon as possible to evaluate for concomitant adrenal insufficiency prior to initiation of thyroid hormone replacement. While awaiting the results of the serum cortisol measurement, it is advisable to empirically initiate high-dose hydrocortisone. This therapy may be discontinued if the serum cortisol level is found to be normal or high. In patients with adrenal insufficiency, administering thyroid hormone prior to glucocorticoids could precipitate an adrenal crisis by augmenting cortisol metabolism.

Following the administration of glucocorticoids, intravenous thyroid hormone replacement should be initiated. Treatment with levothyroxine is universally recommended. Although controversial, some experts suggest administering liothyronine concomitantly. Once clinically improved, the patient can be transitioned to oral levothyroxine.

Hypotension can generally be resolved over a matter of hours with the administration of fluids and treatment of the hypothyroidism. Persistent hypotension can be treated

CONT.

with a vasopressor drug. The initiation of norepinephrine is premature in this patient.

KEY POINT

- In patients with myxedema coma, intravenous hydrocortisone should be administered before thyroid hormones to treat possible adrenal insufficiency.

Bibliography

Ono Y, Ono S, Yasunaga H, Matsui H, Fushimi K, Tanaka Y. Clinical characteristics and outcomes of myxedema coma: analysis of a national inpatient database in Japan. J Epidemiol. 2017 Mar;27(3):117-122. Epub 2017 Jan 5. PMID: 28142035.

Item 75   Answer: C

Educational Objective: Recognize limitations of hemoglobin A_{1c} measurements.

The most appropriate management for this patient is to initiate ferrous sulfate. This patient has iron-deficiency anemia, a hypoproliferative anemia, which has been shown to erroneously increase the hemoglobin A_{1c} level due to an increase in the proportion of older erythrocytes. Hemoglobin A_{1c} testing measures hemoglobin glycation as a consequence of glucose exposure over the preceding 8 to 12 weeks. Given the patient's age and relatively few comorbidities, her goal hemoglobin A_{1c} level should be less than 6.5% to 7%. Her hemoglobin A_{1c} level is above this goal, but her fingerstick blood glucose data are within her fasting goal of 80 to 130 mg/dL (4.4-7.2 mmol/L) and within her 2-hour postprandial goal of less than 180 mg/dL (10 mmol/L) per the American Diabetes Association (ADA) guidelines. Initiating iron supplementation to correct her iron deficiency anemia will increase erythrocyte turnover and shift the proportion toward younger cells, thus allowing a more accurate measurement of glycemic exposure by the hemoglobin A_{1c} to guide therapeutic decisions.

The patient's fasting blood glucose values are within her goal range of 80 to 130 mg/dL (4.4-7.2 mmol/L) per the ADA guidelines. Initiating basal insulin based solely on the elevated hemoglobin A_{1c} value with her current fasting blood sugars will increase her risk of hypoglycemia. Similarly, the risk of hypoglycemia is increased by initiating empagliflozen. Increasing the accuracy of the hemoglobin A_{1c} measurement by correcting her iron deficiency anemia should be addressed before considering other drug therapy.

Hemoglobin A_{1c} measurements may be unreliable not only in the setting of anemia, but also in the presence of certain hemoglobinopathies or kidney or liver disease. For example, hemoglobin A_{1c} values may be falsely elevated in patients with hemoglobin F or low with hemoglobin S. However, this patient has an explanation for the discordant hemoglobin A_{1c} and blood glucose results, and the iron deficiency anemia should be the focus of management. Additionally, newer methods of measuring A_{1c} are not altered by the presence of the most common hemoglobinopathies. Therefore, a hemoglobin electrophoresis is not indicated at this time.

KEY POINT

- Iron-deficiency anemia can erroneously increase the hemoglobin A_{1c} level due to an increase in the proportion of older erythrocytes.

Bibliography

Sacks DB. A1C versus glucose testing: a comparison. Diabetes Care. 2011;34:518-23. [PMID: 21270207] doi:10.2337/dc10-1546

Item 76   Answer: D

Educational Objective: Treat low-risk papillary thyroid cancer.

No additional treatment is needed. The incidence of thyroid cancer has increased over the last four decades with much of this change attributable to a rise in the diagnosis of small noninvasive papillary thyroid carcinomas. The incidence of papillary microcarcinoma (<1 cm) is 5% to 15% in the United States based on autopsy series. Low-risk papillary thyroid cancer is that which is confined to the thyroid gland, completely resected at surgery, does not demonstrate aggressive pathologic features (lymphovascular invasion or tall cell variant), and has not metastasized. The risk of disease-related death is less than 1%, and the risk of structural disease recurrence is 1% to 2% for low-risk unifocal papillary microcarcinomas. Patients receiving either lobectomy or thyroidectomy have similarly excellent outcomes. Therefore, resection of the remaining thyroid lobe would not be required for this patient.

Suppression of thyroid-stimulating hormone (TSH) with levothyroxine therapy may also be used to improve morbidity and reduce mortality, particularly in patients with persistent disease or distant metastases. The necessary degree of TSH suppression varies according to the risk of cancer progression and comorbidities of the patient. Patients with persistent disease typically require lowering of their TSH level to less than 0.1 µU/mL (0.1 mU/L), whereas patients who are disease-free with a low risk of recurrence should maintain a TSH level of 0.3 to 2.0 µU/mL (0.3-2.0 mU/L). This is typically accomplished without the use of thyroxine suppressive therapy.

Patients with distant metastases have improved survival with successful radioiodine therapy, whereas administration of radioactive iodine may decrease the likelihood of recurrent disease in those patients with nodal metastases. Radioactive iodine (^{131}I) therapy offers this patient no appreciable benefit since her prognosis is already excellent and such therapy would result in substantial unnecessary costs and radiation exposure.

KEY POINT

- Lobectomy is the treatment of choice for low-risk papillary thyroid cancer that is confined to the thyroid gland, completely resected at surgery, does not demonstrate aggressive pathologic features (lymphovascular invasion or tall cell variant), and has not metastasized.

Bibliography

Vaccarella S, Franceschi S, Bray F, Wild CP, Plummer M, Dal Maso L. Worldwide thyroid-cancer epidemic? The increasing impact of overdiagnosis. N Engl J Med. 2016 Aug 18;375(7):614-7. doi: 10.1056/NEJMp1604412. [PMID: 27532827]

Item 77   Answer: B

Educational Objective: Diagnose diabetes insipidus.

The most appropriate diagnostic test for this patient is urine and serum osmolality measurement. Central diabetes insipidus (DI) results from inadequate production of antidiuretic hormone (ADH) by the posterior pituitary gland. In the presence of ADH, aquaporin water channels are inserted in the collecting tubules and allow water to be reabsorbed. In the absence of ADH, excessive water is excreted by the kidneys. Excretion of more than 3 liters of urine per day is considered polyuric. Frank hypernatremia is unusual because patients develop extreme thirst and polydipsia, and with free access to water, can maintain serum sodium in the high normal range. When patients do not drink enough to replace the water lost in the urine, due to poor or absent thirst drive or lack of free access to water, they develop hypernatremia. A low urine osmolality in the setting of a high serum osmolality and high serum sodium in a patient with polyuria is diagnostic of DI. Patients with craniopharyngiomas are at higher risk of developing central DI.

Desmopressin challenge is not appropriate at this time. Prior to initiating desmopressin, one must confirm the diagnosis of DI by measuring urine and serum osmolality. Once confirmed, desmopressin can be administered and urine osmolality remeasured to assure that administration of desmopressin resulted in an increase in urine osmolality. After desmopressin is given, urine concentrates to more than 800 mOsm/kg in central DI, less than 300 mOsm/kg in nephrogenic DI, and between 300 and 800 mOsm/kg in partial DI.

Measurement of urine electrolytes is not helpful in the diagnosis of DI.

A water deprivation test should not be performed in this patient. He already has hypernatremia so further water deprivation could result in serious hypernatremia. In the setting of hypernatremia, a urine and serum osmolality are the best tests to confirm the diagnosis of DI. A water deprivation test can be pursued when the diagnosis is unclear. Urine osmolality above 800 mOsm/kg H_2O is a normal response to water deprivation, indicating ADH production and peripheral effect are intact. A serum osmolality above 295 mOsm/kg with inappropriately hypotonic urine (urine osmolality-serum osmolality ratio <2) during fluid deprivation confirms DI.

KEY POINT

- A low urine osmolality in the setting of a high serum osmolality and high serum sodium in a patient with polyuria is diagnostic of diabetes insipidus.

Bibliography

Prete A, Corsello SM, Salvatori R. Current best practice in the management of patients after pituitary surgery. Ther Adv Endocrinol Metab. 2017;8:33-48. [PMID: 28377801] doi:10.1177/2042018816687240

Item 78   Answer: D

Educational Objective: Diagnose thyroid storm.

The most likely diagnosis is thyroid storm. Thyroid storm is characterized by severe thyrotoxicosis associated with systemic decompensation. Presentation often follows a precipitating event, such as non-thyroid surgery as in this patient's case. Clinical manifestations include high fever, altered mental status and seizures, tachycardia, atrial fibrillation and heart failure, and hepatic dysfunction. A diagnostic system, such as the Burch and Wartofsky Point Scale, can support the diagnosis with scores greater than or equal to 45 being highly suggestive. The patient's thyroid function tests should be assessed to confirm recurrent hyperthyroidism and aggressive treatment should be initiated in the ICU. Management includes treatment of any precipitant illness, supportive care, and thyrotoxicosis-directed therapy including β-adrenergic blockers (esmolol infusion), antithyroid drug therapy, intravenous glucocorticoids, and potassium iodide. Plasmapheresis and emergent thyroidectomy are utilized in patients who cannot be sufficiently managed with medical therapy alone.

Adrenal crisis is not the most likely diagnosis. Although autoimmune primary adrenal failure occurs more commonly in patients with other autoimmune disorders, patients with adrenal crisis usually present with hypotension, hyponatremia, and hyperkalemia, in addition to gastrointestinal manifestations. This diagnosis cannot explain the patient's hyperthermia, lid lag, thyromegaly, brisk reflexes, or tremor.

Malignant hyperthermia is an uncommon cause of severe hyperthermia that occurs in genetically susceptible individuals upon exposure to a volatile anesthetic such as halothane or isoflurane. Symptoms begin intraoperatively or in postoperative recovery, not 3 days following surgery. Features include mixed respiratory and metabolic acidosis, muscle rigidity, hyperkalemia, and rhabdomyolysis. This diagnosis does not explain the patient's thyrotoxicosis-related findings. Finally, the patient lacks muscle rigidity, a pathognomonic finding in malignant hyperthermia.

Myxedema coma is also unlikely. Although patients with myxedema coma may experience cardiac dysfunction and mental status changes, this patient is presenting with signs and symptoms of thyroid hormone excess, not deficiency. She has a history of Graves disease in remission after treatment with antithyroid drug therapy. She has not received radioactive iodine or thyroidectomy and thus the development of hypothyroidism at this point would be unusual.

KEY POINT

- Thyroid storm is a severe manifestation of thyrotoxicosis with life-threatening secondary systemic decompensation; it occurs most commonly with underlying Graves disease coupled with a precipitating factor such as surgery.

Bibliography

De Leo S, Lee SY, Braverman LE. Hyperthyroidism. Lancet. 2016;388:906-18. [PMID: 27038492] doi:10.1016/S0140-6736(16)00278-6

Item 79   Answer: D

Educational Objective: Manage early type 2 diabetes mellitus with metformin monotherapy.

The American Diabetes Association (ADA) recommends a hemoglobin A_{1c} goal of less than 6.5% to 7% in patients who are early in the disease course and with few comorbidities. This patient meets these criteria and should aim for tighter glycemic control than he is currently achieving with 3 months of lifestyle modifications alone. Pharmacologic therapy should now be added to his lifestyle modifications. The American College of Physicians recommends a hemoglobin A_{1c} level between 7% and 8% in most patients with type 2 diabetes. More stringent targets may be appropriate for patients who have a long life expectancy (>15 years) and are interested in more intensive glycemic control with pharmacologic therapy despite the risk for harms, including but not limited to hypoglycemia, patient burden, and pharmacologic costs. The ADA and the American College of Physicians (ACP) recommend metformin as first-line therapy for all patients with type 2 diabetes without contraindications. This recommendation is based on data from multiple studies demonstrating the effectiveness and safety of metformin. In addition, metformin is inexpensive.

The patient has had a reduction in his weight and hemoglobin A_{1c} with lifestyle modifications alone over a 3-month period. Despite this, he remains above his hemoglobin A_{1c} goal of less than 6.5% to 7%. Therefore, continuing his current management protocol would not be appropriate. Achieving glucose goals early in the disease course can reduce the risk of developing microvascular and possibly macrovascular complications in the future. He will require the addition of pharmacologic agents at this time to reach his glycemic target.

Empagliflozin has the ability to improve glycemic control while also reducing blood pressure and weight. Empagliflozin is considered second-line therapy after metformin by ADA and ACP.

Liraglutide also has the ability to improve glycemic control while also reducing weight. There are studies also demonstrating a reduction in blood pressure with liraglutide use. Liraglutide is considered second-line therapy after metformin by the ADA and ACP.

If the patient does not achieve his hemoglobin A_{1c} target after 3 months of lifestyle modifications and metformin, dual therapy with metformin and liraglutide or metformin and empagliflozin could be considered.

KEY POINT

- Metformin is first-line therapy for all patients with type 2 diabetes without contraindications.

Bibliography

Barry MJ, Humphrey LL, Qaseem A. Oral pharmacologic treatment of type 2 diabetes mellitus. Ann Intern Med. 2017;167:75-76.doi:10.7326/L17-0234. [PMID: 28672387]

Item 80   Answer: B

Educational Objective: Manage diabetic ketoacidosis.

The most appropriate management for this patient is to decrease the insulin drip rate and add intravenous (IV) dextrose. This patient continues to have anion gap acidosis and should remain on IV insulin therapy to suppress ketogenesis until this resolves. His current blood glucose level below 200 to 250 mg/dL (11.1-13.9 mmol/L) increases his risk for hypoglycemia with continued IV insulin therapy. This risk can be mitigated by transitioning his IV fluids to 5% dextrose with 0.45% normal saline at 150 to 250 mL/h to maintain his glucose between 150 and 200 mg/dL (8.3-11.1 mmol/L) until his diabetic ketoacidosis resolves. Reducing the insulin drip rate to maintain his blood glucose between 150 and 200 mg/dL (8.3-11.1 mmol/L) will also decrease the risk of hypoglycemia while still suppressing ketogenesis.

If he continues at the current insulin drip rate or if he does not have the addition of IV dextrose, he has an increased risk of developing hypoglycemia now that his blood glucose is less than 200 mg/dL (11.1 mmol/L).

Insulin deficiency and urinary potassium losses induce shifts in potassium from the intracellular to extracellular compartments. This can result in low or normal serum potassium levels in the setting of depleted potassium stores. Potassium shifts back from the extracellular to intracellular compartments with resultant hypokalemia as insulin administration corrects the hyperglycemia, anion gap acidosis, and hyperosmolality associated with diabetic ketoacidosis. To avoid cardiac complications, serum potassium must be greater than 3.3 mEq/L (3.3. mmol/L) before initiating IV insulin. Once potassium is 3.3 mEq/L (3.3 mmol/L) or higher and IV insulin has been initiated, 20 to 30 mEq (20-30 mmol/L) of potassium chloride will usually need to be added to each liter of IV fluid to maintain a serum potassium level of 4.0 to 5.0 mEq/L (4.0-5.0 mmol/L). He is at risk of developing hypokalemia if his potassium supplementation is discontinued at this time.

Although subcutaneous insulin would provide insulin to suppress ketogenesis, the IV insulin drip provides greater flexibility in dose adjustments than subcutaneous insulin. Once the patient's anion gap acidosis has resolved, transitioning from the insulin drip to a subcutaneous insulin regimen should occur.

KEY POINT

- In patients with diabetic ketoacidosis, intravenous insulin therapy should be continued until complete resolution of the anion gap acidosis; as acidosis improves, it may be necessary to reduce the insulin infusion rate and add intravenous dextrose to prevent hypoglycemia.

Bibliography

Fayfman M, Pasquel FJ, Umpierrez GE. Management of hyperglycemic crises: diabetic ketoacidosis and hyperglycemic hyperosmolar state. Med Clin North Am. 2017;101:587-606. doi: 10.1016/j.mcna.2016.12.011. [PMID:28372715]

Item 81   Answer: C

Educational Objective: Treat type-2 amiodarone-induced thyrotoxicosis.

The most appropriate initial management for this patient is to prescribe prednisone. Amiodarone is an antiarrhythmic medication with high iodine content and prolonged half-life of approximately 40 days. Thyrotoxicosis affects 5% of patients taking amiodarone and can occur at any time during or up to 9 months after treatment. Type 1 (hyper-thyroidism) amiodarone-induced thyrotoxicosis occurs in patients with underlying multinodular goiter or latent Graves disease and is associated with increased vascularity on color flow Doppler ultrasonography. Type 2 (destructive thyroiditis) usually affects those without thyroid disease and is not associated with increased vascularity on color flow Doppler. Mixed forms can also be seen and making the correct diagnosis can be difficult. The patient's clinical presentation is most consistent with type 2 amiodarone-induced thyrotoxicosis given the absence of structural thyroid disease (no nodules or goiter), absent thyroid-stimulating hormone (TSH) receptor antibody, and absent parenchymal flow seen on Doppler ultrasound. Moderate- to high-dose prednisone is an effective treatment that can be gradually tapered over 1 to 3 months.

Discontinuation of amiodarone would not yield any immediate clinical benefit due to its prolonged half-life elimination. The decision to discontinue amiodarone depends on the patient's cardiac status, availability of effective alternatives, and type of thyrotoxicosis, with treatment cessation being more important in type 1 than type 2.

Methimazole is most effective in treating type 1 (hyperthyroidism) amiodarone-induced thyrotoxicosis, which occurs in patients with Graves disease or thyroid nodules. Since this patient's presentation is most consistent with type 2 amiodarone-induced thyrotoxicosis (destructive thyroiditis), prednisone is the preferred treatment.

Performing thyroid scintigraphy with radioactive iodine uptake is not indicated. Amiodarone has a very high iodine content, which results in high serum iodine levels. This iodine competes with the radioactive isotope used for the test (^{123}I or ^{131}I) resulting in very low radioactive iodine uptake (<1%) in most patients. This test does not discriminate well between type 1 and 2 amiodarone-induced thyrotoxicosis and is not clinically useful.

KEY POINT

- Type 2 amiodarone-induced thyrotoxicosis (destructive thyroiditis) can be treated with moderate- to high-dose prednisone that can be gradually tapered over 1 to 3 months.

Bibliography
Danzi S, Klein I. Amiodarone-induced thyroid dysfunction. J Intensive Care Med. 2015;30:179-85. doi: 10.1177/0885066613503278. Epub 2013 Sep 24. [PMID: 24067547]

Item 82   Answer: D

Educational Objective: Diagnose the cause of rapid-onset hirsutism.

A pelvic ultrasound is the most appropriate management for this patient. Although androgen-secreting ovarian tumors are rare, they should be considered in patients with abrupt, rapidly progressive, or severe hyperandrogenism as well as in women with marked hyperandrogenemia (total testosterone >150 ng/dL [5.2 nmol/L]). Given this patient's rapid onset of hirsutism coupled with significantly elevated total testosterone level, a pelvic ultrasound is the best next step in evaluation to assess for a possible ovarian tumor.

Adrenal vein sampling is a procedure used to confirm whether autonomous adrenal hormone production is unilateral or bilateral. It is most commonly performed in the evaluation of primary aldosteronism. Adrenal vein sampling is needed in most patients to determine the source of aldosterone secretion when imaging is unrevealing and to confirm lateralization when imaging demonstrates an adrenal adenoma. For this patient, adrenal CT is more appropriate to exclude an adrenal cortisol-secreting and/or androgen-secreting neoplasm and may be appropriate if the pelvic ultrasound is unrevealing. There is no indication for this procedure at this time in this patient.

Cushing syndrome (CS) results from elevated levels of cortisol. Clinical findings that are highly specific for CS include centripetal obesity, facial plethora, abnormal fat deposition in the supraclavicular or dorsocervical ("buffalo hump") areas, and wide (>1 cm) violaceous striae. Evaluation for CS is most appropriate in patients who have specific signs and symptoms of CS, rather than in patients who are diffusely obese, have nonpathologic striae, and are having trouble losing weight because endogenous CS is such a rare condition with a costly evaluation algorithm. At least two first-line tests should be abnormal before the diagnosis is confirmed. Initial tests include the overnight low-dose dexamethasone suppression test, 24-hour urine free cortisol, and late-night salivary cortisol. Since the patient has none of the specific findings of CS, a 24-hour urine cortisol test is not indicated.

In addition to weight loss, combined hormonal oral contraceptives are first-line agents for treatment of polycystic ovary syndrome. Polycystic ovary syndrome is a diagnosis of exclusion; given this patient's rapid onset of hirsutism coupled with degree of her total testosterone elevation, an androgen-secreting tumor must be considered.

KEY POINT

- An androgen-secreting ovarian tumor should be considered in patients with abrupt, rapidly progressive, or severe hyperandrogenism as well as in women with marked hyperandrogenemia (total testosterone >150 ng/dL [5.2 nmol/L]).

Bibliography
Mihailidis J, Dermesropian R, Taxel P, Luthra P, Grant-Kels JM. Endocrine evaluation of hirsutism. Int J Womens Dermatol. 2017;3(1 Suppl):S6-S10. doi: 10.1016/j.ijwd.2017.02.007. eCollection 2017 Mar. [PMID:28492032]

Item 83   Answer: D

Educational Objective: Treat type 2 diabetes mellitus with metabolic surgery in an obese patient.

This patient should be referred for metabolic surgery. The gastrointestinal tract plays an important role in glucose homeostasis and serves as an important physiologic target for improving glycemic control. Short- and mid-term data from randomized controlled trials of metabolic surgery demonstrated greater improvements in glycemic control and cardiovascular risk factors compared with optimized medical therapy and lifestyle modifications. Retrospective cohort studies and prospective observational studies suggest a reduction in cardiovascular deaths and lower incidence of cardiovascular events in patients undergoing metabolic surgery. Metabolic surgery should be recommended to patients with type 2 diabetes who have class III obesity (BMI ≥ 40) independent of glycemic control and diabetes treatment regimen and to patients with type 2 diabetes with class II obesity (BMI 35.0-39.9) who fail to meet their glycemic goals despite optimizing medical therapies and lifestyle modifications. In addition, patients with class I obesity (BMI 30.0-34.9) who do not meet their glycemic goals despite optimizing medical therapy should be considered for metabolic surgery. The patient has class II obesity with an inability to meet her hemoglobin A_{1c} goal of less than 7% on her current medical regimen. Further modifications to her current regimen may either exacerbate hypoglycemia and accelerate weight gain or not reach her glycemic goal.

Although sitagliptin, a dipeptidyl peptidase (DPP)-4 inhibitor, is a weight neutral oral agent that could potentially improve her hemoglobin A_{1c} level by 0.95% to 1.1%, it would not achieve her target hemoglobin A_{1c} of less than 7%.

Pioglitazone, a thiazolidinedione (TZD), improves insulin sensitivity and hemoglobin A_{1c} by 0.9% to 1.1%. The addition of pioglitazone in this patient would likely not achieve her target hemoglobin A_{1c} goal and could potentially induce additional weight gain, a known side effect of this drug class.

Increasing the patient's insulin doses may improve her hemoglobin A_{1c} to goal, but it will exacerbate her hypoglycemia and promote additional weight gain.

KEY POINT

- Metabolic surgery demonstrates greater improvements in glycemic control and cardiovascular risk factors compared with optimized medical therapy and lifestyle modifications.

Bibliography

Rubino F, Nathan DM, Eckel RH, Schauer PR, Alberti KG, Zimmet PZ, et al; Delegates of the 2nd Diabetes Surgery Summit. Metabolic surgery in the treatment algorithm for type 2 diabetes: a joint statement by International Diabetes Organizations. Diabetes Care. 2016;39:861-77. [PMID: 27222544] doi:10.2337/dc16-0236

Item 84   Answer: C

Educational Objective: Diagnose osteomalacia.

The most likely diagnosis in this patient is osteomalacia causing bone pain or fracture of the pelvis or proximal right lower extremity. An insidious, protracted course involving enigmatic pain is typical of osteomalacia, which may be dismissed by patients or symptomatically treated by health care providers. Chronically low levels of vitamin D can lead to rickets in children and osteomalacia in adults. Vitamin D deficiency is caused by factors such as intestinal malabsorption due to gastrointestinal disorders or restricted access to sunlight. In promoting absorption from the gut, vitamin D enables proper bone mineralization by maintenance of calcium and phosphorus levels. Vitamin D also modulates the actions of osteoblasts and osteoclasts to ensure proper bone growth and remodeling. The more common forms of osteomalacia related to malabsorption or dietary factors are characterized by low 25-hydroxyvitamin D (calcidiol), low calcium and phosphate, and elevated parathyroid hormone (PTH) (secondary hyperparathyroidism) and alkaline phosphatase levels. Depending on the duration and severity of vitamin D deficiency, the serum concentration of 1,25-dihydroxyvitamin D may be normal, low, or high and is not helpful in the diagnosis of most forms of osteomalacia.

Osteitis fibrosa cystica is due to abnormally high bone turnover that can occur after prolonged exposure of bone to sustained high levels of PTH in hyperparathyroidism. It is associated with very high bone turnover, expansion of osteoid surfaces, and exuberant bone resorption resulting in an increased risk of fracture. Patients can be asymptomatic, or they may have bone pain. Classic skeletal changes on radiograph may include subperiosteal resorption of bone, most prominently at the phalanges of the hands. Osteitis fibrosa cystica is most commonly seen in patients with chronic kidney failure and is rarely associated with severe primary hyperparathyroidism.

Osteogenesis imperfecta (OI) comprises four genetic syndromes characterized by autosomal dominant or recessive mutations in *COL* genes, leading to abnormalities in the structure of type I collagen. OI is associated with bone fractures, short stature, body deformity, hearing loss, and dental deformity. A classic feature of OI is blue sclerae (reflecting visibility of the underlying choroid), but it is not sensitive or specific to OI. The biochemical profile is usually normal in OI.

Postmenopausal osteoporosis is a diagnosis of exclusion, made only after having evaluated and eliminated other causes of low bone mineral density such as osteomalacia. Patients with osteoporosis have a normal biochemical profile.

KEY POINT

- Osteomalacia related to malabsorption or dietary factors is characterized by low 25-hydroxyvitamin D, calcium, and phosphate levels and elevated parathyroid hormone and alkaline phosphatase levels.

Bibliography

Uday S, Högler W. Nutritional rickets and osteomalacia in the twenty-first century: revised concepts, public health, and prevention strategies. Curr Osteoporos Rep. 2017 Aug;15(4):293-302. doi: 10.1007/s11914-017-0383-y. Erratum in: Curr Osteoporos Rep. 2017 Aug 14; [PMID: 28612338]

Index

Note: Page numbers followed by f and t indicates figure and table respectively. Test questions are indicated by Q.

A

A

NAME AND ADDRESS (Please complete.)

_____
Last Name   First Name   Middle Initial

_____
Address

_____
Address cont.

_____
City   State   ZIP Code

_____
Country

_____
Email address

B

Order Number
(Use the 10-digit Order Number on your
MKSAP materials packing slip.)

C

ACP ID Number
(Refer to packing slip in your MKSAP materials
for your 8-digit ACP ID Number.)

ACP®
American College of Physicians
Leading Internal Medicine, Improving Lives

**Medical
Knowledge
Self-Assessment
Program® 18**

TO EARN *CME Credits and/or MOC Points* YOU MUST:

1. Answer all questions.
2. Score a minimum of 50% correct.

TO EARN *FREE* INSTANTANEOUS *CME Credits and/or MOC Points* ONLINE:

1. Answer all of your questions.
2. Go to **mksap.acponline.org** and enter your ACP Online username and password to access an online answer sheet.
3. Enter your answers.
4. You can also enter your answers directly at **mksap.acponline.org** without first using this answer sheet.

To Submit Your Answer Sheet by Mail or FAX for a $20 Administrative Fee per Answer Sheet:

1. Answer all of your questions and calculate your score.
2. Complete boxes A-H.
3. Complete payment information.
4. Send the answer sheet and payment information to ACP, using the FAX number/address listed below.

D

Required Submission Information if Applying for MOC

Birth Month and Day   ABIM Candidate Number
M M D D

COMPLETE FORM BELOW ONLY IF YOU SUBMIT BY MAIL OR FAX

Last Name   First Name   MI

Payment Information. Must remit in US funds, drawn on a US bank.
The processing fee for each paper answer sheet is $20.

☐ Check, made payable to ACP, enclosed

Charge to ☐ **VISA** ☐ **MasterCard** ☐ **AMERICAN EXPRESS** ☐ **DISCOVER**

Card Number _____

Expiration Date _____/_____ Security code (3 or 4 digit #s) _____
    MM YY

Signature _____

Fax to: 215-351-2799

Mail to:
Member and Customer Service
American College of Physicians
190 N. Independence Mall West
Philadelphia, PA 19106-1572

1 Ⓐ Ⓑ Ⓒ Ⓓ Ⓔ
2 Ⓐ Ⓑ Ⓒ Ⓓ Ⓔ
3 Ⓐ Ⓑ Ⓒ Ⓓ Ⓔ
4 Ⓐ Ⓑ Ⓒ Ⓓ Ⓔ
5 Ⓐ Ⓑ Ⓒ Ⓓ Ⓔ

6 Ⓐ Ⓑ Ⓒ Ⓓ Ⓔ
7 Ⓐ Ⓑ Ⓒ Ⓓ Ⓔ
8 Ⓐ Ⓑ Ⓒ Ⓓ Ⓔ
9 Ⓐ Ⓑ Ⓒ Ⓓ Ⓔ
10 Ⓐ Ⓑ Ⓒ Ⓓ Ⓔ

11 Ⓐ Ⓑ Ⓒ Ⓓ Ⓔ
12 Ⓐ Ⓑ Ⓒ Ⓓ Ⓔ
13 Ⓐ Ⓑ Ⓒ Ⓓ Ⓔ
14 Ⓐ Ⓑ Ⓒ Ⓓ Ⓔ
15 Ⓐ Ⓑ Ⓒ Ⓓ Ⓔ

16 Ⓐ Ⓑ Ⓒ Ⓓ Ⓔ
17 Ⓐ Ⓑ Ⓒ Ⓓ Ⓔ
18 Ⓐ Ⓑ Ⓒ Ⓓ Ⓔ
19 Ⓐ Ⓑ Ⓒ Ⓓ Ⓔ
20 Ⓐ Ⓑ Ⓒ Ⓓ Ⓔ

21 Ⓐ Ⓑ Ⓒ Ⓓ Ⓔ
22 Ⓐ Ⓑ Ⓒ Ⓓ Ⓔ
23 Ⓐ Ⓑ Ⓒ Ⓓ Ⓔ
24 Ⓐ Ⓑ Ⓒ Ⓓ Ⓔ
25 Ⓐ Ⓑ Ⓒ Ⓓ Ⓔ

26 Ⓐ Ⓑ Ⓒ Ⓓ Ⓔ
27 Ⓐ Ⓑ Ⓒ Ⓓ Ⓔ
28 Ⓐ Ⓑ Ⓒ Ⓓ Ⓔ
29 Ⓐ Ⓑ Ⓒ Ⓓ Ⓔ
30 Ⓐ Ⓑ Ⓒ Ⓓ Ⓔ

31 Ⓐ Ⓑ Ⓒ Ⓓ Ⓔ
32 Ⓐ Ⓑ Ⓒ Ⓓ Ⓔ
33 Ⓐ Ⓑ Ⓒ Ⓓ Ⓔ
34 Ⓐ Ⓑ Ⓒ Ⓓ Ⓔ
35 Ⓐ Ⓑ Ⓒ Ⓓ Ⓔ

36 Ⓐ Ⓑ Ⓒ Ⓓ Ⓔ
37 Ⓐ Ⓑ Ⓒ Ⓓ Ⓔ
38 Ⓐ Ⓑ Ⓒ Ⓓ Ⓔ
39 Ⓐ Ⓑ Ⓒ Ⓓ Ⓔ
40 Ⓐ Ⓑ Ⓒ Ⓓ Ⓔ

41 Ⓐ Ⓑ Ⓒ Ⓓ Ⓔ
42 Ⓐ Ⓑ Ⓒ Ⓓ Ⓔ
43 Ⓐ Ⓑ Ⓒ Ⓓ Ⓔ
44 Ⓐ Ⓑ Ⓒ Ⓓ Ⓔ
45 Ⓐ Ⓑ Ⓒ Ⓓ Ⓔ

46 Ⓐ Ⓑ Ⓒ Ⓓ Ⓔ
47 Ⓐ Ⓑ Ⓒ Ⓓ Ⓔ
48 Ⓐ Ⓑ Ⓒ Ⓓ Ⓔ
49 Ⓐ Ⓑ Ⓒ Ⓓ Ⓔ
50 Ⓐ Ⓑ Ⓒ Ⓓ Ⓔ

51 Ⓐ Ⓑ Ⓒ Ⓓ Ⓔ
52 Ⓐ Ⓑ Ⓒ Ⓓ Ⓔ
53 Ⓐ Ⓑ Ⓒ Ⓓ Ⓔ
54 Ⓐ Ⓑ Ⓒ Ⓓ Ⓔ
55 Ⓐ Ⓑ Ⓒ Ⓓ Ⓔ

56 Ⓐ Ⓑ Ⓒ Ⓓ Ⓔ
57 Ⓐ Ⓑ Ⓒ Ⓓ Ⓔ
58 Ⓐ Ⓑ Ⓒ Ⓓ Ⓔ
59 Ⓐ Ⓑ Ⓒ Ⓓ Ⓔ
60 Ⓐ Ⓑ Ⓒ Ⓓ Ⓔ

61 Ⓐ Ⓑ Ⓒ Ⓓ Ⓔ
62 Ⓐ Ⓑ Ⓒ Ⓓ Ⓔ
63 Ⓐ Ⓑ Ⓒ Ⓓ Ⓔ
64 Ⓐ Ⓑ Ⓒ Ⓓ Ⓔ
65 Ⓐ Ⓑ Ⓒ Ⓓ Ⓔ

66 Ⓐ Ⓑ Ⓒ Ⓓ Ⓔ
67 Ⓐ Ⓑ Ⓒ Ⓓ Ⓔ
68 Ⓐ Ⓑ Ⓒ Ⓓ Ⓔ
69 Ⓐ Ⓑ Ⓒ Ⓓ Ⓔ
70 Ⓐ Ⓑ Ⓒ Ⓓ Ⓔ

71 Ⓐ Ⓑ Ⓒ Ⓓ Ⓔ
72 Ⓐ Ⓑ Ⓒ Ⓓ Ⓔ
73 Ⓐ Ⓑ Ⓒ Ⓓ Ⓔ
74 Ⓐ Ⓑ Ⓒ Ⓓ Ⓔ
75 Ⓐ Ⓑ Ⓒ Ⓓ Ⓔ

76 Ⓐ Ⓑ Ⓒ Ⓓ Ⓔ
77 Ⓐ Ⓑ Ⓒ Ⓓ Ⓔ
78 Ⓐ Ⓑ Ⓒ Ⓓ Ⓔ
79 Ⓐ Ⓑ Ⓒ Ⓓ Ⓔ
80 Ⓐ Ⓑ Ⓒ Ⓓ Ⓔ

81 Ⓐ Ⓑ Ⓒ Ⓓ Ⓔ
82 Ⓐ Ⓑ Ⓒ Ⓓ Ⓔ
83 Ⓐ Ⓑ Ⓒ Ⓓ Ⓔ
84 Ⓐ Ⓑ Ⓒ Ⓓ Ⓔ
85 Ⓐ Ⓑ Ⓒ Ⓓ Ⓔ

86 Ⓐ Ⓑ Ⓒ Ⓓ Ⓔ
87 Ⓐ Ⓑ Ⓒ Ⓓ Ⓔ
88 Ⓐ Ⓑ Ⓒ Ⓓ Ⓔ
89 Ⓐ Ⓑ Ⓒ Ⓓ Ⓔ
90 Ⓐ Ⓑ Ⓒ Ⓓ Ⓔ

91 Ⓐ Ⓑ Ⓒ Ⓓ Ⓔ
92 Ⓐ Ⓑ Ⓒ Ⓓ Ⓔ
93 Ⓐ Ⓑ Ⓒ Ⓓ Ⓔ
94 Ⓐ Ⓑ Ⓒ Ⓓ Ⓔ
95 Ⓐ Ⓑ Ⓒ Ⓓ Ⓔ

96 Ⓐ Ⓑ Ⓒ Ⓓ Ⓔ
97 Ⓐ Ⓑ Ⓒ Ⓓ Ⓔ
98 Ⓐ Ⓑ Ⓒ Ⓓ Ⓔ
99 Ⓐ Ⓑ Ⓒ Ⓓ Ⓔ
100 Ⓐ Ⓑ Ⓒ Ⓓ Ⓔ

101 Ⓐ Ⓑ Ⓒ Ⓓ Ⓔ
102 Ⓐ Ⓑ Ⓒ Ⓓ Ⓔ
103 Ⓐ Ⓑ Ⓒ Ⓓ Ⓔ
104 Ⓐ Ⓑ Ⓒ Ⓓ Ⓔ
105 Ⓐ Ⓑ Ⓒ Ⓓ Ⓔ

106 Ⓐ Ⓑ Ⓒ Ⓓ Ⓔ
107 Ⓐ Ⓑ Ⓒ Ⓓ Ⓔ
108 Ⓐ Ⓑ Ⓒ Ⓓ Ⓔ
109 Ⓐ Ⓑ Ⓒ Ⓓ Ⓔ
110 Ⓐ Ⓑ Ⓒ Ⓓ Ⓔ

111 Ⓐ Ⓑ Ⓒ Ⓓ Ⓔ
112 Ⓐ Ⓑ Ⓒ Ⓓ Ⓔ
113 Ⓐ Ⓑ Ⓒ Ⓓ Ⓔ
114 Ⓐ Ⓑ Ⓒ Ⓓ Ⓔ
115 Ⓐ Ⓑ Ⓒ Ⓓ Ⓔ

116 Ⓐ Ⓑ Ⓒ Ⓓ Ⓔ
117 Ⓐ Ⓑ Ⓒ Ⓓ Ⓔ
118 Ⓐ Ⓑ Ⓒ Ⓓ Ⓔ
119 Ⓐ Ⓑ Ⓒ Ⓓ Ⓔ
120 Ⓐ Ⓑ Ⓒ Ⓓ Ⓔ

121 Ⓐ Ⓑ Ⓒ Ⓓ Ⓔ
122 Ⓐ Ⓑ Ⓒ Ⓓ Ⓔ
123 Ⓐ Ⓑ Ⓒ Ⓓ Ⓔ
124 Ⓐ Ⓑ Ⓒ Ⓓ Ⓔ
125 Ⓐ Ⓑ Ⓒ Ⓓ Ⓔ

126 Ⓐ Ⓑ Ⓒ Ⓓ Ⓔ
127 Ⓐ Ⓑ Ⓒ Ⓓ Ⓔ
128 Ⓐ Ⓑ Ⓒ Ⓓ Ⓔ
129 Ⓐ Ⓑ Ⓒ Ⓓ Ⓔ
130 Ⓐ Ⓑ Ⓒ Ⓓ Ⓔ

131 Ⓐ Ⓑ Ⓒ Ⓓ Ⓔ
132 Ⓐ Ⓑ Ⓒ Ⓓ Ⓔ
133 Ⓐ Ⓑ Ⓒ Ⓓ Ⓔ
134 Ⓐ Ⓑ Ⓒ Ⓓ Ⓔ
135 Ⓐ Ⓑ Ⓒ Ⓓ Ⓔ

136 Ⓐ Ⓑ Ⓒ Ⓓ Ⓔ
137 Ⓐ Ⓑ Ⓒ Ⓓ Ⓔ
138 Ⓐ Ⓑ Ⓒ Ⓓ Ⓔ
139 Ⓐ Ⓑ Ⓒ Ⓓ Ⓔ
140 Ⓐ Ⓑ Ⓒ Ⓓ Ⓔ

141 Ⓐ Ⓑ Ⓒ Ⓓ Ⓔ
142 Ⓐ Ⓑ Ⓒ Ⓓ Ⓔ
143 Ⓐ Ⓑ Ⓒ Ⓓ Ⓔ
144 Ⓐ Ⓑ Ⓒ Ⓓ Ⓔ
145 Ⓐ Ⓑ Ⓒ Ⓓ Ⓔ

146 Ⓐ Ⓑ Ⓒ Ⓓ Ⓔ
147 Ⓐ Ⓑ Ⓒ Ⓓ Ⓔ
148 Ⓐ Ⓑ Ⓒ Ⓓ Ⓔ
149 Ⓐ Ⓑ Ⓒ Ⓓ Ⓔ
150 Ⓐ Ⓑ Ⓒ Ⓓ Ⓔ

151 Ⓐ Ⓑ Ⓒ Ⓓ Ⓔ
152 Ⓐ Ⓑ Ⓒ Ⓓ Ⓔ
153 Ⓐ Ⓑ Ⓒ Ⓓ Ⓔ
154 Ⓐ Ⓑ Ⓒ Ⓓ Ⓔ
155 Ⓐ Ⓑ Ⓒ Ⓓ Ⓔ

156 Ⓐ Ⓑ Ⓒ Ⓓ Ⓔ
157 Ⓐ Ⓑ Ⓒ Ⓓ Ⓔ
158 Ⓐ Ⓑ Ⓒ Ⓓ Ⓔ
159 Ⓐ Ⓑ Ⓒ Ⓓ Ⓔ
160 Ⓐ Ⓑ Ⓒ Ⓓ Ⓔ

161 Ⓐ Ⓑ Ⓒ Ⓓ Ⓔ
162 Ⓐ Ⓑ Ⓒ Ⓓ Ⓔ
163 Ⓐ Ⓑ Ⓒ Ⓓ Ⓔ
164 Ⓐ Ⓑ Ⓒ Ⓓ Ⓔ
165 Ⓐ Ⓑ Ⓒ Ⓓ Ⓔ

166 Ⓐ Ⓑ Ⓒ Ⓓ Ⓔ
167 Ⓐ Ⓑ Ⓒ Ⓓ Ⓔ
168 Ⓐ Ⓑ Ⓒ Ⓓ Ⓔ
169 Ⓐ Ⓑ Ⓒ Ⓓ Ⓔ
170 Ⓐ Ⓑ Ⓒ Ⓓ Ⓔ

171 Ⓐ Ⓑ Ⓒ Ⓓ Ⓔ
172 Ⓐ Ⓑ Ⓒ Ⓓ Ⓔ
173 Ⓐ Ⓑ Ⓒ Ⓓ Ⓔ
174 Ⓐ Ⓑ Ⓒ Ⓓ Ⓔ
175 Ⓐ Ⓑ Ⓒ Ⓓ Ⓔ

176 Ⓐ Ⓑ Ⓒ Ⓓ Ⓔ
177 Ⓐ Ⓑ Ⓒ Ⓓ Ⓔ
178 Ⓐ Ⓑ Ⓒ Ⓓ Ⓔ
179 Ⓐ Ⓑ Ⓒ Ⓓ Ⓔ
180 Ⓐ Ⓑ Ⓒ Ⓓ Ⓔ